MILK
The Deadly Poison

Robert Cohen

Argus Publishing, Inc.
Englewood Cliffs, NJ

ISBN: 0-9659196-0-9   616.39 COH

Library of Congress Catalog Card Number: 97-094585

Additional copies of this book are available for bulk purchases. For more information, please contact: ARGUS Publishing, Inc., 301 Sylvan Avenue, Englewood Cliffs, NJ, 07632, or call 201-871-5871, FAX 201-871-9304.

Manufactured in the United States of America

First Printing January 1998
Printed with soy based inks on recycled paper

INTERNET ACCESS: http://www.NOTMILK.com

3

This work is dedicated to all people throughout the world who endure a variety of symptoms and diseases without recognizing the dietary root of their suffering. May they learn to recognize that the fountain of youth for themselves, their children and future generations might be revealed after eliminating just one food from their diets.

Acknowledgments

Jane Heimlich, you provided the spark.

Robert Collier of Monsanto and Richard Teske of FDA, together you helped to light the fuse.

Betty Martini, you became my teacher, and Barbara Mullarkey, you scrutinized my work. Together you two fueled the fire.

Richard Kurtz, you saw to it that the fire was never extinguished.

Rudy Shur, the embers were glowing when your breath of oxygen accelerated the fire with renewed vigor.

Lisa, my researcher and editor...and wife, you fanned the flames.

Jennifer, Sarah, Elizabeth, Nat and Dot...you stood back and allowed that burning flame to consume every part of my life, as it had to, and now it burns bright.

Contents

FOREWORD
by Jane Heimlich, author of *What Your Doctor Won't Tell You*

One of my earliest memories is my father coaxing me to drink milk. "Calling all cars, calling all cars--Jane hasn't finished her milk." You may be applying the same pressure to your children. After all, isn't milk "the most perfect food on earth?" Nutritionists reiterate that we need the calcium in milk to keep our bones strong. At present, celebrities pose with milk mustaches.

You may not want to hear this but what you've been told all your life about milk is an outright lie. Your glass of milk, even low fat, is awash in fat (the equivalent of three slices of bacon), cholesterol, antibiotics, bacteria, and--the most distasteful ingredient--pus.

I suspected that milk was a health disaster back in the Spring of '94. At that time, while researching an article for *Health & Healing*, a newsletter with a half million subscribers, I learned that the Food & Drug Administration had approved the use of a genetically engineered hormone called "recombinant bovine growth hormone" (rBGH). The alleged purpose of the hormone, a $500 million investment on the part of the Monsanto Company, is to increase a cow's milk output. Considering the glut of milk for the past decade, economic justification for using rBGH remains a mystery.

Injecting hapless cows with a growth hormone raised a red flag for me. In my 20 plus years of health reporting, I've found that when a company interferes with Mother Nature, this cold-blooded exploitation, invariably for economic gain, brings suffering and disease.

This was clearly the case with the bovine growth hormone. I knew that, over the years, pasteurization and homogenization had destroyed most of the natural goodness of milk. The growth hormone was the supreme insult. As dairymen reported, this hormone made our cows sick, namely developing mastitis, thus requiring enormous doses of antibiotics. For this reason, 95 percent of dairy farmers initially refused to inject their cows with rBGH; later, many caved in under pressure.

A more disturbing consequence of the bovine growth hormone is that it increases levels of a powerful growth hormone, IGF-I. IGF-I is a key factor in the growth and proliferation of cancer.

Despite the health threats posed by the bovine growth hormone, I was one of the few health writers taking a critical view of the situation. Starting in 1994, the media assured us that milk from treated and untreated cows is virtually the same. Here they were dutifully quoting the FDA, the American Medical Association, and the World Health Organization. Few bothered to investigate why a growing number of dairy farmers and environmental watchdogs were bitterly opposed to its use.

I wasn't impressed by these scientific assurances from on high. From reporting on alternative medicine, I knew too well how the medical establishment can lie through its teeth. Mainstream doctors continue to label chelation therapy, a life-saving treatment for heart disease, as "quackery," despite its over 30 year track record as a safe and effective treatment.

What was needed to bring the deleterious effects of rBGH to the fore was an intrepid scientist who could confront scientists from these prestigious organizations, speak their language, interpret scientific data, and reveal the facts about the true nature of the bovine growth hormone.

Enter Robert Cohen, with rich experience in biological research and a risk taker--one of his pursuits is mountain climbing. A call came from Mr. Cohen shortly after my July '94 article appeared. A boyish voice crackling with energy. Cohen divulged his suspicions that the FDA's approval of the bovine growth hormone represented not only collusion between Monsanto and the FDA, but a cover-up of epic proportions by the scientific establishment. His three-year fact-finding journey proved him chillingly right.

Reading this book, you will learn that milk contributes to heart disease and increases your risk of breast cancer. You will learn that milk is a poor source of calcium and why, and that milk is a prime cause of allergies and much more. You will learn that milk can even kill your infant.

Cohen doesn't expect you to accept these shocking findings on faith. He takes you by the hand as he uncovers layers of scientific fraud perpetuated by the FDA, with assistance from *JAMA*, *Science News*, and even the Cadillac of scientific publications, *Science*. In digging for scientific facts, Cohen found that the web of deception concerning the bovine growth hormone involved not only key players--FDA and Monsanto--but reached members of Congress as well as a respected medical authority turned Monsanto lobbyist. At times this book reads like a detective story.

Eventually our indefatigable scientific sleuth uncovered the smoking gun--incontrovertible evidence showing that laboratory animals treated with rBGH developed cancer, but he could not induce the FDA to reconsider their approval of the hormone.

My husband, Dr. Henry Heimlich, devisor of the Heimlich maneuver, had a similar experience dealing with the American Red Cross (ARC). Following his discovery that the Maneuver, applying upward pressure to the diaphragm caused the choking object to pop out, he implored the ARC to stop teaching the public to administer back blows to a choking victim, which only drives the object deeper into the airway. Stymied by scientific fraud and bureaucratic blindness, he took his life and death issue to the public.

Robert Cohen has taken the same tack. Reading this meticulously documented book, written in a lively informal style and punctuated with irreverent humor, I feel sure you will be convinced, as I am, that milk is hazardous to your health. Don't worry about what you're going to put on your cereal. Cohen offers plenty of nondairy milk suggestions.

Share the author's findings with your family members and friends. Buy a copy for anyone you care about. Take its message to heart.

Preface

In the summer of 1994, an article in a health newsletter reviewed the most controversial drug application in the history of America's Food and Drug Administration (FDA). Monsanto Agricultural Company had isolated the naturally occurring bovine growth hormone. They then found a way to combine that hormone with microorganisms, merging genetic material from cows and *E. coli* bacteria to achieve a new product, which, when injected back into cows would result in an increase in milk production. That new hormone was called recombinant bovine somatotropin (rbST). An investigation of that new hormone and of milk and dairy products released a Pandora's box of demons and dilemmas that milk producers had wished had never been exposed. As a result of that subsequent investigation, many questions were asked. The answers to those questions will place America's entire dairy industry in jeopardy.

It is probable that milk consumption is the foundation of heart disease and the explanation for America's number one killer. While there is much debate about dietary cholesterol, by the time the average American reaches the age of fifty-two, he or she has consumed in milk and dairy products the equivalent cholesterol contained in 1 million slices of bacon. Could milk be the reason that one out of eight American women will develop cancer of the breast? Do cancers grow because of the powerful growth hormones found in milk? Should more research be performed to investigate childhood allergies occurring as a result of the body's reaction to bovine milk proteins? Twenty-five million American women over the age of forty have been diagnosed with bone crippling arthritis and osteoporosis. These females have been drinking, on average, in excess of two pounds of milk per day for their entire adult lives. What could possibly keep these women and their doctors blind to the fact that drinking milk has not prevented osteoporosis? Perhaps their lack of vision is biased by the millions of dollars of revenue strategically invested to buy ads in magazines accompanied by articles extolling the virtues of calcium in milk. Wouldn't they be surprised, after reviewing scientific research, to learn that the calcium in milk is not adequately absorbed and that milk consumption is the probable cause of osteoporosis?

A growing number of Americans are turning away from milk and eliminating dairy products from their diets. Many attentive parents are noting that when milk and dairy products are eliminated, so too are their disease-causing symptoms such as colic and colitis, earaches, colds and congestion in their young. Many children develop diabetes. Research indicates that one bovine protein in milk destroys the insulin-producing beta cells of the pancreas. Sixty percent of America's dairy cows have leukemia virus. Is it prudent to eat the flesh or drink body fluids from diseased animals? Pasteurization is intended to kill bacteria and viruses in milk. However, in 1985, Chicago experienced a terrible accident when a milk processing plant incorrectly pasteurized one day's output of milk and four people died and 150,000 were made sick due to salmonella poisoning. That tainted milk might have contained live leukemia virus, tuberculosis virus and vast assortments of other infectious organisms. No records were kept to monitor subsequent cases of encephalitis, meningitis or leukemia.

At one time, the FDA allowed farmers to treat their cows with low levels of bacteria killing drugs resulting in a relatively small amount of antibiotics in milk. Government scientists recognized that consumers should not be drinking a fluid containing high levels of antibiotics. In 1990, the one part per hundred million antibiotic residue in milk standard was increased one hundred times to one part per million. Today, farmers are permitted to give their animals increased levels of antibiotics. Ultimately, after cows graze in fields treated with pesticides, their milk contains a toxic and near lethal brew of chemicals.

Beer bellies are indeed making a comeback in America. As a society, we have never been more overweight. According to the *Food Consumption, Prices and Expenditures, 1996, Statistical Bulletin Number 928*, published by the United States Department of Agriculture (USDA), the average American consumed 24 gallons of beer in 1994. That works out to just under 8 1/2 ounces of beer per day per person. Total milk and dairy products consumed per capita in 1994 equaled 26 ounces per day, more than triple the amount of beer. One 12 ounce glass of beer contains 144 calories and no fat. On the other hand, a 12 ounce glass of milk contains 300 calories and 16 grams of fat. It seems that beer is taking a bad rap. Protruding stomachs on overweight people should be called milk bellies, not beer bellies.

If one eats a steak containing powerful growth hormones, those hormones are destroyed in the stomach by strong digestive acids and enzymes. In drinking milk, the wisdom of mother nature ensures the survival of these protein hormones. The powerful stomach acids are diluted by liquid milk, and the strength of the acid environment, measured in pH, changes to a less acidic condition and the hormones are not destroyed. Most scientists have not considered this process. Mothers faced with children with tummy-aches certainly do. They serve warm milk to their child who painlessly goes to sleep because the acid in the child's stomach is diluted and the suffering is ended.

America's suffering has just begun. The FDA is supposed to act as a fiduciary to American health needs. Unfortunately, this agency is influenced by special interest groups including private industry pharmaceutical companies. FDA regulators and scientists often find employment in private industry, rewards for services rendered. The reverse is also true. Scientists and attorneys working for these companies often find employment at FDA. One such case occurred in 1990 when the bovine growth hormone was genetically engineered. Monsanto, the manufacturer of rbST, faced many hurdles during the application process of their new drug. Somehow, Monsanto's top scientists were hired by FDA to review their very own research. Monsanto's attorney was also hired by FDA to write the labeling laws for the new drug. Simultaneous to these career moves, Monsanto lobbyists were paying enormous sums of money to members of the Congressional Agriculture Committee, the Dairy Livestock and Poultry Subcommittee. This group of 12 congressmen was at the time considering a bill designed to label milk that came from cows treated with this new genetically engineered hormone. As the dollars poured in, these congressmen stalled the legislation in committee where the bill died when the 1994 session of Congress expired. The bill never even made it to a congressional vote.

America was told that milk from rbST-treated cows was identical to the milk that had been enjoyed for generations. This statement was untrue. After cows were injected with this hormone, their milk contained increased levels of another hormone, insulin-like growth factor-I (IGF-I), the most powerful growth hormone occurring in nature. The greatest biological coincidence of all time had occurred. IGF-I was identical between cows and humans. No other hormone known to science is identical between another species of animal and humans. IGF-I is the lone exception, containing 70 amino acids in the same gene sequence in humans and bovines. When we drink milk we are taking in the most powerful growth hormone naturally produced by our own bodies. However, the survival of this growth hormone in milk is safeguarded by naturally occurring mechanisms unique to milk.

Milk hormones exert growth effects on humans. Milk proteins exert allergenic effects. Fat and cholesterol contribute to an overweight society. Antibiotics in milk destroy the immunoreactive properties of those same antibiotics when they are needed. Cancer, heart disease, asthma, allergies, and so much more, are all made possible by milk.

"Everyone that useths milk is unskillful in the word of righteousness, for he is a babe. But solid food belongeth to them that are of full age, even those who by reason of use have their senses exercised to discern both good and evil."

King James Version of The Holy Bible, HEBREWS: 5:13-14

"To my thinking, there is only one valid reason to drink or use milk products. That is just because we simply want to. Because we like it and because it has become part of our culture. Because we have become accustomed to its taste and texture. Because we like the way it slides down our throat. Because our parents did the very best they could for us and provided milk in our earliest training and conditioning. They taught us to like it. And then probably the very best reason is...ICE CREAM! I've heard it described, '...to die for'."

Robert M. Kradjian, M.D., Surgeon and Author of **Save Yourself From Breast Cancer,** *Berkley Books, New York, 1994.*

Chapter 1
Wholesome Milk: The Dairy Industry Message

Hundreds of millions of dollars are invested each year by the Dairy Industry and milk processors to insure that Americans will drink milk and eat dairy products. Some of those dollars are used to pay for advertising and some of those dollars are donated to congressmen and senators who vote on issues affecting the Dairy Industry. Some of those dollars are paid to the American Dietitians Association (ADA) which promotes the use of milk and dairy products. Some of those dollars are granted to universities to finance research that supports the marketing message of the Dairy Coalition. Adult Americans would react with repugnance when faced with the suggestion of drinking human breast milk. How about milk from man's best friends, his cats and dogs? Instinctively, one knows that there are substances in milk which are intended for the young of each specific species. Yet, we continue to drink milk from cows. That practice has been made acceptable. We drink a tall glass of milk, unaware that we also are consuming powerful growth hormones, enormous quantities of dietary cholesterol, fat, allergenic proteins, insecticides, antibiotics, viruses and bacteria.

Milk and dairy products represent the major portion of America's diet. According to the United States Department of Agriculture (USDA), in 1995, the average American ate 394 pounds of vegetables and 121 pounds of fresh fruit. The average American ate 192 pounds of flour and cereal products. Each person also ate 193 pounds of meat, poultry and fish. Last, but not least, the average American ate or drank 584 pounds of milk and dairy products. (1) To summarize: dairy, 584 pounds; vegetables, 394 pounds; meat, 193 pounds; flour, 192 pounds; fresh fruit, 121 pounds. That totals to over four pounds of food per day per person, and nearly forty percent of that is dairy. That's one very lopsided food pyramid!

Breakfast without cereal moistened with milk would be extremely boring. Late evening cookies without milk would be unsatisfying. In between breakfast and late night snack we eat yogurt and pizza and cream cheese on bagels. Ice cream is the perfect dessert to any meal. Cheese, butter, sour cream and cottage cheese. It would be difficult to give up dairy products. Just to insure that we do not, the Dairy Industry invests their money to continually let Americans know that milk tastes good and the intake of milk and dairy products must be continued to insure good health.

"A big surprise right under your nose!" (2) That's the message promoted by the National Fluid Milk Processors, the marketing arm of America's Dairy Industry. The directive is clear: Milk mustaches are stylish. Drink milk and you're beautiful! Gorgeous models, actors, actresses, sports heroes, even President Clinton and Bob Dole have posed for milk advertisements, all asserting, the milky white goo artificially applied to their upper lip, that drinking milk is healthful and wholesome. Who would argue with such an overwhelming endorsement? Billboards spanning America ask the question, "Got milk?" Film director Spike Lee peers down at cars passing on the roads and highways with his "milkstache" proclaiming the same wholesome announcement droning on radio and television, printed in black and milky-white in newspapers and magazines. Americans love milk. Americans need milk. African-Americans, Caucasians, male and female, young and old. Wholesome milk. American as apple pie.

This skillfully marketed message is constantly reinforced. If you require more information, the invitation is to call 1-800-WHY MILK. When you do, free advice is offered and a week later you will receive the Dairy Industry prospectus. You call, and soon two brochures show up in your mailbox. One declares, "Real Men Drink Milk." (3) Cal Ripken, Jr., of the Baltimore Orioles is a "Real Man." He's on the cover. Ripken broke Lou Gehrig's record for consecutive major league baseball games played, and at this writing he's still going strong. Steve Young, quarterback of the San Francisco Forty-Niners is on the cover too. Film director Spike Lee adds his face to the cover, and rounding out the foursome is singer Tony Bennett.

Cal Ripken, Jr., holding a baseball bat, smiles from inside the front cover and is quoted, "With all the skim milk I drink, my name might as well be Calcium Ripken, Jr." Ripken is joined by New York basketball star Patrick Ewing who asks, "Have you seen me sweat? I must lose 10 pounds a game. And from what I hear it's not just about losing water. It's about nutrients. That's why I drink milk. 2 percent. It's got nine essential nutrients my body needs, like calcium and potassium. I thought about telling the boys in Chicago, but it's about time they lost something."

I am a New York Knick fan and a devotee of Patrick Ewing. He plays a great game and is an intense competitor. Unfortunately, Ewing is a lousy interview. When he's not avoiding press conferences altogether, he usually answers all questions with a one or two word response. Those who truly know Patrick would be stunned by his milk remarks, which cumulatively add up to a full season's worth of comments, playoffs included. This athlete must truly love milk!

The logo of the National Osteoporosis Foundation is shown on the back cover of this brochure. In large letters one reads, "ADVICE FROM THE EXPERTS." In small letters we're advised, "Pour it, don't pop it. Calcium supplements do not contain the range and balance of the nutrients that milk provides...Besides, experts recommend a 'food first' approach for getting the essential nutrients your body needs." Food first? Elsewhere on the back page the experts tell us, "Popeye was wrong." These health conscious experts go on to warn, "Spinach isn't the only answer. It may contain some calcium, but spinach also contains certain substances that bind with calcium and lessen its absorption. Other leafy greens provide some calcium, but in smaller amounts."

Milk: What a Surprise!

The larger of the two brochures displays a beautiful woman with perfect features, eyebrows with nary a hair out of place, skin without a blemish, pearly white teeth and a smile that warms the heart, a face capable of launching 10,000 ships. And, of course, that MILK MUSTACHE that has been so carefully applied, make-up on top of make-up glued onto a model's upper lip, a sight that men must truly find irresistible because it epitomizes and highlights all that is sensual with the ideal American woman.

Why Milk? America's Misconceptions

The Dairy Industry thinks that it's time to "set the record straight about milk." Their message, "When you take another look at one of Mother Nature's most delicious drinks, milk may surprise you." I couldn't have said that any better myself! In all fairness, their story first. The National Fluid Milk Processor Promotion Board (NFMPPB) asks, "Why have many people stopped drinking one of the most nutrient-dense, natural foods around?" In answering their own question they explain that it must be just a "simple misunderstanding."

This is brought to you word for word from the folks at NFMPPB:

Myth: Milk is high in fat and calories.
Fact: Skim and 1% milk have little or no fat with all of the calcium and other nutrients found in whole milk. And fewer calories too.
Myth: Milk is just for kids.
Fact: Our bodies need the calcium and nutrients in milk as much when we're 70 as when we're 7. Adults, especially women, need 1000-1500 mg of calcium each day. That's the amount in three to five 8 fl oz glasses of milk.
Myth: Adults can get all the calcium they need from supplements.
Fact: Calcium supplements and calcium-fortified drinks don't provide the range of nutrients found in milk- like vitamin D, potassium and phosphorus - that help our bodies use calcium efficiently. And, the National Institutes of Health says that calcium-rich foods, like dairy products, are the preferred source of calcium.

A naked model on page 9 of the brochure has a message written on her back, "The beauty of strong bones." Page 8 informs the reader that, "More than 20 million American women suffer from osteoporosis, a painful, bone-weakening disease." Thank goodness, the text explains, "In fact, milk is one of the best and richest sources of calcium. It's also one of the easiest, most natural and delicious ways to meet your daily calcium requirement."

Advice From the Experts

The NFMPPB brochure was "developed with the help of a variety of experts, including top chefs, registered dietitians, leading physicians and scientists." The back cover lists an impressive scientific advisory panel of doctors and nutritionists.

Susan I. Barr, Ph.D.

Susan Barr, Ph.D., is the first "expert" listed on the "ADVICE FROM THE EXPERTS" page. Dr. Barr is an associate professor of nutrition at the University of British Columbia. Dr. Barr was kind enough to welcome questions and offer advice about milk. When responding to an e-mail request, Barr wrote to me, "I'd hesitate to identify myself as an 'expert' on nutrition and milk---but it is an area I do work in...fire away and I'll try to respond within a reasonable length of time." (4) I wrote back, "The NFMPPB calls you an expert. Anyway, here are my questions..." I'm still waiting for a response from Susan Barr, Ph.D. and milk expert. Why is she listed on the back cover of the "Milk, What a Surprise" brochure, under the heading, "Advice from the Experts"?

Barr is a member of the National Institute of Nutrition (NIN) of Canada, whose purpose and function is to advance the knowledge and practice of nutrition in Canada. In the summer of 1995, NIN issued a report titled, "Dairy Products in the Canadian Diet." This report concludes:

> Dairy products in the amounts recommended by *Canada's Food Guide to Healthy Eating* provide a wide range of nutrients essential to Canadians of all ages. These nutrients play a crucial role in the maintenance of health and the prevention of the diseases that are the heaviest burden on the health and well-being of our population: cardiovascular diseases, cancers, osteoporosis and hypertension. However, choosing lower-fat products more often is important, given the relationship of fats or certain types of fats with some of these diseases. To ensure an adequate vitamin D intake and to maintain fat intake within the recommended levels, fluid milk should probably contribute at least one half of the recommended number of servings." (5) Here are some interesting statements in the article:

1) Dairy products are a significant source of fat, saturated fats and cholesterol, all of which have been shown to increase blood cholesterol and the risk of cardiovascular disease.

2) Epidemiological studies suggest a relatively strong association between dietary fats and colorectal cancer.

3) A few studies have reported a positive association between milk intake and ovarian cancer.

Suzanne Oparil, Ph.D.

Suzanne Oparil, Ph.D., is a professor of medicine at the University of Alabama. According to the NFMPPB, she is the current president of the American Heart Association. She also serves as a national advisor to the American Dietetic Association's Nutrition and Health Campaign for Women. Great credentials, and she's listed under "ADVICE FROM THE EXPERTS" on the back cover of the milk brochure. I wrote to Oparil and asked, "I wished to discuss milk, milk hormones and other factors in milk as they may affect heart disease. America had been told that Dr. Oparil was THE expert. Was I in error?" Oparil wrote to me and indicated that she "has no appropriate expertise." (6)

Robert P. Heaney, M.D.

We are told by the milk processors that Robert P. Heaney, M.D., is also in the select group of experts whose advice one should follow. (7)   Although Dr. Heaney must have, at one time, believed that milk provided the best form of dietary calcium, he no longer believes what the NFMPPB brochure represents. Heaney recently was asked whether milk is the best form of calcium, and replied, "That is not the case." Dr. Heaney is also listed as a calcium expert and Professor of Medicine at Creighton University School of Medicine in Omaha, Nebraska. This milk expert has accepted the evidence in a recent study published in the June, 1995 issue of *The American College of Nutrition*. That paper reveals that people absorb only 25 percent of calcium in milk while absorbing 42 percent of the calcium in apple juice. One wonders if Heaney still is considered an "Expert" by the Dairy Industry?

How Much Milk Do We Drink?

The United States Department of Agriculture (USDA) publishes a pamphlet containing annual data of food consumption by Americans. The information in this 1997 publication includes data from 1970 through the last year available, 1995. The Summary (page vii) reveals, "Increased use of low-fat and skim milk instead of whole milk has been substantial. However, the overall use of milkfat did not fall, because cheese consumption soared." (8)

The USDA calculations for dairy products are somewhat misleading. Milk by any other name is milk. However, cheese is not milk. It is a concentrated form of milk. An individual eating one pound of milk every day will consume 365 pounds of milk in a year. Therefore, an individual eating 365 pounds of cheese or ice cream or butter is consuming equal weight in pounds but different profusions of concentrated dairy factors. Dairy farmers and food processors are paid by the pound, not by liquid measure. People eat pounds of cheese and drink pounds of milk. How much milk does the average American drink? To understand the dairy influence on diet we must consider the conversions factors.

It takes 21.2 pounds of milk to make one pound of butter, so the 4.5 pounds of butter each American consumed in 1995 converts to 95.4 pounds of milk used to make that butter.

10 pounds of milk to make one pound of hard cheese.

12 pounds of milk to make one pound of ice cream.
2.1 pounds of milk to make one pound of evaporated milk.
11 pounds of milk to make one pound of non-fat dry milk.
7.4 pounds of milk to make one pound of dry whole milk.

The USDA publishes the conversion factors and the average annual consumption totals for each product. In 1995, each American ate 15.9 pounds of ice cream. Since each pound of ice cream requires 12 pounds of milk, the total milk products eaten (fat, cholesterol, milk proteins, etc.) would be equal to 12 X 15.9 or a total of 190.8 pounds of milk. The following data are based upon a total 1995 population of 260,341,000 Americans. The USDA reveals that the average American consumed 584 pounds of milk and dairy products in 1995. The amount of milk needed to manufacture the dairy products that Americans actually ate (ice cream, butter, cheese, etc.) was far greater than USDA statistics indicated.

1995 Per Capita Dairy Consumption In Pounds

Food Item	Pounds Eaten	Conversion Factor	Milk Consumption*
Butter	4.5	21.2	95.40
Whole Milk	72.1	1.0	72.10
2% Milk	69.1	1.0	69.10
1% Milk	22.0	1.0	22.00
Skim Milk	33.7	1.0	33.70
Flavored Milk	10.4	1.0	10.40
Cream	8.7	1.0	8.70
Cheese	27.7	10.0	277.00
Cottage Cheese	2.6	4.0	10.40
Ice Cream	15.9	12.0	190.80
Ice Milk	7.6	6.0	45.60
Sherbet	1.3	4.5	5.85
Other Frozen Products	4.8	1.0	4.80
Condensed Milk	6.4	2.1	13.44
Dry Whole Milk	0.4	7.4	2.96
Nonfat Dry Milk	3.8	11.0	41.80
Dried Whey	3.5	8.0	28.00

*Milk consumption after conversion

Annual Total Dairy (consumption)............932.05 lbs

By dividing the number of pounds of milk and dairy consumed each year by the average American (932.05) by the number of days in one year (365), we discover that it took 2.55 pounds of milk to supply the daily intake of dairy of that typical American. Consequently, in 1995, 10 million cows had to produce 663 million pounds of milk every day to insure that each man, woman and child in the United States would have a milk mustache. USDA reveals that 152 billion pounds of milk were produced by America's dairy cows in 1995. That's 416,000,000 pounds per day.

The Milk Discrepancy

The numbers do not add up! The United States Department of Agriculture reports that 416 million pounds of milk are produced each day and the consumption numbers published by the same agency work backwards to reveal that 663 million pounds of milk are produced daily. We're missing 247 million pounds of milk per day. Where did it go? Why is it missing? One can understand that when all of the milk fat in whole milk is made into butter, something is left behind. That something, no-fat protein milk, is used to make dried no-fat milk powder which is added as filler to many different commercial products. USDA does not detail the loss, nor do they note the discrepancy.

There probably is an overlap of various products, depending upon milk equivalency calculations which are calculated on milkfat content. USDA does not publish complete data, and detailed and rigorous calculations for these data are virtually impossible. Perhaps there should be an accounting.

Consider this. America's dairy farmers pay 15 cents to the Dairy Marketing Board for every hundred pounds of milk they produce. This means that if USDA is correct, and 416 million pounds of milk per day are produced, then the Dairy Marketing Board collects $228 million dollars a year to "market" milk and dairy products. However, if 663 million pounds of milk are produced daily, then the Dairy Industry receives $364 million dollars per year. How much income does the Dairy Industry receive from dairy farmers. Is it $228 million or $364 million? Does anybody, other than the Dairy Industry, audit those numbers? A message left on the 1-800 WHY MILK hotline regarding this discordance of numbers was not returned.

Why Milk?

Milk has been called the most perfect food on earth. Who calls it that? The Dairy Industry? Madison Avenue? Our mothers? Their mothers? Seven generations of mothers! From childhood we accept the myth and practice the tradition that milk is essential for growth and good health. Look back at the chart. It takes 21.2 pounds of milk to make one pound of butter. Simple math...5 1/4 pounds of milk to make one stick of butter. Divide that stick of butter into 5 pieces. One piece is used to fry your eggs and butter your toast, or approximately one pound (or approximately one pint) of milk.

American parents use milk to make breakfast a 30 second affair. A portion of cereal sprinkled into a bowl, dusted with sugar and softened in nice, cold wholesome milk insures a "healthy" nourishing breakfast is eaten by Junior before school. Eggs take a few minutes to prepare. Every child would like a Western omelet, two slices of buttered whole wheat toast, freshly squeezed juice. If only mom or dad had the time. Rip, pour, open, flow, sprinkle, snap-crackle-pop, and off to school.

Dietitians, family doctors, school nurses agree milk helps build strong bodies and is an important part of every American's diet. The National Institutes of Health agree. So does the *Journal of the American Medical Association*. Wholesome milk. It provides calcium and phosphorous and sodium. It gives you protein and carbohydrates and fat. It adds Vitamins A and C and D to your diet. It tastes great alone and better with a chocolate brownie. It's a requisite ingredient with a bowl of dry cereal. It makes a great bedtime snack with cookies for children. A warm glass of milk cures tummy aches.

Milk makes coffee palatable for millions. It's in hot chocolate and chocolate pudding and squirts as whipped cream on ice cream, covered with a caramel sauce made with milk. We grate cheese on our pasta and cover our pizzas with gooey mozzarella. We eat fermented milk with bacteria and yeast as yogurt for good health. We spread butter on our toast, use it to sauté onions and peppers. Our chicken-ala-king and cream of mushroom soup would be less tasty without the dairy influence. Could one eat a bagel and lox without cream cheese? Life would be so boring without dairy products. A sandwich without Swiss or American or Provolone? Never! Practically un-American!

The information in this book is going to provide:

A REALLY BIG SURPRISE!

When they read this book the farmers who milk and feed their cows are going to be surprised. So are the truck drivers who haul 50,000 pound tanks of milk from farm to processor. The supermarket managers who carefully planned and situated their milk cases as far from the front door as possible...they'll be in for a big surprise. So will consumers who buy gallons of milk each week to insure the good health of their families. Doctors who should know better...are going to be surprised, and dietitians who should know better, but don't, why they'll have their surprise too! Perhaps the most surprised folks will be those to whom we've entrusted our health needs. The people at FDA, the scientists and administrators at the USDA. These people act as our fiduciaries and they do know better. The scientists who have the actual research evidence that refutes Dairy Industry publicity know better. These people are aware of bits and pieces of the evidence.

There is another group of people who should know better, but money gets in their way. We elect them to Congress but they take bribes, PAC money, from the Dairy Industry to "look the other way" and know nothing but the way to the bank. Finally, there are the research scientists who have changed milk by genetically engineering it. These men and women employed by pharmaceutical companies do know better and are going to have one unfortunate surprise when their secrets are revealed. They've taken "wholesome milk," which was never really intended to be consumed by humans, and they've changed it so remarkably that it doesn't come close to resembling the white fluid which comes directly from the udder of a cow.

Milk, What a Surprise!

"People think that it must be fun to be a super genius, but they don't realize how hard it is to put up with all the idiots in the world."

Calvin (to Hobbes), CALVIN & HOBBES,
Bill Watterson

"Isn't your pant's zipper supposed to be in the front?"

Hobbes (in response to Calvin), CALVIN & HOBBES,
Bill Watterson

"Sometimes I lie awake at night, and I ask, "Where have I gone wrong?" Then a voice says to me, "This is going to take more than one night."

Charlie Brown, PEANUTS,
Charles Schultz

Chapter 2

A Brief History of Milk in America

Milk in the twenty-first century will be quite different from the milk that was produced in the seventeenth century. When the Pilgrims milked their animals almost 380 years ago, they were fortunate to receive even one quart of milk per day from each cow. Many changes over the centuries have improved that yield and today's milk production per cow has been increased by a factor of 50. Our founding fathers and mothers sat on a stool and placed a bucket under their cow and yanked on her udders until there was enough milk to be churned into the equivalent of one stick of butter. That butter was stored so that the concentrated fat would provide nourishment for Pilgrims to survive harsh New England winters. Since the 1620s improved management techniques and new ways of processing and storing milk have altered the dairy industry. Today milk is refrigerated, pasteurized and homogenized. Animals are injected with antibiotics which control the levels of bacteria in their milk. Their feed has changed. Cows used to graze in fields and eat grass. Today their diets are supplemented with bone meal and blood meal and ground body parts from the byproducts of slaughterhouse renderings.

Cows have been cross-bred, in-bred, selectively bred (and served between two pieces of bread with special sauce). It is only a matter of time before the best producing cows are cloned. News of the first cloned bull (appropriately named

"Gene") was divulged six months after the fact on August 6, 1997. Cows are also injected with genetically engineered versions of their own growth hormones. These new hormones allow the animal to produce greater amounts of milk. The new milk is different from the old milk. Each procedure has changed the taste and consistency of milk. Each change has generated controversy from those who protested the altering of previously "wholesome" milk. Food purists criticized pasteurization, a process that saved the dairy industry. Without pasteurization, milk quickly spoils as bacteria multiplies. On November 5, 1993, FDA approved the use of a genetically engineered recombinant bovine growth hormone. Natural growth hormones were taken from dairy cows and recombined with the genetic material of bacteria, then implanted inside of *E. coli* bacteria. The resulting bacteria produced large amounts of bovine growth hormones which are processed. The procedure was commercially viable for farmers and represented the beginning of a new food industry, genetic engineering. We've come a long way since Colonial times. Native Americans had no cows and drank no milk. They witnessed the Pilgrims landing and ate the Pilgrim's butter. Our dairy industry all began with Miles Standish and the Mayflower.

Miles Standish? Every school-aged child knows who Miles Standish was. He was the captain and cruise director of the good ship Mayflower which landed at Plymouth Rock, Massachusetts, on December 21, 1620. Actually, he wasn't really the captain. He wasn't even a Pilgrim! But he was a leader among men, and when the Pilgrims did land at Plymouth Rock he became their leader. The actual captain of the Mayflower, for trivia buffs and history students, was Christopher Jones. [1]

Why anybody would travel to New England in the winter is a question nobody thought of asking. The Pilgrims had very little for which to be thankful. That first bitter winter they had limited food supplies, poor clothing and crudely built housing. During the months preceding spring, fifteen of the eighteen married women died as did twenty-two of thirty-eight men. Nearly all the children under two died. Interestingly, only one of the eight single women died. The other seven must have used some special resource, unreported by Pilgrim historians, to survive. Even Miles Standish lost his wife, Rose. However, he quickly married one of the hardy unattached lasses. Because of this great trauma of death from starvation, something had to be done to assure the survival of the colony.

Two years earlier, Pilgrims had established a settlement at Jamestown, Virginia. The South was warmer than Massachusetts. Pocohantas married John Rolfe and he learned how to cure tobacco. Dutch traders captured African slaves from a Spanish ship and sold them to the tobacco growers as cheap labor. [2] Subsequent ships brought cows to the New World which the Jamestown colonists found to their liking. There are no records of milk use or milk production. However, there are records of barbecues. There was no need to store the fat from these cows because there was no harsh winter. Instead, the fat was used to self-baste baked and broiled cow parts.

The First Dairy Cows in America

Meanwhile, back at the fort in Plymouth, Massachusetts, Pilgrims were shivering, diseased and dying of starvation. History does not record whose idea it was to get some of those cows. Finally, in March 1624 they came to Plymouth on the ship, *Charity,* which delivered three cows and a bull to the grateful pilgrims. (3) Within a generation every family in America had a dairy cow. Everybody knows the look of a butter churn. Milk was churned into butter. Few records were kept of how much butter or ice cream was consumed or how much cheese was produced. We are only left with evidence of the existence of butter churns.

Sophisticated techniques and technological advances in animal husbandry were not yet developed. Dairy cows weren't cross-bred in the seventeenth century. Genetic engineering and dairy herd management were un "herd" of, if you'll excuse the expression. One can assume that cows in the 1600s yielded as much milk as cows in the 1300s. Will and Ariel Durant, those historians who wrote the epic series of tomes, *The Story of Civilization,* reveal that a typical dairy cow in the 1200s yielded but a quart of milk per day. In the *Age of Faith,* history of life in the Middle Ages, the Durants wrote:

> Dairy farming was unprogressive; the average cow in the thirteenth
> century gave little milk, and hardly a pound of butter per week. (4)

Making butter requires 21.2 pounds of milk for each "finished" pound of butter. One quart of milk weighs 2.15 pounds. (5) A dairy cow in Plymouth Rock, Massachusetts, might yield his Pilgrim family "hardly a pound of butter per week." That averaged out to three pounds of milk per day, about three pints or a quart and-a-half.

People who think early Americans drank milk do not consider how little milk cows gave. Nor do they consider the existence of butter churns. Butter churns weren't hood ornaments for Pilgrim's carriages. Pilgrims used them only for one purpose: to churn milk into butter. That three pounds of milk per day would yield only one-half stick of butter. That's it! That's all. Imagine fifteen of the eighteen Pilgrim wives dying during the first winter. Imagine the same proportion of the mothers in your community dying from starvation over the winter. Imagine half of the fathers in your city or town dying over the winter because there was not enough food to eat. You'd need emergency rations to survive. Fat from milk, stored underground, saved for the winter months. Drink milk? Milk mustaches? Got milk? No way! One-half stick of butter per day, one pound of butter per week, carefully and strenuously churned by a Pilgrim and stored for the cruel New England winter.

Did the Pilgrims drink milk in the summer? Did milk store well? Of course not. Milk was loaded with bacteria which quickly spoiled, making it undrinkable. By churning the milk into butter and storing it underground, the fat was saved until it was needed. Milk was first pasteurized in 1864, but Louis Pasteur's work wasn't introduced in America until 1897. (6) Had Miles Standish landed in the Hamptons in July 1620 (like New York State's first settlers did) or waited for the winter to end before sailing to America, the Pilgrims could have had nine months of good weather to build, plan, and plant crops and survive winter without devastation and death. Instead, their experience made it necessary for every family to carefully store food through the bountiful months so that they might survive the hardships of winter. Butter became their insurance policy. It became necessary for every New England family to own a dairy cow. In a few years, that's just what happened.

The Actual Reason For Thanksgiving

Imagine the depression of imminent death by starvation. You come to a new world without food and shelter, you haven't bathed in three months and are wearing the same clothes in which you started your voyage. It's December of 1620 and it's snowing, you've sent a landing party ashore and they've stolen corn from some very angry Abenaki Indians (7) who would like nothing better than to shoot their arrows at you. (Which they did!) Didn't the Pilgrims bear in mind the Eighth Commandment, "Thou shalt not steal?" Obviously not! They left England, seeking religious freedom, or so our children are taught, and immediately broke one of God's commandments by stealing food from the Indians. Thank goodness for modern day revisionist history and historians and school teachers who twist the truth to relieve our conscience.

How would you handle such fear? By spring, half of your fellows are dead. At last, summer arrives and you discover the great bounty of the New World. You store enough food to guarantee the survival of your entire colony for the next winter. That's reason enough to give thanks! That's a reason to throw a party! However, the death and despair could have been avoided.

Fate and Fat: The Dairy Connection

The Pilgrims had actually planned for the harsh winter of 1620. They sailed from Holland to London to Southampton, England, where they boarded the *Mayflower*, bringing along their provisions. There was one big problem. At this point in their journey, they were broke and they could not pay their bills. Owing 100 English pounds, they couldn't sail until they paid this bill. So they sold some of their provisions, a calculated gamble which put them at the mercy of diminished resources and divine providence. Unfortunately, their resources were inadequate. The bet didn't work. Historian William Bradford relates:

> So they were forced to sell off some of their provisions to stop
> this gap, which was some three or four-score firkins of butter,
> commodity they might best spare, having which provided too
> large a quantity of that kind. (8)

They sold their insurance policy, their food for the winter, their butter, and with it the lives of half of their number. A letter written on August 3, 1620, to the "beloved friends" of these Pilgrims explained:

> We are in such a strait at present, as we are forced to sell away our
> provisions to clear the haven and withal to put ourselves
> upon great extremities, scarce having any butter...we are willing
> to expose ourselves to such eminent dangers as are like to
> ensue, and trust to the good providence of God... (9)

They sold the concentrated fat which would have helped them to survive in New England. Had they not sold this treasure, they would have most certainly not starved and suffered the trauma of seeing half their number perish. Would a three day Thanksgiving have been called for, the following year? All because they sold their butter. How much butter did they intend to bring to the New World? Some "three to four-score firkins." William Bradford, author of *Of Plymouth Plantation*, said that the Pilgrims sold approximately 4,040 pounds of butter. That meant that every man woman and child was rationed 40 pounds of butter each. By today's standards, in order to produce those 4,040 pounds of butter they would have required 85,648 quarts of milk. A herd of 100 cows, each producing one quart of milk per day would have taken nearly eight months to produce that much milk. Now, that's a lot of churning! So, that's why Miles Standish, today's symbolically appointed leader of the Mayflower Pilgrims, gets a share of the credit. Without his poor planning and great leadership the Pilgrims might not have landed in New England in the winter. Without such a mistake, the Pilgrims would not have faced such hardships. They would have had time to harvest the natural resources of their new land. The Pilgrims could have survived on fat from butter from dairy cows. Thank you, Miles Standish.

How Times Change: Milk Yield Per Cow

By the mid-1800s, the average cow yielded just under two quarts of milk each per day. By 1960, that yield was over nine quarts per animal per day. Today, thanks to new techniques including increased use of antibiotics, genetically selective breeding, and, my own personal favorite, genetic engineering, cows can yield up to 50 quarts of milk/day, with the average dairy cow producing 18,000 pounds per year, or 24 quarts daily.

Pasteurization

In 1856, Louis Pasteur began experiments resulting in a new technology that rewarded Pasteur by borrowing his name. Thank goodness this process was not developed by my great-grandfather on my mother's side, Simon Lipshitz. Then we would have milk that was, well, use your imagination! There'd be enormous confusion with respect to its wholesomeness, although there would be poetic justice in such a label and warning. Amid great controversy, Chicago passed the first American compulsory pasteurization law in 1908. Most current day Americans have never tasted real milk. Fresh from the udder, milk foams at body temperature. When chilled, the taste changes. Londoners have acquired the taste for warm beer in British pubs. Warm beer, warm milk. Acquired tastes. Pasteurized milk is heated milk. It has been cooked to kill the bacteria, then quickly chilled. Tuberculosis epidemics, botulism, myriads of diseases spread through the milk supply made pasteurization necessary. Yet, the essence of milk changed. Pasteurization destroys vitamins and enzymes. In 1908, doctors, dietitians and health activists condemned the process.

Imagine taking delicate strawberries and cooking them. Watermelon? Yeech. Note the difference between fresh apple cider and commercially prepared and bottled apple juice. Taste the crisp burst of flavor from a luscious apple, and follow that with a mouthful of cooked apple sauce. What have we done to milk by pasteurizing it? We've killed the goodness and flavor. But if we hadn't gone to such extremes, we would have witnessed the end of the dairy industry. Unpasteurized "wholesome" milk was the ideal environment for bacteria to rapidly multiply.

Homogenization

In 1932, a procedure of adding artificially produced vitamin D into milk was developed. Technological advances soon insured that milk would not separate. Homogenization, a process begun in 1919, became the standard and not the exception. In 1964, plastic milk containers were first commercially introduced. Later, labeling laws required mandatory nutrition information on every container of milk sold.

Politics and Science

When mankind began to tamper with nature's own substance again in the 1990s, controversy followed. Genetic engineering? There was a movement to label the milk containing the new genetically engineered hormones. Scientists, politicians and admen with marketing propensity determined policy. The public won't buy a milk with warnings that it has been genetically engineered, they assumed. To hell with the public's right to know!

In an incredible act of political intrigue Monsanto's attorney resigned from his law firm to go to work for the FDA. "Genetically engineered milk is indistinguishable from normal wholesome milk," wrote Michael Taylor. Michael Taylor was the attorney, a partner at King & Spalding, a powerful Washington law firm. Overnight, Taylor became one of the "powers" at FDA. Once there, he would continue to work in his new capacity for his old client, Monsanto. Taylor wrote the labeling laws which lied to the citizens of America. "The milk from cows treated with genetically engineered bovine growth hormone is indistinguishable from normal milk," said Taylor. Although Congress investigated this conflict of interest, he was subsequently rewarded by being named the acting under-secretary of food safety at the Department of Agriculture. Before joining King & Spalding in 1981, Taylor served as executive assistant to the commissioner of FDA. He then practiced food and drug law for ten years at King & Spalding before re-joining FDA. After his stint at FDA he went to the USDA. As of November 1996, Taylor was back at the firm.

So, today the public does not know whether the milk they buy has been treated with a genetically recombined hormone, recombined with *E. coli* bacteria, or whether the milk is the same "wholesome" stuff they've been drinking since childhood. The average milk production of a dairy cow in India is under three quarts per day with the average per capita milk consumption equal to 3 ounces per day. In the USA, the average dairy cow produces 24 quarts per day. Pasteurization, homogenization and genetic engineering. We've changed milk.

The Milk Controversy

My children are the reason I developed an interest in milk. One day in August 1994, I read a column written by Jane Heimlich, a health and nutrition writer for Julian Whitaker's *Health and Healing* newsletter. Her column explored all aspects of the controversy surrounding the first genetically engineered product developed for our food supply. This new hormone, recombinant bovine somatotropin (rbST) also was named recombinant bovine growth hormone (rbGH). (10) The Monsanto Agricultural Company of St. Louis, Missouri, had found a way to combine the genetic material from a naturally occurring cow hormone with bacteria. This new technology allowed Monsanto scientists to grow this new version of the naturally occurring hormone inside of a specially developed strain of bacteria so that the growth factor could be inexpensively mass produced.

The bacteria were then "harvested" with sophisticated new techniques, and the hormone collected. The new drug called re-combinant bovine somatotropin (rBST) would then be injected into cows. The rBST-treated cows then would produce more milk. The controversy revealed that there might be problems with the milk. This was the first I had heard of it. I called the publisher of this newsletter and soon connected with Jane Heimlich. The more I learned, the more concerned I became for my children. I certainly could control the milk my children consumed. It was summer, but there were personnel working at the Board of Education at the public school which they attended. After a few phone calls I learned that their school was negotiating with a new milk supplier. They were about to sign a contract to buy milk from a company that was buying milk from dairies that treated their cows with this new hormone. I protested this decision by writing letters, making phone calls, and successfully stalled this decision. Instead, the school bought milk from a supplier who stated that his dairy farmers do not use the new hormone and he would not accept milk from cows treated with rBST. That was good enough for me. I had won a minor skirmish. Soon there'd be more battles.

My Credentials

At Long Island University's Southampton College I studied physiological psychology under Robert K. Orndoff, Ph.D., whom I consider my mentor. I selected psychobiology as my major to prepare for a career in biological research. I loved the challenge of exploring a hypothesis, designing experiments to test it, and solving the riddles, the maze of variables and influences associated with the scientific investigation of living organisms and life processes. I was soon immersed in laboratory research in the field of psychoneuroendocrinology, studying the influence of hormones on brain chemistry and subsequent mammalian behavior. I performed surgery on hundreds of laboratory animals and learned how slight details, easily overlooked, can drastically affect a research project, or nullify it altogether. Undergraduate students, correctly instructed in performing proper research techniques or experimental protocols, learn that very subtle cues may modify and manipulate behavior.

I have worn many hats in my life, done many things. Life has been a series of games and adventures, an exciting roller coaster ride. I've scuba dived with sharks. I've piloted a plane. I've climbed a mountain. I attended the Culinary Institute of America. I've been in the restaurant business. I worked for a major real estate company in Englewood Cliffs, New Jersey, KAMSON, where I was head of new development. I worked for one of the finest men on this planet,

Richard Kurtz. In that capacity, I once attempted to negotiate a deal with George Steinbrenner's chief counsel, to purchase the New York Yankees and build a baseball stadium in the New Jersey Meadowlands. Henry Aaron, a man I much admire, would have been our General Manager.

I was a lab assistant in a biological research laboratory where I performed brain surgery on laboratory animals. We are all unique individuals. We are all the sum of our previous experiences. All of my life experiences have made me into a unique individual. I possess many skills. Those skills allow me to write this book. I can communicate with scientists, understand complicated scientific data, and I can translate scientific experience into concepts easily understood by non-scientists. I believe that all of my life has been a journey to take me where I now am.

I Wanted To Be A Scientist

All I really wanted out of life, at age 20, was to be a scientist. I was attending Southampton College, part of Long Island University, in New York State's Hamptons. What a wonderful place to go to school! I studied under Robert K. Orndoff. For two years, I was a psychology major. After taking physiological psychology with Orndoff, I switched my major to psychobiology. I never wanted to be a doctor. I simply wanted to do biological research. I studied genetics and endocrinology and took a pre-med curriculum that included courses in histology and mammalian physiology. After I changed my psychology major to psychobiology, I conducted research on laboratory animals in the field of psychoneuroendocrinology. I learned how hormones acted on the brain and affected mammalian behavior. As an undergraduate student I was privileged to be able to conduct research in a small college. Orndoff had graduated from Berkeley with a most prestigious group of advisors including three Nobel Prize winners on his Orals Committee. He had a favor to call in and his influence and my performance would have succeeded in getting me accepted as a Berkeley graduate student, had I so wished.

How "Science" Can Go Wrong

In performing research, a scientist must endeavor to eliminate any variables which compromise that research. It's usually a good idea, when treating one group of animals with a drug or device, to use a control group. Without a control group one can never know what the effects of that drug would be on the "untreated" group. This makes sense! Undergraduate students are taught proper research techniques. They learn that very subtle cues can modify and manipulate a subject's behavior. For example, if the subjects were human, the researchers might treat attractive volunteers differently and those biases would compromise the effects of the drug and the results of the study. One researcher, world renowned Frank Beech, Ph.D., of Berkeley, would not allow women to work in his lab. Dr. Beech correctly reasoned that women menstruate and animals react to the chemical smells, called pheromones, from these women. These chemical messengers alter an animal's behavior and any data collected from research would have been compromised by daily hormonal differences during a woman's menstrual cycle.

All Important: Critical Details

An example of how unanticipated variables can betray a scientist illustrates the care that must be taken in designing and conducting studies. Here is what occurred in one study in which I participated. By telling you about this mistake, and revealing my techniques, and subsequent discovery of a serious error, you might accept my credentials and excuse the fact that I have no M.D. or Ph.D. after my name. I helped to design a study intended to discover how the female hormone, estrogen, worked inside of an animal's body. Where does estrogen go, what tissues does it affect? Working with rats I injected a radioactive form of estrogen (tritiated estradiol benzoate) into two dozen animals. I carefully sacrificed these animals ("sacrificed," a politically acceptable way of saying I killed them) and using surgical techniques mastered from previous experience, I carefully separated various organs and tissues for testing. (I had previously operated on hundreds of animals, performing ovario-hysterectomies, ligating renal arteries in kidney hypertension studies, implanting electrodes in various areas of the brain, among other things). I was proficient at isolating various tissues including thigh muscle, organs and brain tissues.

Using a machine called a scintillation spectrometer which measured the radioactive samples of estrogen, I was able to calibrate how, where and in what amounts estrogen was bound to various organs and tissues. The study provided enlightenment into previously conceived areas of knowledge. I was excited, until a dreaded word emerged from deep within my consciousness. A word never to be uttered by a surgeon or a doctor treating a patient. A word to strike fear in the hearts of scientists and lab personnel everywhere. "Mistake!" We had made a mistake! I hadn't considered a variable so critical as to negate six months of planning and compromise all results of the study. I rushed to check, and found my worst fears confirmed. Rat Chow! Purina Rat Chow! Made from alfalfa! Oh, no! Alfalfa contains a substance that is almost identical in steroid structure to estrogen.

I tell this story to demonstrate how critical every detail of a research project is. It was my responsibility to identify and eliminate all possible extraneous variables, but I overlooked the powerful influence of dietary hormones. The last thing scientists or pharmaceutical companies want is to have their work questioned or compromised. Twenty-four years would pass before I applied my scientific training and knowledge and love of reading journal articles and interpolating complicated scientific data to the milk controversy generated by Monsanto's new genetically engineered hormone.

I doubt that many doctors or scientists have the opportunity, or more specifically, the time and desire to spend two years reading, analyzing every aspect of research, contacting hundreds of labs and scientists, putting together a complete picture of how milk hormones work and affect the human body. When people go to work they do their jobs and then leave those jobs to go home. They have hundreds or thousands of different tasks and assignments over a two-year period. I had one. They went home for a weekend. I worked seven days per week. I read and studied and analyzed.

The approval of the genetically engineered milk hormone was the most controversial in the history of the Food and Drug Administration. The amount of research submitted by Monsanto, 55,000 pages, overwhelmed FDA reviewers. Monsanto invested $500 million in developing this new drug and food additive. I became the one person in America to meet with the FDA on the scientific merits of this controversy and on April 21, 1995, I was invited to the Center for Veterinary Medicine and discussed many of the issues in this book with FDA scientists.

In college I enjoyed reading scientific journals. In order to be current with the latest research and techniques one has to read such journals every day. For a doctor or practicing scientist, this is nearly impossible. For a motivated investigator seeking the solution to a mystery this is a labor of love. During the summer of 1994, I read a column written by Jane Heimlich in a medical newsletter. (11) Heimlich, author of the best selling book, *What Your Doctor Won't Tell You,* is the wife of the world famous Henry Heimlich, M.D., inventor of the "Heimlich Maneuver," the anti-choking technique that has been used to save thousands of lives. Jane writes a column in Dr. Julian Whitaker's *Health and Healing Newsletter,* published by Philips Publishing. This medical newsletter has a circulation of 500,000 readers and is one of the most popularly read and respected newsletters in America. They'll send you promotional information if you call them at 1-800-777-5005.

Jane Heimlich's Column

Reprinted with the permission of Julian Whitaker, Jane Heimlich and Philips Publishing.

Is Your Milk Safe to Drink?

Care to increase your health risks? That's what you (or your child or grandchild) will be doing when you drink a glass of milk, or eat ice cream, butter, cheese or beef that comes from cows treated with the genetically engineered hormone called, "recombinant bovine growth hormone" (rBGH).

The synthetic growth hormone, also called Bovine Somatotropin, increases cow's milk output by as much as 20%. The drug became available to farmers on February 3, 1994, and is expected to earn an annual $500 million in the U.S. for Monsanto, the giant chemical company which is the first to sell it. (Considering the glut of milk for the past decade, economic justification for using rBGH remains a mystery.)

But the Food and Drug Administration (FDA), which approved rBGH Nov. 5, 1993, says that hormone-treated milk is "not significantly different" from untreated milk. The safety of rBGH has been endorsed by the American Medical Association, the National Institutes of Health, and the American Dietetic Association, among others. rBGH is not approved in Canada, Japan, Australia, New Zealand and Europe.

Dairy Farmers Protest rBGH

Despite official U.S. approval, 95% of dairy farmers are refusing to inject their cows with rBGH, says Pete Hardin, editor/publisher of The Milkweed (the farmers' milk market report), Brooklyn, Wisc. In response to consumer demand, over 250 milk producers, distributors, companies and supermarket chains are in the process of certifying their products free of rBGH.

Four states (Vermont, Minnesota, Wisconsin and Maine) have passed laws making it legal for rBGH-free companies to label their products as such. (According to the FDA, a company can only state that its milk comes from untreated herds if it also says: "no significant difference has been shown" between milk from treated and untreated cows.)

My deep concern about rBGH is that this new and poorly tested drug poses serious health risks to humans, aside from the fact that it's apt to make cows sick and cause them to suffer.

The single most disturbing aspect of rBGH, from a human safety standpoint, concerns Insulin-like Growth Factor-I (IGF-I), which is linked to breast cancer. IGF-I occurs naturally in human beings as well as cows, but rBGH injections cause substantial and sustained increases of IGF-I levels in milk, says Samuel S. Epstein, M.D., professor of occupational and environmental medicine at the Illinois School of Public Health.

Worse yet, "IGF-I is not destroyed by pasteurization, survives the digestive process, is absorbed into the blood, and produces potent growth-promoting effects," according to Epstein.

Epstein says it is highly likely that IGF-I helps transform normal breast tissue to cancerous cells, and enables malignant human breast cancer cells to invade and spread to distant organs.

Increases the Risk of Infections - and Drug use - in Dairy Cows

As clearly stated in the package insert that Monsanto sends with the drug, Posilac (trade name for rBGH) increases risk of mastitis (an infection of the udder), and "has been associated with increases in somatic cell counts." (In plain words, pus.)

Increased risk of infections (almost 80% in rBGH-treated herds), says Consumers Union biochemist, Michael K. Hansen, Ph.D., means farmers have to treat their cows with more drugs, a fact also mentioned in the drug-package insert. (Consumers Union, New York, is the publisher of Consumer Reports Magazine.)

Upping the use of antibiotics already is a serious concern, because, according to a Government Accounting Office August 1992 study, a majority of antibiotics are not approved for use on dairy cows - and testing for antibiotics by milk inspectors is extremely lax.

What the FDA calls "safe levels" of antibiotic residues have been shown to increase the growth of drug-resistance in bacteria. So, if you develop salmonella, a virulent infection, antibiotics may have no effect.

Incredible as it sounds, the FDA's assumption that rBGH is safe for humans is based upon short-term rat experiments done by Monsanto-sponsored scientists, not independent ones. Contrary to FDA conclusions, biochemist Dr. William von Meyer, president of Fairview Industries (a firm conducting genetic and biochemical research), Middleton, Wisc., found that these rats showed significant bone growth and changes in liver size.

The only human study involving rBGH was a 50-year-old experiment in which dwarfs were given BGH to see if they would grow. They did not.

Make Your Views Known About rBGH

Concerned about rBGH in our milk products? Here's what you can do:

* Contact the manager of your supermarket, and ask if the store sells milk and dairy products that come from cows not treated with rBGH. If he or she hedges on the issue, say you'll buy your milk products elsewhere.

* If you can't locate a source for rBGH-free dairy products, investigate milk alternatives, which are healthier than cow's milk (as described in the July 1993 issue of Health and Healing). My favorite is Original Lite Rice Dream, a 1% fat drink made from brown rice (quart size costs $1.99 to $2.40). Another

option is Edensoy Original (a liter costs $1.99 to $2.59). You'll find them in health food stores.

* *Call the Pure Food Campaign, a national organization (800/253-0681) that is fighting rBGH in milk, to get in touch with local coordinators.*

* *Ask your local news editor to cover the bovine growth hormone issue, or write a letter to the editor. Or call-in a local radio talk show to discuss the issue, and give the Pure Food Campaign's 800 number.*

* *Contact members of your local school board and ask them to pass a resolution prohibiting the use in school meal programs of milk or dairy products that come from rBGH-injected cows. Thus far, 73 school districts have passed such resolutions.*

* *Contact your state and nationally elected officials and tell them you want labels on products treated with rBGH. (Your public library or the League of Women Voters can supply names and phone numbers.)*

Like any good teacher, Heimlich's job was to inspire her students. This column inspired me to learn more and investigate the milk controversy. I did not immediately give up milk as a result of Heimlich's exposition and commentary. However, subsequent investigation suggested that genetic engineering just made a bad product significantly worse.

"Whoso would be a man, must be a nonconformist. He who would gather immortal palms must not be hindered by the name of goodness, but must explore if it be goodness. Nothing is at last sacred but the integrity of your own mind..."

Ralph Waldo Emerson - "Self Reliance" - 1844

Chapter 3

Milk Has Changed: Genetic Engineering

O ur milk has been altered and only a relatively small sample of America's population is aware of the change. Some people have heard of BST (bovine somatotropin) or BGH (bovine growth hormone). BST and BGH are two different acronyms for the same hormone that is naturally present in milk. Some consumers have become very discriminating purchasers, refusing to drink milk containing hormones, unaware that all milk carries growth hormones. Milk naturally embodies hormones.   Those natural hormones have been genetically engineered and combined with genetic material from bacteria. When a hormone is recombined with genetic material from another species of animal, the resulting hormone has the letter "r" placed before it. Therefore, BST becomes rBST and BGH becomes rBGH. Milk from cows injected with rBST or rBGH contains more hormones.   There is much misunderstanding on this controversial issue.   The reason for this misunderstanding lies (an appropriate word) with the Food and Drug Administration (FDA) which informed America that rBST-treated milk and normal wholesome milk were indistinguishable.

Many researchers, doctors and activists protested the research and questioned the numerous contradictions in the scientific data that were published by FDA.   There were also conflicts of interest between FDA and the drug's manufacturer.   The conflicts resulted in a Congressional request for an investigation, but the subsequent recommendations made to Congress were ignored.   In addition, cows treated with these new hormones were getting sick. The milk contained more hormones and increased levels of bacteria.   Calves birthed to the cows were born with genetic deformities. FDA withheld much of the data from investigators, despite Freedom of Information Act requests.

A small group of extremely dedicated nonconformists were named in the Jane Heimlich milk column. Each, a true American hero. They included Pete Hardin, editor of the dairy industry newsletter, *The Milkweed*, Sam Epstein, Ph.D., professor, cancer researcher and author of numerous books and scientific articles, and Michael Hansen, Ph.D., scientist, writer and lecturer from the Consumers

Union, publisher of *Consumers Reports Magazine*. Rounding out the foursome was Dr. William von Meyer, president of Fairview Industries, a firm conducting biochemical and genetic research. I spoke to these men, each and every one an acknowledged and respected authority in his field regarding the subject of milk and/or genetic engineering.

In order to balance my education and make an unbiased judgment, I also called the Monsanto Agricultural Company in St. Louis, Missouri. I was directed to speak with Robert Collier, Ph.D. Collier was friendly and obviously well versed on all of the issues. This well-published scientist and spokesman for Monsanto offered to send me a package of scientific studies and I accepted his offer. The next day a large priority mail package was delivered to my home. I discussed Jane Heimlich's column with Collier. I related four major areas that troubled me. These were no small concerns. I asked, "Was BST improperly tested? Did BST cause serious problems to cows? Were additional levels of antibiotics found in the milk because sick cows had to be doctored to combat increased occurrences of mastitis? Was there an increased risk of cancer to users of dairy products containing this new genetically engineered hormone?" He flippantly dismissed my concerns. Collier explained that the Board of Education of the Chicago school system considered this controversy in contemplating a ban on milk from cows treated with this hormone. He offered to send me the same studies and papers which Chicago had used to decide that the "new milk" was as safe as wholesome milk and indistinguishable from the milk of untreated cows. On August 25, 1994, I wrote a letter to Collier thanking him for sending me the following documents: (1)

1) NIH (National Institutes of Health) Technology Assessment Conference Statement
2) OTA (Office of Technology Assessment) Report
3) FDA (Food and Drug Administration) Juskevich and Guyer's August 24, 1990 *Science* publication
4) Executive Branch (White House) Study of BST
5) Inspector General Audit of BST Issues
6) NIH Panel Conclusions
7) GAO (Government Accounting Office) Report, 1990
8) Commission of European Community Reports
9) IGF-1 (Insulin-like growth factor-I) paper
10) WHO (World Health Organization) Committee on Food Additive Monographs
11) WHO 1993 Evaluation of Drug Residue Report

How FDA "Ended" the Milk Controversy

In order to end the debate surrounding the genetically engineered milk hormone, FDA published an article in the journal, *Science* (2) This August 24, 1990 paper was intended to end the controversy. Instead, it added fuel to the fires of protest of men like Epstein, Hansen, Hardin and von Meyer. Their voices would soon be joined by Jeremy Rifkin of the Pure Food Campaign. Each of the documents supplied by Monsanto's Collier relied on data and "facts" contained in the *Science* article. A review made clear that this FDA paper was the "LANDMARK" document to which all other agency reports referred. Thorough understanding of this article is critical to understanding the issues. This wasn't easy reading. So, to my desk I went, armed with calculator to interpolate the data. My background allowed me to read through and understand it in about three days. This was challenging to me. Laypersons in the Chicago school system trying to grasp the complex scientific issues would find the terminology and complexities of the *Science* paper nearly impossible! Yet they had a vital decision to make affecting the health and futures of thousands of students.

The Journal, *Science*

A press release from the peer-review journal *Science* reveals that each weekly issue is read by an estimated 500,000 persons. (3) It is published by the American Association for the Advancement of Science (AAAS) which has more than 143,000 members. The magazine was established by Thomas Edison in 1880 and has been the official journal of the AAAS ever since. Articles appearing in this journal represent the leading edge of scientific inquiry and research, and these articles are reviewed before publication by experts in the related subject field. The reviewers are supposed to be independent of any conflicts of interest and their identities are kept confidential. Once the articles are published, the information is laid bare to 500,000 other reviewers consisting of the world's scientific community.

Science is found in libraries, schools and research facilities. Often, publication of an article in *Science* is of such importance to a researcher that it can guarantee academic success and establish reputation. Of the hundreds of scientific peer-reviewed journals, *Science* is considered by many in the world of science to be one of the most prestigious.

FDA's Motivation to Publish in *Science*

Very simply, in order to end the controversy about genetically engineered hormones, FDA took an unprecedented action. For the first time in their history, they assigned the task of reviewing and summarizing the BST research to two FDA employees, Judy Juskevich, Ph.D., and Greg Guyer, Ph.D. These two scientists immortalized their names in the scientific community by writing a paper to which all others referred. Although this paper was accessible to 500,000 readers, and is now available in the archives of most of America's libraries, there are many who would prefer not to see it in print in its entirety. Had I written this paper for a high school biology class, I probably would have failed miserably. Not only were references incorrectly cited, but data were erroneously recorded, inaccurately reported, and conclusions were incorrectly reached. Very few of *Science's* readers detected these errors. Only a handful of critics saw anything wrong and of that small group only this author recognized that wholesome milk also contained the same powerful and dangerous growth hormones. Fraud was shaped in the world's most respected journal by a government agency, and the scientific community was asleep. Not even the independent peer-reviewers caught on, whomever they might have been.

As a result of this paper, Monsanto was granted approval for rBST. FDA commissioner, David Kessler, and other FDA employees testified before Congressional committees to a number of conclusions that were outright lies. The greatest lie, told by FDA, the *Journal of the American Medical Association*, National Institutes of Health, the World Health Organization, repeated by dozens of scientific agencies, thousands of newspapers and magazines, was:

Genetically engineered milk is identical to untreated milk. (4)

To list every reference to this lie would be to catalogue every newspaper in America. In Chapter Seven, our media, the "fourth estate," will be rigorously cited and criticized for letting this mistake become part of America's collective consciousness. Like the bold writing etched into the pedestals of monuments, the above statement was imprinted into the collective consciousness of America. Yet, even in the abstract (introduction and synopsis) of the paper, the authors told the truth in revealing that the two milks were different. According to Juskevich and Guyer, and supported by substantial and overwhelming research:

> Recombinant bGH (rBST) treatment produces an increase
> in the concentration of insulin-like growth factor-I (IGF-I)
> in cow's milk.

Jane Heimlich was concerned about IGF-I. She linked this hormone in milk to breast cancer. Genetic engineering produced more of this hormone in milk. FDA said that there was no difference, contradicting their own article, which appears with appropriate commentary.

As the author, I am your guide. A scientific paper can be as mysterious as a jungle, unyielding in its secrets to those who have not previously traveled its paths. In order to be able to see the trees and the root systems and the fauna living in harmony with the flora, I will present the forest in its entirety, pausing occasionally to point out what might ordinarily have been missed.

For the remainder of this chapter, two distinct style types will be used in order to allow the reader to examine the exact words presented by the two FDA scientists, Judy Juskevich and Greg Guyer, in their landmark *Science* paper, published on August 24, 1990. That paper will be presented in *italics.*

The Juskevich & Guyer Paper

Abstract

Scientists in the Food and Drug Administration (FDA), after reviewing the scientific literature and evaluating studies conducted by pharmaceutical companies, have concluded that the use of recombinant bovine growth hormone (rBGH or rBST) in dairy cattle presents no increased health risk to consumers. Bovine GH is not biologically active in humans, and oral toxicity studies have demonstrated that rBGH is not orally active in rats, a species responsive to parenterally administered bGH. Recombinant bGH treatment produces an increase in the concentration of insulin-like growth factor-I (IGF-I) in cow's milk. However, oral toxicity studies have shown that bovine IGF-I lacks oral activity in rats. Additionally, the concentration of IGF-I in milk of rbGH-treated cows is within the normal physiological range found in human breast milk, and IGF-I is denatured under conditions used to process cows' milk for infant formula. On the basis of estimates of the amount of protein absorbed intact in humans and the concentration of IGF-I in cow's milk during rbGH treatment, biologically significant levels of intact IGF-I would not be absorbed.

Translation: Scientese to Laymanese

Papers published in scientific journals are meant to be shared and meticulously critiqued by the entire scientific community. In theory, a scientist in Great Britain or Katmandu should be able to replicate the published studies of research performed in the United States and end up with similar results.

Therefore, experimental data and support for scientific arguments must be available for review, especially if conclusions are drawn and the authors expect those conclusions to be given credibility. The scientific community is not sitting in church listening to a preacher recite gospel from the great book. Many scientists are from the good state of Missouri, and if another scientist is bold enough to make a conclusion, he had better be prepared with data to answer upon demand a petition to "Show me!"

After reading the Juskevich and Guyer paper, I had many concerns and I went to FDA and Monsanto and said, "Show me." That's when the real "game" began. Their response was, "We do not have to show you. We are insulated and protected by law to the secrecy of our data. You'll never see it." As a scientist I was offended, then outraged. I felt that I had every moral and ethical right to examine the raw data. I wasn't interested in learning trade secrets. I wanted to know the actual weights of 32 different tissue and organ samples from 360 animals in just one experiment. I wanted 11,520 pieces of raw data so that I could perform rigorous statistical analyses and either confirm or reject the conclusions of the scientists. How could they logically deny me access to these data?

It took me one year to learn just how they would deny access to that data. My nuncupative requests were denied. Then formal Freedom of Information Act Requests were denied. An appeal to the Department of Health and Human Services was subsequently denied. A request to a Federal Court also proved unsuccessful in yielding the data. The United States was not concerned with a food additive that caused cancer in laboratory animals. They were concerned only with protecting the rights of companies manufacturing these poisons.

THEY SAID:	rBGH is not orally active in rats.
THAT MEANS:	When rats are fed rBGH nothing happens to them.
I SAID:	Why then does the data indicate that the average spleen size of animals that were injected with this hormone increase by 46 percent and that there were also increases in animals ingesting rBGH orally?
THEY RESPONDED:	That's not statistically significant.
I SAID:	Let me examine the actual raw data.
THEY SAID:	That's not possible.
I SAID:	Why not?
THEY SAID:	Because the raw data is a trade secret and if we release the truth, Monsanto will suffer harm.
THEY SAID:	The concentration of IGF-I in milk of rbGH-treated cows is within the normal physiological range found in human breast milk.
I SAID:	Adults don't drink human breast milk. Neither do most children over the age of two.

FDA: "Nursing (Breastfeeding) Doesn't Work"

FDA said many things I contradicted. That led to our meeting at the Center for Veterinary Medicine (FDA's scientific and investigative branch in Rockville, Maryland) on April 21, 1995. At that meeting, the FDA scientists unanimously agreed that milk proteins are "burned" in the stomach and rendered harmless, inactivated by digestive enzymes. I asked, "Do you gentlemen believe then, that a nursing mother passes nothing onto her infant child?   No hormones, no immunological factors?" They put together their collective scientific intellect and responded, "Perhaps nursing offers some psychological and nurturing benefit, but nothing more."   The Juskevich and Guyer paper appears, as written, with highlighted notes from this author.

Juskevich & Guyer

Growth hormone (GH) is a protein produced in the pituitary gland of all animals and is an important endocrine factor for normal lactation and growth in mammals. It was known as early as the 1930s that injection of dairy cows with bovine pituitary extracts increased milk yield, and this increase was eventually attributed to bovine growth hormone (bGH; also called bovine somatotropin or bST). The limited supply and the impurity of pituitary-derived bGH, however, precluded its commercial use on dairy farms. The advent of biotechnology in the 1980s has allowed the production of large quantities of pure bGH through recombinant DNA processes. Subsequently, several pharmaceutical firms have developed rbGH for administration to dairy cows to increase milk yield and the efficiency of milk production and are currently conducting studies necessary for evaluation of these products by the FDA.

Bovine GH treatment increases milk production by affecting several physiological processes (1*). In general, there is an increased mammary uptake of nutrients used for milk synthesis accompanied by altered metabolism in other tissues, which results in the increased availability of these nutrients for milk synthesis. These changes in tissue metabolism initiated by bGH involve both direct effects and indirect effects mediated by insulin-like growth factors (IGFs).

Some consumers have become concerned about the use of rbGH in dairy cows as a result of reports from the news media of allegations of potential hazards. Although FDA scientists have determined that milk and meat from rbGH-treated animals are safe for human consumption (2*), questions have remained in the mind of the consumer regarding the regulatory process within the FDA that permits marketing of food products from animals used in investigational studies and the scientific basis for decisions regarding the human safety of such *products. The purpose of this article is to address these concerns by briefly explaining the approval process within the FDA and to summarize the scientific information used by the agency to evaluate the human safety of these products.*

New Animal Drug Regulation

The FDA has the responsibility of enforcing the Federal Food, Drug, and Cosmetic Act (FD&C Act), and the enforcement authority for animal drugs is delegated to its Center for Veterinary Medicine (CVM). Before approving a new animal drug, the FDA requires that the pharmaceutical company demonstrate that food products from treated animals are safe for human consumption. In addition, the company must show that the drug is effective and safe for the animal, and that the manufacture of the drug will not adversely affect the environment. These general requirements are outlined in the Code of Federal Regulations (3*). The efficacy and target animal safety studies must include trials in several different geographical locations in the United States under typical conditions of use. To conduct clinical studies with investigational drugs, the pharmaceutical companies must establish an Investigational New Animal Drug (INAD) application with the FDA, through which the agency controls the use of the not yet approved compound in food animals. The label for the compound indicates that the drug is investigational and that the animals treated with the drug must not be used for human food unless this use is expressly authorized by the FDA.

Under an INAD application, pharmaceutical companies may conduct the human food safety studies required for approval of their product. The results of these studies may be submitted to the CVM while the compound is still undergoing investigation. CVM scientists review the human food safety data and establish an appropriate period for drug withdrawal before slaughter, or a discard period for milk, which ensures that no unsafe residues are present in the food products. At that point, the FDA may authorize the use in human food of products from animals treated in investigational studies. Initially, investigators were required to discard milk while cows were being treated with rbGH and for 4 days or longer after the end of rbGH treatment and were not allowed to slaughter the cows for human consumption for 15 days after the last treatment. The pharmaceutical companies later completed the human food safety studies, and the results demonstrated that a withdrawal period was not required. Under conditions of the INAD regulation, the FDA then permitted milk and meat from rbGH-treated cows to be marketed with no withdrawal period. Because the FDA requires the pharmaceutical companies to submit all studies they conducted on their products, the agency continues to receive human food safety information even after the requirements have been met.

The FDA's current human food safety requirements for protein drugs such as bGH are discussed below. Guidelines for conducting safety studies for nonprotein drugs will not be discussed here but can be obtained from CVM (4*).

Data Quality Assurance

The pharmaceutical companies provide descriptions of the human food safety studies and summaries of results, but ultimately it is the FDA that decides on the integrity of the data. The FDA has established specific guidelines ("Good Laboratory Practices") to ensure that the data obtained from the pharmaceutical companies provide accurate and reliable information (5*). The companies also submit the raw data from all safety studies that will form the basis of approval of the product; the submission permits CVM scientists to confirm the accuracy of the results and conclusions. CVM scientists may also order data audits and inspections of specific studies to aid in evaluating the adequacy of the data.

A "Freak" Amino Acid was Produced by Monsanto

This paper was written in 1990. As part of their 55,000 page application to FDA, Monsanto was required to, and did submit a chart (see page 68) identifying every amino acid on the 191 amino acid chain structure of BST. (5) On that chart, amino acid #144 was represented as being lysine. It was not. Monsanto made a mistake. During the gene transcription process, a freak amino acid was created. A Monsanto scientist, Bernard Violand, published evidence of this mistake in the July 1994 issue of the journal *Protein Science*. (6) The mistake resulted in the production of a substance unlike the naturally occurring bovine protein. Amino acid #144, lysine, was incorrectly transcribed as a "freak" amino acid called, epsilon-N-acetyllysine. Shades of Jurassic Park! Shades of Frankenstein! Monsanto had created a "Frankenfood!" FDA allowed that food to enter our food supply. Monsanto has never officially admitted this error. I called Richard Teske, Ph.D., the hands-on director of research at CVM in May 1995 and told him of this error. Dr. Teske seemed to me to be unconcerned. No FDA action was taken.

I reminded Teske that one amino acid difference produces conditions such as sickle cell anemia or Alzheimer's disease. This error compromised all of the research performed and submitted to FDA. The Monsanto publication revealed that the error was discovered and a process developed which filtered out the freak amino acid. Unfortunately for Monsanto, $300 million worth of research was invalidated. Fortunately for Monsanto, they had friends at FDA. Microbiologists are aware that one amino acid difference in a protein can result in hundreds of known diseases including sickle cell anemia and forms of Alzheimer's disease. How many unknown diseases? Unknown!

Juskevich & Guyer

Safety Requirements for Protein Products

With the advent of recombinant DNA techniques to produce easily purified proteins in recombinant DNA techniques (**AUTHOR'S NOTE: It wasn't so easy as evidenced by the gene transcription error**) *in large quantities, the investigation of protein products for use in food animals increased dramatically. The chemical nature, biological activity, and potential for harmful residues are better understood for protein products than for new chemical entities that are generally developed for use in food animals. The scientific literature provides a good background for understanding the biological effects of these products, and the knowledge about digestion of proteins in the human gastrointestinal tract provides information on their potential for harmful residues. The FDA's "Guideline for Toxicological Testing (4*) provides for alternatives to the general tests outlines, depending on the potential exposure of people to residues and the possible biological effects of the compound, and the CVM has determined that these alternatives are more appropriate for protein products.*

The FDA does not believe that protein hormones survive digestion so we've relieved Monsanto from the responsibility of performing further toxicological studies. Furthermore, we are going to review, in a scientific manner, why such proteins are digested in the stomach. When I met with FDA scientists they repeated a very important "GIVEN" which was accepted by all men of science. Here's what FDA believes. When we eat food, pepsin, hydrochloric acid, and other strong digestive enzymes act upon that food, rendering any protein hormones inactive. These scientists were astonished that I couldn't understand this basic precept of science. On the other hand, I was astonished that these men of science were so stubbornly pig-headed, that they could not see how easily these proteins did survive digestion.

I said, "If I held out my hand and it contained a little red pill with 3000 nanograms of the most powerful growth hormone in your body, and offered it to you, would you swallow that pill?" (A nanogram is equal to one-billionth of a gram. Many chemical messengers function on a very tiny scale, called a nano-molecular level. Most people understand that minute quantities of chemicals such as the hallucinogenic substance, LSD also work on a nano-molecular level). The scientists laughed. Of course they would not be foolish enough to take a pill containing the most powerful growth hormone in the human body. Now, that was a given. "Yet," I continued, "the hormones in that pill would not work. They would certainly be destroyed by the acid in your stomach. So would those same hormones contained in a steak or hamburger. They are naturally destroyed." Everybody agreed with me.

"Now for the milk," I went on. "When you drink a glass of milk, what happens?" I paused for effect. "I'll tell you what happens. The milk mixes with everything inside of your stomach. There's acid and mucous and undigested food. It's a complex and heterogeneous soup. Before drinking the milk, the pH scale (the level of acidity) of the gastric environment is between 1.8 and 2.0. After drinking a 12 ounce glass of milk, the gastric environment changes. The acid becomes weaker. The milk has a buffering effect. The gastric environment and everything contained in the stomach now has a pH. of 6...And what happens at a six?" I asked. No answer came from the scientists.

Nearly four months later, I received a letter from Teske, now the Acting associate director for policy at the CVM. On page two of his three page letter, Teske wrote, "At pH 6 bovine milk xanthene oxidase encapsulated in liposomes (fat molecules) is protected from degradation by gastric juices (pepsin). This is not surprising since pepsin is virtually inactive at pH 6." (7) Teske admitted, in "scientese," that proteins which would normally be destroyed in the stomach are protected by milk. Milk changes the stomach's acidity, buffering it from an acidic 1.8 to a more basic 6.0.

Medical science does not yet realize the significance and implications of this observation. Perhaps I was invited because I do not have credentials. I remember another who didn't have credentials either. He yelled to the crowd, "The Emperor is not wearing any clothes." Nobody believed him...at least not in the very beginning. Milk is loaded with hormones to promote growth. They survive digestion because milk itself acts as an enzyme inhibitor, buffering the acid in the stomach and changing the acidity by decreasing it from a very acidic 1.8 to a more neutral 6.0. FDA ignored this and falsely explained that protein hormones are destroyed. In a subsequent chapter, enormous scientific evidence, published in peer-reviewed journals, will demonstrate the survival mechanisms and implications of the durability of these protein hormones, particularly IGF-I.

Juskevich & Guyer

Human Food Safety Considerations - Protein Digestion

Ingested rbGH would be expected to be degraded in the human gastrointestinal tract in the same manner as other proteins. In adults, protein digestion products generally enter the blood almost entirely as free amino acids. Peptides may enter cells if their molecular weight is less than 250 (6*), and the extent to which a peptide enters the blood intact also depends on the rate of absorption and rate of intracellular hydrolysis. In neonates, the activity of various digestive enzymes ranges from 10 to 100% of adult levels. However, *neonates and even pre-term infants, have the complement of enzymes necessary to digest protein efficiently, although digestive capacity is limited (7*).*

Absorption of Intact Proteins

Initially, uptake of intact proteins was considered to be limited to neonates and the mechanism of uptake has been studied in several species (8*). The transport of intact proteins across the intestinal wall in mature animals has not been extensively studied; however there is evidence that proteins may be absorbed intact. (9*, 10*). In humans, this evidence relies on the presence of circulating antibodies to food proteins; however, no adverse reactions have been observed in the majority of individuals in response to protein absorption (11*).

The authors clearly contradict themselves by offering evidence that proteins may be absorbed intact. Juskevich and Guyer are absurd in the use of the English language...it's easy to miss the significance of their words until one reads them over and over again. For example, they say, "No adverse reactions have been observed IN THE MAJORITY OF INDIVIDUALS in response to protein absorption." I would guess that the majority of individuals have not been tested. Have you? No? Neither have I. Now, if they had correctly stated, "no adverse reactions have been observed in individual responses to protein absorption," they would not have been so ludicrous. They would have still have been wrong, just not incongruous in their attitude. Two Connecticut researchers, Kurt Oster, M.D., and Donald Ross, Ph.D., observed that every one of their heart attack patients suffered atrial damage as a result of a bovine enzyme which survived digestion. (8)

Juskevich & Guyer

Whether full-term human neonates absorb a substantially greater amount of intact protein than older children and adults is still equivocal. The gut of the newly born infant is impermeable to a large variety of antibodies administered in colostrum or milk (12*); however, absorption of foreign proteins must take place to some extent, as evidenced by the appearance of specific antibodies against proteins (13*). The time of closure of gut permeability to proteins (gut closure) in the newborn has not been determined, but may occur before birth (14*) or as long as 3 months after birth (14*, 15*). Because the time of gut closure appears to be quite variable among species, studies performed in other animals cannot be easily extrapolated to humans (8*, 10*, 16*).

The conflicting results of studies to determine the extent of intact protein absorption by human neonates demonstrate the complexity of the system being studied. A variety of factors are involved, including the type of protein being studied, gestational age of the neonate, and perhaps feeding regimen (14*, 17-

19*). However, uptake of macromolecules into intestinal epithelial cells does not appear to be any more significant in the full term neonate than in the adult. Estimates of the amount absorbed are on the border of 1:10,000 to 1:50,000 of the protein load given orally (11*).

Yes, that may be true when those gentle proteins are dropped into a cauldron (your stomach) containing powerful acids. When the acid is neutralized those protein hormones may not be broken down into their basic components.

Juskevich & Guyer

Most protein and polypeptide drugs will have minimal activity, at most, when administered orally. However, it would be inappropriate to assume that a compound does not have oral activity simply because it is a protein. For example, two polypeptide-releasing factors, synthetic thyrotropin-releasing factor (TRF; a tripeptide) and synthetic gonadotropin-releasing hormone (GnRH; a decapeptide) display some oral activity (20*) because of their low molecular weights or their high specific activities, or both. The molecular weights of synthetic TRF and GnRH are approximately 330 and 1,100 daltons, respectively; in contrast; the respective molecular weights of bGH and IGF-I are approximately 22,000 and 7,800 daltons.

Growth Hormone

The effects of GH can be considered at two levels: the effects on cell proliferation and protein synthesis and the effects on metabolic factors (1*, 21-26*). In vivo and in vitro studies have demonstrated that GH exerts direct effects on some processes and indirect effects, mediated by insulin-like growth factors, on other processes. In some tissues GH may first induce differentiation of precursor cells and then increase production of IGFs in the differentiated cells, resulting in a mitogenic effect (22*, 27*). The physiological effects of GH are manifested in (I) anabolic effects (such as nitrogen accretion in growing animals and milk synthesis in lactating animals), (ii) effects on electrolytes (phosphorus, sodium, potassium and calcium), (iii) effects on carbohydrate metabolism, (iv) effects on lipid metabolism, and (v) growth of cartilage and bone.

Bovine Growth Hormone: Human Food Safety

The evaluation of the human food safety of bGH was based on several factors: bGH is biologically inactive in humans, rbGH is orally inactive, and rbGH and bGH are biologically indistinguishable.

The amino acid sequence differences between normally occurring bGH and genetically engineered rbGH were known to FDA. How could they write that these two proteins were "biologically indistinguishable?" Lies, lies and more lies. BGH may be biologically active in humans. That has never been determined. There is strong evidence that it might. In order to illustrate why, an explanation and understanding of how chemical messengers work in animals (including humans) is required. Our bodies are made up of trillions of cells. These cells communicate with each other by a combination of weak electrical impulses and by different chemicals. Many of these actions and mechanisms are well understood.

One example of these hormones is adrenaline, that chemical sprayed from glands located on top of kidneys (adrenal glands) which allowed cavemen to fight or run from that bear in his cave. This chemical allows strong men and women to become stronger and faster during emergencies. Another example is testosterone, that male hormone which elicits aggressive behavior in males. One more example is estrogen, the female hormone. Combinations of testosterone and estrogen elicit various sexual behaviors. Growth hormones cause cells to grow. They initiate or increase the incidence of a process called cellularity. In the presence of growth hormones, cells exhibit increased activity, which may include the movement of chromosomes to begin a mitosis, the process taught in high school biology classes.

Chemical messages or hormones usually work only on very specific cells or parts of cells. They first must find an area on a cell to which they can attach or bind. Nicotine, the active substance in tobacco, is a messenger. So is heroin. Both of these chemicals work by attaching to very specific areas, or groups of cells, in a tiny organ located in the brain. This organ is about the size of a thumbnail. It's called the hypothalamus. Within the hypothalamus there is an area known as the median forebrain bundle where heroin and nicotine both work. Many scientists refer to the median forebrain bundle as the addiction center.

On a microbiological level, these chemical messengers attach to cells. This process of attachment has been referred to as binding. The area of the cell in which a chemical attaches is referred to as a binding site. Each chemical is different and each site is different. An analogy can be made to illustrate this process as being comparable to a lock and a key. One key will not open up every lock. A specific key (chemical) can fit into a specific lock (binding site) and "open up" a specific action or response.

Ask your endocrinologist, "Doctor? Is it true that the mammary tissue of cows does not contain binding sites to BGH or BST, the bovine growth hormone?" Then ask, "If there are no binding sites for bovine growth hormones in mammary tissue, then how the heck does it work?" That should get the doctor thinking. There's no book yet that can answer this question, yet, that mechanism can be explained. The action of the bovine growth hormone on mammary tissue is assisted and completed with the help of another receptor. BST binding is actually mediated by IGF-I and IGF-I receptors. What follows is a model of simplification.

There exists a key (BST) with no lock. No door can be opened. The BST key is used to open up the IGF-I lock and various actions occur in those mammary tissues. This is about milk. When cows are injected with a genetically engineered version of BST, the binding occurs on a micro-cellular level at the IGF-I receptor.

IGF-I, a protein hormone, is identical in both humans and cows. It is exactly the same! Both hormones contain 70 amino acids in the same gene sequence. If IGF-I in mammary tissues in cows allows the bovine growth hormone to function, by allowing it to bind to the IGF-I receptor, can we not assume that the same receptor in humans would also allow the bovine growth hormone to bind? Perhaps that's why so many American women and men, drinking so much milk containing so many growth hormones, gain enormous weight, and end up resembling cows.

The Proof of the Pudding

Remember Monsanto spokesman, Robert Collier, Ph.D., who mailed me an enormous amount of scientific material? As early as 1977, P.V. Malvern, a co-publisher of scientific papers and associate of Collier's, wrote:

> Bovine milk has been reported to contain trace levels of
> BST although it is not clear how it enters the milk, since
> no BST receptors have been identified on the surface of
> the mammary gland. (9)

In 1987, Collier and Malvern studied the binding of bovine proteins. Malvern reported:

> The lactating mammary glands of dairy cows do not appear
> to have receptors for somatotropin (somatotropin being the
> "ST" in bovine somatotropin), receptors for IGF-I and -II
> have been identified in the mammary tissues of pregnant
> cows. (10)

In 1989, Collier presented a paper at a conference in Fougeres, France. Commenting on the previous study, Collier and Hammond wrote:

> Since somatotropin (bovine growth hormone) does not
> appear to have a direct affect on mammary secretory tissue,
> it is conceivable that the galactopoietic effect of somatotropin
> may be mediated, at least in part, through IGF-I, since this
> somatomedin has a stimulatory effect on mammary growth. (11)

I treasure the word, *galactopoietic*. It refers to milk, but it also refers to galaxies...the big picture. Why do scientists sometimes miss the big picture? If these bovine hormones do not have their own receptors, so the bovine hormones must bind to IGF-I receptors in order to function, and these receptors are identical in humans and cows, then the human receptors can make the bovine hormones work too! How did these Monsanto scientists miss this one? They had to see it. How did FDA reviewers miss this? Somebody missed the big picture. Let's continue with the Juskevich and Guyer *Science* paper. We were considering human food safety.

This FDA paper was most pivotal in influencing FDA to issue a determination that milk hormones do not work in humans. Although the genetically engineered hormone was still four years away from being formally approved, the milk from test herds was deemed safe for human consumption and was allowed to enter America's milk supply. This same genetically engineered hormone caused the spleens of lab animals to increase in size by 46 percent, this same hormone with a "freak" amino acid. This is the same hormone that caused cancer in every one of the animals treated with rBST in one study which FDA has and refuses to release. (12) Milk -- what a surprise, indeed!

Juskevich & Guyer

Species Specificity

On the basis of studies in the 1950s, it was concluded that, although the physiological effects of GH (Growth Hormone) *could be demonstrated in animals, pituitary GH preparations from animals were not effective in humans (24* 28* 29*). GH derived from human cadavers is effective...*

Effective? Children treated with these hormones developed a rare brain-destroying condition similar to an Alzheimer's-type of disease called Jacob-Creutzfeldt. (13) How could these FDA reviewers claim that these hormones were effective? Moore reveals this problem in the very first paragraph of his publication. If the authors did not see the paper, one could overlook and excuse their ignorance. However, these authors cite this very article as reference #47 in their report. C'mon! The importance of the reference citing Jerome Moore's paper was to demonstrate that, although the 181st amino acid in the BST and rBST chain was different, that really did not matter.

In his second paragraph, Moore reveals that one amino acid difference in the middle of a chain can have serious consequences resulting in different actions of a hormone. However, he and the FDA investigators didn't know that Monsanto had made an error in amino acid #144, and had created a freak amino acid, subsequently published by Bernard Violand's Monsanto publication of 1994.

Juskevich & Guyer

...but GH derived from bovine (30*), ovine, whale (31*) and porcine (32*) pituitaries is ineffective in humans. Although bGH and human GH (hGH) both have 191 amino acids, the amino acid sequence differs by approximately 35% (33*). A reflection of this difference is the demonstration that bGH does not compete with hGH for binding sites in membranes from human tissues, including liver, indicating that bGH does not bind to GH receptors in human tissues (34*).

Monsanto scientists were perplexed by the fact that cow growth hormone doesn't work by binding to receptors in mammary tissue of cows either, yet it works by binding with the IGF-I receptor which is identical in cows and humans.

Juskevich & Guyer

The finding that GH from non-primate species is ineffective in humans led to the application of the term "species specific." Although it is apparent from animal studies that this terminology is not technically correct (for example, bGH is effective in rats), the terminology has continued to be used with the understanding that it implies a difference in sensitivity as one goes up the phylogenetic tree, with humans and monkeys being unresponsive to GH from lower species.

Fragment Activity

To obtain a more plentiful source of GH for human therapy, attempts were made to produce a growth factor from animal-derived GH that would be active in humans. Chymotrypsinized bGH produced no anabolic or metabolic effects in patients (31*). Limited tryptic digests of bGH retained some of the activity of intact bGH when administered parenternally to hypophysectomized rats (30*, 35-37*), but there was a progressive loss of growth-promoting activity in the rat as the number of hydrolyzed peptide bonds were split (38*). Recombined fragments have approximately 10% of the activity of bGH in rats (37*). In patients, parenteral administration of tryptic digests of bGH produced some of the metabolic effects seen after administration of hGH. However, large doses were required, and variable and opposite effects were observed (35*, 39*).

Toxicity Studies of bGH

On the basis of background information obtained from the scientific literature, studies were designed by the CVM to demonstrate further the human food safety of rbGH. Initially, each sponsoring company conducted an oral toxicity study with their particular rbGH product. The primary sequence of these products was either the same as or differed only slightly from pituitary-derived bGH, because of the recombinant DNA techniques used by each of the companies. Differences occur only at the NH2-terminus end of the protein.

Remember the freak amino acid, epsilon-N-acetyllysine? FDA did not know about this error because it was never reported by Monsanto. FDA went to great lengths to demonstrate that the difference in the "end" amino acid was not significant. In doing so, FDA revealed that a difference in the "middle of an amino acid chain" might produce serious consequences.

American Cyanamid's rbGH product has three additional amino acids, Met-Asp-Gln. Eli Lilly & Company's (Elanco) product contains the following additional amino acids, Met-Phe-Pro-Leu-Asp-Asp-Asp- Asp-Lys. Monsanto Agricultural Company's product has a single amino acid substitution of Met for Ala on the NH2-terminus end, and the Upjohn Company's product is identical to pituitary-derived bGH.

Upjohn conducted a 26-day oral toxicity study in which normal rats were treated with rbGH at 0, 0.5, 5.0, or 50.0 mg/kg of body weight per day by gastric intubation; a separate group was given rbGH at 50 micrograms per rat per day by subcutaneous injection (40*). Monsanto conducted two studies: a 28-day study in which normal rats were treated with rbGH at o, 0.06, 0.6, or 6.0 mg/kg per day by gavage (41*) and a 90 day study in which normal rats were treated with rbGH at 0, 0.1, 0.5, 5.0. or 50 mg/kg by gavage, and a separate group was treated with 1 mg/kg per day by subcutaneous injection (42*).

The biggest lie of all was exposed when FDA admitted that the data from the above experiments were not rigorously reviewed. A letter from Richard Teske revealed that organ weights were so unusual as to be rejected. Enormous spleen growths were considered to be not statistically significant. Teste and ovary weights were "unreal." The study continued in a "reverse withdrawal phase." FDA admitted that charts were not labeled properly.

Richard Teske's Letter

Dear Mr. Cohen,   *August 10, 1995*

This is to follow-up on the meeting between you and representatives of the Center for Veterinary Medicine (CVM), held at your request on April 21, 1995, to discuss some of your concerns about the safety of rbST. Your concerns centered around:

(A)   during the fermentation process for production of raw rbST the bulk rbST produced is contaminated with rbST containing modified lysine amino acid at chain position 144;

(B)   whether IGF-1 levels are increased in the milk from cows treated with rbST and your contention that since IGF-1 is a "key factor in the growth and survival of tumors" any increase in IGF-1 levels in milk should be considered to represent a public health risk; and

(C)   the effects of rbST on spleen weights in rats.

With respect to your concern about the contamination of raw rbST with rbST-like material containing modified lysine amino acid at chain position 144, Mr. Marnane explained that the contaminant was removed during purification of the final bulk rbST product. You indicated that since the work identifying the contaminant was not published until 1994 the rbST produced prior to that time would have been contaminated and therefore different. Mr. Marnane explained that the purification process used from the start of production (including that produced for experimental purposes) removed this contaminant.

With respect to your concern about IGF-1 levels in milk from rbST-treated cows, we explained that the very small increase in milk IGF-1 levels demonstrated by data initially submitted by the sponsor(s) was biologically insignificant when compared with endogenous levels of IGF-1.   Further, there is little or no absorption of IGF-1 entering the gastrointestinal tract whether contained in animal-derived foodstuffs or as a component of saliva.

In addition, you asked Dr. Leighton top review and comment on a paper authored by D.J. Ross, S.V. Sharnick and K.A. Oster titled, Liposomes as a Proposed Vehicle for the Persorption of Bovine Xanthine Oxidase.   As Dr. Leighton explained to you in a subsequent telephone conversation, the authors of this paper demonstrate that at pH 6 bovine milk xanthine oxidase encapsulated in liposomes is protected from degradation by gastric juices (pepsin). This is not surprising since pepsin is virtually inactive at pH 6. (The optimal pH for pepsin is about pH 2.)

Finally, with respect to your concern that the increased spleen weight observed in rats fed rbST should raise questions about the oral activity of rbST, it was explained that since there was no dose-response effect associated with the increased spleen weights, it was concluded that the effect was not biologically significant. It should be noted that an increase in body weight is the most consistent weight parameter for measuring the effect of growth hormone in rats. Even at the highest dose, there was no increase in body weight due to oral treatment of rbST in this study.

In addition, you asked that Dr. Condon re-review the organ weight data in the 90-day rat feeding study to determine if there were any important effects on organ weights attributable to the feeding of rbST. Dr. Condon did re-review the available data. Dr. Condon's analysis did not uncover any additional effects on organ weights. Therefore, the Center's original conclusions concerning the effect rbST on organ weights is unchanged.

I should note that Dr. Condon did uncover some errors in the information as it was presented in Table 2 of the Science *paper. The heading of Table 2 states that 30 rats per sex per treatment group were utilized in the study. While the 90-day study did involve the use of 30 rats per sex per treatment group, only 15 rats per sex per treatment were sacrificed to obtain organ weight data. (Ten rats per sex per treatment were used for blood analysis and the remaining five animals per sex per treatment were scheduled for an effect reversal phase of the study.) This error becomes important if one tries to calculate standard errors from the data presented, exaggerating the importance of differences in data presented in the table.*

The weight of one heart in a negative control male rat was given as being almost 3.5 grams. No other heart weight was over 2 grams for this control group or any other of the rbST oral groups. In Dr. Condon's opinion, this heart weight is an impossible value. When this observation is deleted, the control average weight is 1.602 grams which is essentially identical to the oral rbST groups. Dr. Condon concluded that there is no change in heart weights due to oral administration of rbST.

There is an unresolved issue regarding the average spleen weight for the female negative control group. The correct value could be 0.630 grams rather than 0.585 grams. The available data are not sufficient to determine the correct value. In either case, the effect on spleen weight is not considered to be biologically meaningful.

In conclusion Mr. Cohen, I believe that while our discussion on April 21, 1995, and the two assignments we undertook were, in part, interesting and stimulating, we have found no new information which alters our conclusion that milk from rbST-treated cows is safe.

Sincerely yours,
Richard H. Teske, D.V.M.
Acting Associate Director for Policy Center for Veterinary Medicine

A footnote to this letter adds that, "There were too many questionable weights for ovary and testes for a reliable analyses of these organs."

Here's Where the BS(T) Hit the Fan

FDA reviewers called this study, referenced as #42, as a 90-day study. It was actually a study lasting 180 days, according to Teske's letter, which uses Orwellian "doublespeak" in referring to "an effect reversal phase of the study."

The results were so horrifying that Monsanto, aware that their investment in genetic engineering was about to go down the drain, called in every political and scientific favor. They bribed members of the House of Representatives, congressmen who sat on the Dairy Committee, a subcommittee of the House Agriculture Committee, by paying them PAC money. (Chapter 6) They also made arrangements for their scientists, Margaret Miller, Ph.D., and Suzanne Sechen, Ph.D., to be hired by FDA (more in Chapter 6), and got their own attorney, Michael Taylor, hired by FDA. Taylor rewrote a congressional act (the Delaney Amendment) that was intended to protect Americans from cancer.

FDA reviewer, Judy Juskevich, reached at her home in Halifax, Nova Scotia, Canada, by telephone (14), admitted to me that she never reviewed these data. Instead, she relied upon another FDA employee, Margaret Miller, Ph.D., to summarize the findings. Miller was employed by Monsanto before being hired by FDA to review her own scientific research. This key unpublished study was never reviewed by FDA. One bit of evidence supporting this is the fact that they continue to call this a 90-day study. Another is an admission made to this author by FDA scientists at a meeting on April 21, 1995 that the most important study in the *Science* paper was never reviewed. Confirmation of that admission and indications of enormous evidence of errors in that study are contained in the FDA letter.

Juskevich & Guyer

American Cyanamid conducted a 15-day study in which normal rats were treated with rbGH at 0, 0.1, 1.0, or 10.0 mg/kg per day by gavage (43*). Elanco conducted a 14-day study in which normal rats were given rbGH at 0, 0.05, 0.5, or 5.0 mg/kg per day by subcutaneous injection (44*).

Each study met the FDA's minimum requirements of treating rats with up to 100 times or more of the dose of administered daily to dairy cattle on the basis of milligrams per kilogram of body weight and administration for at least 14 days. Therefore, the high dose chosen for each study varied according to the company's proposed dosage for treatment of dairy cattle. Negative results were obtained with oral administration of rbGH in all studies, and only the details of the study conducted for the longest duration will be presented here. The parameters examined in each study were comparable.

In a 90-day oral toxicity study conducted by Monsanto, rats were treated with rbGH either by gavage or subcutaneous injection (42*). Body weight and food consumption were determined weekly. In addition, blood samples were collected for extensive clinical chemistry and hematology examinations, and urinalysis parameters were determined. Gross pathology and microscopic examination of tissues were conducted on all animals at the termination of the study (45*).

There were no treatment-related deaths or clinical findings. A marked increase in body weight gain and feed consumption was observed from week 2 throughout the treatment phase for rats given subcutaneous injections; differences in mean body weights reached 16% in males and 20% in females by study week 13, compared to the negative control group. Body weights were unchanged after oral administration of rbGH (Table 1). An increase in absolute organ weights accompanied the change in body weight in rats treated with rbGH subcutaneously (Table2). Heart, liver, kidney, and spleen weights increased in both sexes, and in addition, adrenal weight in males and thymus and ovary weights in females increased (42). In contrast, there were no biologically significant increases in organ weights for rats given rbGH orally. Absolute spleen weight increased for males and females given rbGH orally at 0.5 mg/kg per day; however, the increase was not dose related and was most likely an incidental finding.

Incidental finding? When things do not turn out just the way scientists want them to, they're called, "incidental findings." Unbiased scientists have another word for incidental findings...CLUES! The spleen is an important organ. It manufactures red and white blood cells. As part of the lymphatic system the spleen reacts to "foreign invaders" and enormous spleen growth can be a sign of an enormous problem. FDA called these spleen growths "incidental."

Juskevich & Guyer

In rats treated subcutaneously, ratios of organ weight to body weight were increased for spleen and adrenal and decreased for testes in male rats, and increased for heart and spleen and decreased for brain in the female rats. In contrast, increases in ratios or organ weight to body weight were sporadic in the rats administered rbGH orally and were not treatment-related.

No toxicologically significant changes were noted in the clinical chemistry, hematology, or urinalysis parameters determined in rats administered rbGH orally. Significant changes in clinical chemistry and hematology parameters occurred only in the group that received rbGH by subcutaneous injection (42*).

These two FDA reviewers, Juskevich and Guyer, knew too much, considering the fact that they never reviewed this study. Only two individuals knew the full story. They were Margaret Miller and Suzanne Sechen. They knew this study because they reviewed it while they still were employed at Monsanto. It was critically important for Monsanto not to have the study independently reviewed by others at FDA. That's why these two scientists got jobs at FDA. All of the animals treated with rbGH in this study got cancer, even the animals orally ingesting this new hormone. These events were known to Monsanto scientists. Somehow, Monsanto's attorney, Michael Taylor, who was a partner in the law firm of King & Spalding, was hired by FDA to be deputy commissioner of policy where he oversaw the approval process. Despite Freedom of Information Act requests, FDA will not release the name of the individual who hired Miller. Similar requests were made as to how Sechen and Taylor were hired. Since Taylor assumed a senior position, serving directly under the FDA commissioner, one wonders who asked/ordered that commissioner to hire Monsanto's own attorney.

Juskevich & Guyer

There were no statistically significant differences in the distribution half-lives, terminal distribution half-lives, total body clearances, and volumes of distribution between rMet-bGH and a recombinant, naturally occurring variant, rAla-Val-bGH, in lactating Holstein cows (46*). These results indicate that the body does not treat rMet-bGH as a protein distinct from a naturally occurring bGH variant. Similar results have been obtained in another study in which two recombinant forms or hGH were found to have equivalent potency and pharmacokinetics in cynomolgus monkeys (47*). One recombinant form had an amino acid sequence identical to that of the natural pituitary hormone and the other form had an additional NH2-terminal methionine.

Residue Studies of BGH

Residue studies are not normally required for protein products unless: (I) the protein is orally active and a safe concentration is required, (ii) no adequate biological end point can be determined for toxicological testing, or (iii) the product will be used in lactating food animals and has the potential for biological activity in humans. For rbGH, none of the three exceptions applied, therefore, residue testing is not required.

Although rbGH residue studies are not significant for human food safety considerations, some studies have been conducted to determine if bGH concentrations are increased in the milk of rbGH-treated cows. The analytic methods used by the pharmaceutical companies to determine the amount of bGH in the milk were exclusively radioimmunoassay (RIA) procedures. Each company developed its own RIA procedure; none of these procedures could distinguish between the pituitary-derived bGH and rbGH product.

American Cyanamid conducted two studies (48*). In the first study, milk from 22 control cows and 27 cows receiving daily injections of 37.5 mg of rbGH (approximately three times the proposed dose) was assayed for bGH. In the control group, 21 of the 22 cows had detectable levels (greater than or equal to 1.0 ng/ml) of bGH in their milk ranging from 1.1 to 1.7 ng/ml. Concentrations of bGH in the milk from the treated cows ranged from 1.1 to 2.1 ng/ml. The average bGH concentrations in the milk of control cows and rbGH-treated cows were 1.3 *and 1.4 ng/ml, respectively. In the second study, similar results were obtained with 12 cows in which the bGH concentrations in the rbGH-treated cows were in the same range in the untreated cows.*

Groenewegen et. al. (49*) conducted a study with three untreated cows and three cows treated with 10.6 mg. of rbGH per day (approximately the proposed dose) beginning at 28 days postpartum. When comparing the milk samples collected from both groups they found that levels of bGH in milk from rbGH-treated cows (4.2 ng/ml) were not significantly different from those found in nontreated cows (3.3 ng/ml).

Scientists enjoy talking at a level way above laypersons. They discuss chemicals and samples in milliliters which are one-thousandth of a liter. A liter is approximately the size of a quart of milk. Nobody consumes one-thousandth of a liter...a thimble-full? Consequently, in order to make scientific jargon a little easier to swallow, along with the milk, I am going to convert FDA's numbers to liters.

Accordingly, there are 3300 nanograms (which for the sake of simplicity I will refer to as units) of bGH in normal wholesome milk. When a cow is injected with rbGH, the milk contains 4200 units of bGH. I asked my 11-year-old daughter to do the math for me. She subtracted 3300 from 4200 and got a difference of 900 units. She then divided the difference, 900, by the level in normal milk, 3300, and came up with an increase of more than 26 percent. When you give a cow a shot of genetically engineered bovine growth hormone, her milk will contain a 26 percent increase in the level of bGH. FDA says that there is "no significant increase." Why does FDA want America to believe that 26 percent is not a significant increase? Which container would you drink? The one with 3300 units or the one with 4200 units? I hope you select the bottle of water or orange juice or even soda.

Juskevich & Guyer

Although these very limited studies suggest that milk concentrations of bGH do not increase significantly as a result of the treatment of dairy cows with rbGH at the proposed doses, the need to pursue more definitive studies has already been stated as unnecessary because bGH is biologically inactive in humans and orally inactive.

Additionally, it has also been determined that at least 90 % of bGH activity is destroyed upon pasteurization of milk (47*). Therefore, bGH residues do not present a human food safety concern.

Scientific Fraud and FDA

FDA had just committed the greatest scientific fraud in the history of mankind. They left the evidence, plain as day, and nobody caught on. Besides the obvious conspiracy there is a re-compounding of conspiracies here...add the conspiracy of ignorance. There have been, throughout our history, instances of scientific fraud that were perpetrated upon mankind for a variety of reasons. Academic pressures can be enormous, financial pressures are great motivators. It's easy to explain and understand why scientists sometimes cheat. They're only human.

Gregor Mendel, the father of genetics, actually cheated. Mendel, a monk, cross-bred peas by mixing their pollens and altering their characteristics. He kept a journal, which when analyzed, revealed data that were too perfect for what probably occurred in nature. The 1993 edition of the *Information Please World Almanac* contains an article on scientific fraud that includes evidence of fraud committed by the founder of the modern scientific method, Galileo, the father of modern astronomy, Kepler, John Dalton, a noted chemist, and Sir Isaac Newton, father of physics. (15)

The Groenewegen fraud, upheld by FDA (revealed on the following page), can be designated as number one on that list. Paul Groenewegen is in good company. His name appears as the senior author of the most influential article in the BST controversy and as a senior author he receives most of the credit and fault for the publication bearing his name. Groenewegen, an undergraduate at the time of his study, was chosen by Brian McBride, his professor, to be "point man" for this fraud. His professor and co-author had close ties with Monsanto.

Juskevich & Guyer:

"It has also been determined that at least 90% of bGH activity is destroyed upon pasteurization of milk. Therefore, bGH residues do not present a human food safety concern." (4)

The Litmus Test

Let this above quote be the litmus test for determining whether or not everything I've written in this book is nonsense, or whether FDA should be disbanded and we start anew. Juskevich and Guyer attributed the 90 percent destruction citation to reference #47. Upon review of the references, that would be J.A. Moore's publication in the *Journal of Endocrinology*. A few months after first reading this portion of the Juskevich and Guyer paper, I received a copy of Moore's paper. There was absolutely no mention of pasteurization and 90 percent destruction of BGH.

Was it possible that Juskevich and Guyer made this up or miscited the reference? The same reference appeared in numerous reports from prestigious agencies like the *Journal of the American Medical Association*, the World Health

Organization, and the National Institutes of Health. Could 500,000 readers of *Science* have also missed this? Nah!

Moore was incorrectly cited! The study was actually performed by Paul Groenewegen. Today Groenewegen is a swine (pig) specialist for the Ralston Purina Company in Guelph, Ontario. When his study was accepted by the American Institute of Nutrition on November 21, 1989, Paul was an undergraduate student at the University of Guelph in Ontario, Canada. Groenewegen's co-authors were Brian McBride, John H. Burton and Theodore Elsasser. McBride and Burton have a long history of working closely with Monsanto, having published numerous papers together, underwritten by Monsanto research money. Many papers have been co-published with Monsanto's chief cow researcher, Dale Bauman, of Cornell University.

Scientists often reveal their relationships with each other by publishing papers together. These three published one such paper together, sponsored by the International Dairy Federation, in 1994. (16) Elsasser was employed by the United States Department of Agriculture. He also has close ties to Monsanto and has published with Hammond, a Monsanto scientist who published papers with Robert Collier. (17) McBride has strongly supported the introduction of the genetically engineered hormone in Canada. Monsanto, the dairy industry, the paid scientists, and USDA are all members of one big happy family.

I spoke to Paul Groenewegen on a number of occasions, both at his home and in his car. (18) The last time that I spoke with Paul I asked him to take responsibility for his paper. His response, which I respect, is that the data from his study stand on their own, exactly as they were published and he is not responsible for the actions of FDA. Groenewegen tried very hard to demonstrate that pasteurization or heat treatment destroyed BST in milk. (19) This was important to Monsanto. Groenewegen heated his milk in a Safeguard Home Milk and Cream Pasteurizer (Model P-300, Janesville, Wisconsin). He heated his milk for 30 minutes at 71 degrees Centigrade. FDA concluded that 90 percent of the BST in milk was destroyed.

The Fraud

On page 515 of his publication, Groenewegen informs us of the correct protocol for heating and pasteurizing milk. USDA calls for milk to be pasteurized at either (a) 63 degrees Centigrade for 30 minutes, (b) 72 degrees Centigrade for 15 seconds or (c) 89 degrees Centigrade for 1 second. We may never know why Groenewegen heated his milk samples for 30 minutes at 71 degrees Centigrade.

Pasteurization Methods and Temperature Conversions

METHOD #1 = 30 minutes at 63 Centigrade = 145 degrees Fahrenheit
METHOD #2 = 15 seconds at 72 Centigrade = 162 degrees Fahrenheit
METHOD #3 = 1 second   at 89 Centigrade = 192 degrees Fahrenheit

     Groenewegen's exaggerated method was designed to destroy all traces of the genetically engineered bovine hormone. He heated the milk for 30 minutes at a temperature intended for the 15 second pasteurization process. Even with the high heat for 30 minutes, this scientists attempt to destroy the bST had failed.

     The data on page 517 of their publication, Table 3, reveal that they destroyed 18 percent of the bST in normal untreated milk, and 19 percent of the BST in milk from cows treated with BST. They could not destroy the bST. That must have been their mission. Why else would they heat the milk for 30 minutes at a high temperature reserved for a 15 second heat treatment? They then "spiked" the milk. This is their word, "spike." They added artificial bST to normal milk and bST-treated milk and then heated it again. Then, amazingly, they added 146 times the level of naturally occurring bST in powdered form to the milk and heated it. The powdered rbST in milk was destroyed! They saved the day for Monsanto. The experiment worked. These men of science could claim that heat treatment destroys bST. In their concluding discussion, these scientists determined:

1)   Heat treatment effectively reduced the immunoreactive quantities of bST in milk.

2)   Milk from bST-treated cows contains immunoreactive bST at a level that is not different from that found in control cows.

     Their data indicates otherwise. Milk from bST-treated cows contains 26 percent MORE bST than milk from control cows.

Juskevich & Guyer

Effects of rbGH Treatment of Cows on Milk Composition

     The effects of rbGH treatment on the major components of milk, when presented, are minor and primarily occur early in the treatment period before the cow's intake of dry matter is adjusted. Milk composition of treated cows is well within the normal variation observed during the course of a lactation. Changes in milk fat and protein composition depend on the cow's energy and nitrogen balances, respectively, and generally are temporary effects. The principal carbohydrate in milk, lactose, is not altered by rbGH treatment, and there are no *consistent changes in the milk content of calcium, phosphorus and other minerals, or several vitamins (1*, 50*). Thus, rbGH treatment appears to have no significant impact on the nutritional quality of milk.*

In Juskevich and Guyer's abstract they said that bST-treated milk contains higher concentrations of IGF-I. Miller tested cows over every possible cycle and energy balance and determined that the average increase of IGF-I in milk is 78 percent. I accept Miller's number.

Juskevich & Guyer

Insulin-Like Growth Factors

Because it is known that IGFs mediate many of the effects of GH and concentrations of IGFs are regulated by GH (51-53*), the FDA considered it important to determine the potential impact of IGFs on the human food safety of rbGH. Two main types of IGFs have been defined by their structural and immunological properties and receptor activity (52*) : IGF-I, a 70 amino acid polypeptide, which is identical to somatomedin-C (54*), and IGF-II, a 67-amino acid polypeptide. IGF-I was chosen as the sole representative of growth factors influenced by GH, because it is the major factor mediating the effects of GH and is more potent than IGF-II. Several reviews have been published on the biological actions of IGFs (23*, 53*, 55*, 56*).

Because production of IGFs was initially thought to be primarily in the liver, IGF's were believed to act solely by an endocrine mechanism, producing their effects at a site distant from its production. However, a study by D'Ercole et. al. (57*) demonstrated that changes in tissue concentrations consistently preceded changes in serum IGF-I after injection of GH, and on this basis it was postulated that IGF-I may also exert its biological effects by an autocrine or paracrine mechanism. Later work confirmed that local production of IGFs appears to be important for producing cellular effects (58*).

The IGFs have acute metabolic and long-term, growth-promoting effects. In vivo, bolus injections of IGF-I and IGF-II cause insulin-like effects on glucose homeostasis and metabolism, but have no effect on lipid synthesis (59*). The fact that IGF-I exerts its long-term growth-promoting effect only when it is administered by subcutaneous infusion, but not when it is administered daily by intravenous or subcutaneous injection (60*), reinforces the theory that IGFs act as local growth factors rather than as circulating mediators or GH effects.

This "reinforces the theory" that there was a pervasive practice of bad science. Bovine IGF-I should not exert remarkable effects on rats. However, bovine IGF-I should work on humans. Why? Human IGF-I and bovine IGF-I are identical in amino acid structure and amino acid sequence.

Juskevich & Guyer

Studies in rats demonstrated that infusion of IGF-I causes a dose dependent increase in body weight, tibial epiphyseal width, and thymidine incorporating activity. However, IGF-II has no effect on body weight and is three times less potent than IGF-I when the other parameters are examined (55*, 61*).

Infusion? Confusion! Rats do not infuse or inject hormones. Nor do we. Juskevich and Guyer got so deep into their assumptions and theory that truth and logic were buried under layers of scientific hodgepodge. People drink milk. Milk buffers gastric pH. Hormones survive digestive processes. Fat molecules in homogenized milk protect these hormones from breakdown. Would it not make sense then to feed animals milk containing these hormones? This type of research has never been considered because, by eliminating all extraneous variables, we eliminate models which represent the reality of real world situations.

Juskevich & Guyer

Serum IGF-I levels in normal humans are lowest in umbilical cord blood (0.33 U/ml) and increase during the first 2 to 4 years (0.4 to 0.85 U/ml) (51*, 62*). Serum levels of IGF-I in adults are in the range of 1.1 to 1.5 u/ml (51) or 200 ng/ml (52), and plasma levels of IGF-II of approximately 650 ng/ml have been reported in adults. The plasma levels of IGF-I are highest in 12-year-old girls and 14-year-old boys, with concentrations reaching two-to threefold those in adults (52). The age-dependent pattern for IGF-II concentrations appears to be different from the pattern for IGF-I. Levels at birth are low but reach almost the normal adult levels in the 1-year-old child (62).

Human milk concentrations of IGF-I were measured during the first 9 days of postpartum (63*) . The mean IGF-I concentration was 17.6 ng/ml at 1 day postpartum, 12.8 ng/ml at 2 days postpartum, and 6.8 ng/ml at 3 days postpartum. After 3 days postpartum, the IGF-I concentration stabilized over the following week at 7 to 8 ng/ml. In a later study (64*), IGF-I concentrations in human milk were measured and ranged between 13 and 40 ng/ml at 6 to 8 weeks postpartum with a mean of 19 ng/ml.

FDA is sloppy in their assumptions about levels of IGF in human serum. By citing a 1977 study *(51*)* and a 1984 study *(62*)*, and, finally, a 1988 study *(64*)*, FDA seems unaware that new technology of DNA mapping was developing different ways of measuring IGF-I over these three dates. It might appear that FDA was simply establishing a wide range so that one day they could define any future readings as: "WELL WITHIN THE RANGE." This is how FDA explained increases in levels of IGF-I in milk from rbST-treated cows. Since then, technology has developed tests. Even in 1988 there was no way to measure IGF-I accurately. Here's why.

The available test only detected a portion of the chain of the 70 amino acid IGF-I protein. The test acted metaphorically like a camera photographing a few boxcars of a train of 70 cars. That picture did not reveal whether or not the IGF-I was bound to other proteins and de-activated or whether it was free to exert a growth "influence." It was not possible until 1994 to measure IGF-I in human serum, when a Danish researcher, Frystyk, quantified the amounts of free and unbound IGF-I in human serum (18). Frystyk found that IGF-I levels in humans were inversely proportional to age and ranged from 950 nanograms per liter in a 20-30-year-old male to 410 ng/L in a 60-year-old male. FDA assumes that the average human body contains 500,000 nanograms of IGF-I. The number of nanograms of free and unbound IGF-I is actually equal to the same amount contained in a 12 ounce glass of normal untreated milk.

Juskevich & Guyer

Insulin-Like Growth Factor-I: Human Food Safety

Although a variety of growth factors may have specific effects on cells and cellular metabolism, IGF-I is the main factor known to be regulated by GH. Human and bovine IGF-I are identical (65*), but treating dairy cattle with rbGH was not expected to cause an increase in IGF-I in concentrations of biological significance to humans.

Juskevich and Guyer wrote "...*not expected to cause an increase...of biological significance to humans...*" This is the way scientists use statistics to mislead. The average human serum contains 500,000 nanograms of IGF-I. A 12-ounce glass of untreated milk contains approximately 3,000 nanograms. To FDA, 3,000 is compared with 500,000 and that is considered to be insignificant. If the amount of IGF-I in milk were to double, FDA would still consider it to be insignificant. If the levels of IGF-I were to increase twenty-fold to 60,000 nanograms that still would be considered insignificant. However, there is considerable lack of logic in their thinking. First, most of the 500,000 nanograms of IGF-I are already bound or attached to other proteins, like keys into locks. The possible growth-initiating effects of these protein hormones have been negated.

An analogy can be made. Do you have glue in your home? Most people would imagine a jar of that "white stuff" with a picture of the cow on the bottle sitting on a shelf in a cabinet. Would there be 1/2 cup of glue then or a 55 gallon drum? To the rigorous scientists at FDA, you would have 55 gallons. They'd use sophisticated techniques to measure the glue in your furniture, the sheetrock in your walls, the bathroom tiles, your rug. There's lots of glue in your house. The doorbell rings and there's an inebriated fellow, barely able to stand, holding a dripping cup of gooey glue. Would you invite him in? I don't think so! His glue would soon bind with your rug. The glue in your furniture and rug will never act like glue again, yet it's still glue. Most of the IGF-I, easily measured, will never act like IGF-I again either. It's the free and unattached IGF-I which should concern all of us. Frystyk had measured the total amount of free IGF-I in a typical adult to be equal to the same amount contained in a 12 ounce glass of milk.

IGF-I contained in meat or in pill form would most certainly be digested and "broken down" into basic amino acids in the stomach. In milk, IGF-I survives digestion and remains biologically active for up to 30 minutes after passing through the stomach! (20) Sure, we produce it naturally in our bodies. However, what great planning to put a growth hormone in milk. What is lactation and nursing all about, if not growth?

Juskevich & Guyer

This perception was based on the mechanism of action of IGF-I, the concentration of IGF-I found in human milk, preliminary information on the concentration of IGF-I in milk or rbGH-treated cows, the way in which milk is processed for infant formula, and our knowledge of protein absorption and digestion in adults and neonates. However, because of the general lack of information in the scientific literature regarding the oral activity of IGF-I, the CVM decided to obtain more information.

Toxicity Studies of IGF-I

Elanco (66*) and Monsanto (67*) have conducted toxicity studies to determine whether IGF-I is active when administered orally. Both IGF-I oral toxicity studies are described in detail because they were conducted in different models, namely, hypophysectomized and normal rats. The IGF-I administered to the rats in both studies was a recombinant product with an identical sequence to the natural IGF-I.

Elanco conducted a 2-week oral toxicity study with rIGF-I in hypophysectomized rats (66*). Rats were treated with rIGF-I at 0.01, 0.1, or 1.0 mg/kg per day by gavage (LD, MD, and HD, respectively) or at 1.0 mg/kg per day by subcutaneous infusion (s.c. group). There were also two negative control groups; one given saline and the other given bovine serum albumin (BSA) by gavage.

Animals receive the drug orally or by injection. FDA reasons that the injected drug has an effect because it bypasses digestive acids in the stomach and enters directly into the bloodstream. On the other hand, the oral drug, unprotected by natural enzymatic inhibitory substances normally present in milk, is burned by stomach acid, rendered inactive.

Juskevich & Guyer

There were no treatment-related deaths or clinical signs. Mean body weight and mean body weight gain for the s.c. group were significantly higher than those for the negative controls, starting on day 3 and continuing throughout the study. At termination, body weights of the males and females in the s.c. group were 15 and 12% greater than those of controls, respectively. Body weight gain of female rats in the LD oral group was significantly lower than that for controls. The mean body weights and body weight gains in all other groups were not statistically different from those of the control group (P>0.05) (66*).

No treatment-related changes in the hematological parameters were observed in any of the groups. A moderate increase (approximately twofold) in absolute neutrophil values was seen in the s.c. group animals which may reflect the mild irritation associated with the subcutaneous minipump implant. Statistically significant changes in clinical chemistry parameters were generally limited to rats in the s.c. group and included decreases in blood urea nitrogen (BUN), creatinine, albumin, total protein, and globulin and increases in inorganic phosphorus and potassium. The only difference noted in rats treated by oral administration of rIGF-I was a biologically insignificant decrease in total protein in the HD males.

FDA will not release the data that they reported to be *"...biologically insignificant."* After FDA reports that there are statistically insignificant increases in numerous data, I formally requested that data to perform my own analyses. Their response was, "Sorry, the data actually are secret. We cannot release them."

Juskevich & Guyer

The only statistically significant differences in organ weights compared to controls were found in the s.c. group and included increased kidney, spleen, adrenal and brain weights in males, and kidney, liver, and spleen weights in females (Table 3) (45*, 66*). Increases in relative organ weights included kidney weight in LD females and kidney, spleen and brain weights in the males and females of the s.c. group. Relative thyroid and parathyroid weight was decreased in MD males. None of the organ weight changes were accompanied by gross or *microscopic changes. There were no compound-related changes in organ weights of animals treated with rIGF-I by gavage.*

*The results of this study **(66*)** demonstrated that subcutaneous infusion of rIGF-I in hypophysectomized rats caused increased body weight; increased neutrophil count; decreased BUN, creatinine, and albumin; and increased relative kidney and spleen weights in both males and females. These changes are attributed to the physiologic effects of IGF-I. In contrast, oral treatment with rIGF-I at doses up to 1 mg/kg per day caused none of the changes seen in the rats treated subcutaneously.*

*A 2-week oral toxicity study with normal rats was conducted for Monsanto Agricultural Company by Hazleton Laboratories **(67*)**. Rats were treated with rIGF-I at 0.02, 0.2, or 2.0 mg/kg per day by gavage (LD, MD, and HD, respectively), or at 0.05 or 0.2 mg/rat per day by subcutaneous infusion (LD and HD s.c. groups, respectively).*

Usually, laboratory animals are given doses of drugs, carefully measured out according to that animal's body weight. That's why mg/kg so often appears. That represents milligrams per kilogram of body weight. If the dose is 1.0 mg/kg and the animal weighs 1 kilogram then it would get 1.0 milligram of chemical. If it weighed 1/2 kilogram it would receive 0.5 milligrams. It's all weight related, with each subject animal receiving a different dose. In this experiment the animals being dosed orally received 0.2 milligrams per rat, as opposed to the other groups receiving weight dependent doses. This is an excellent example of poor laboratory technique!

Juskevich & Guyer

A negative control was included for each route of administration, and one group was treated with alanyl porcine GH as a positive control (pGH-treated group). Treatment was initiated on two consecutive days to accommodate the large number of rats to be implanted with osmotic pumps. The study was planned in blocks of rats so that all treatments were equally presented on each start date. Body weights were recorded twice weekly, and food consumption was recorded weekly.

All rats survived until the termination of the study, and no compound-related clinical signs were seen. A significant increase in body weight was seen throughout the study in males of the LD s.c. group and in both sexes of the HD s.c. and pGH-treated groups (Table 4). These findings were considered to be treatment-related.

The mean body weight for males in the HD oral group was slightly but significantly increased from day 7 of the study; average daily gain was also significantly increased. There was no significant increase in average daily gain in any of the males in the other gavage groups or in any of the females. When examined by block, it appeared that there was an increase in average daily gain only in the male rats of the HD oral group of block 2 (8.41 g/day versus 7.74 g/day for controls) and not in block 1 (8.27 g/day versus 8.10 g/day for controls). It is therefore questionable whether the overall increase in body weight in males of the HD oral group can be attributed to rIGF- treatment.

Significant changes in hematology, clinical chemistry, and urinalysis parameters were noted in both sexes of pGH-treated group (67*). There was a slight but significant decrease in erythrocyte count, hemoglobin, and hematocrit, and a significantly increased platelet count in the females. Evaluation of the clinical chemistry data for this group revealed significantly increased total serum protein, serum albumin, albumin/globulin ratio, calcium, and total bilirubin, and significantly decreased chloride in both sexes. Males also showed a significant increase in creatinine and decrease in inorganic phosphorus and sodium. Females showed a significant decrease in aspartate transaminase. Urinalysis revealed a significant increase in urine osmolality for both sexes.

In contrast to the rats in the pGH-treated group, rats receiving rIGF-i via osmotic minipump showed minimal changes and those only at the high dose. Platelet count and BUN decreased significantly in both sexes, and creatinine decreased significantly in females. The only significant change noted in rats treated with rIGF-I by gavage was a slight decrease in hemoglobin for the females in the MD oral group without concomitant changes in erthrocyte count or hematocrit. No significant changes were seen in the HD oral group rats. The decrease in hemoglobin is not considered to be treatment-related.

When a *"significant change"* was noted in the group orally receiving rIGF-I, this decrease in hemoglobin was *"...not considered to be treatment-related."* By whom? FDA? The pharmaceutical company? FDA concludes that there are no biological effects from oral ingestion, by ignoring all evidence of oral effects!

Juskevich & Guyer

Gross pathology revealed no notable differences between control and treated groups. In the pGH-treated group, significant increases were observed in adrenal (67*), heart, spleen, kidney and liver weights in both sexes (Table 5), and in brain (with brainstem) and ovary weights in females (67*). In the HD s.c. group, significant increases were observed in kidney and heart weights of males and females and in adrenal and brain with brainstem weights in females; liver weight increased and testes weights decreased in males. The only organ weight changes noted in LD s.c. group were increases in kidney and liver weights in males. Liver weights of the HD oral group males were increased. No other *statistically significant organ weight changes were noted for other animals treated with rIGF-I by gavage (P>0.05).*

Changes noted in relative organ weights (67*) are as follows: The pGH-treated group showed an increase in heart and liver weights and a decrease in relative brain weight for both sexes; an increase in adrenal and kidney weights and a decrease in relative testicular weight in males; and an increase in relative spleen weight and a decrease in relative ovary weight in females. The HD s.c. group showed an increase in kidney weight and a decrease in brain weight for both sexes, a decrease in relative testicular weight in males and an increase in relative spleen weights in females. The LD s.c. group showed only a decrease in relative brain weight in males. The only organ weight change noted in rats treated with rIGF-I by gavage was an increase in the relative heart weight for males in the LD oral group.

Epiphyseal widths were increased in females of the HD s.c. group and both sexes of the pGH-treated group. Tibia lengths were increased in the LD s.c. group males and both sexes of the pGH-treated group. In the groups treated with rIGF-I by gavage, epiphyseal widths were decreased in both sexes of the HD group and tibia lengths were increased in the LD and HD group males. These findings (67*) in the oral groups are considered contradictory in terms of effects of IGFs on growth indices and are therefore considered to be sporadic results.

Again, contrary results from oral ingestion are considered to be insignificant and explained away as being *"...sporadic results."* Let me translate what happened here. The tibia is the innermost and larger of the two leg bones located below the knee. Animals taking IGF-I orally experience increased growth in this bone. They became deformed. William von Meyer was the first of many critics to note that FDA's numbers did not add up. The tibia bone is sensitive to levels of growth hormone. This did not worry FDA. After all, who was going to be drinking the milk containing increased levels of IGF-I. Americans, that's who!

Juskevich & Guyer

The results of this study (67*) demonstrate that subcutaneous infusion or rIGF-I in rats produces effects similar to those seen with subcutaneously injected GH. When administered orally, rIGF-I had no effect.

Juskevich and Guyer explained that experimental results were not significant, *"orally...no effect."* FDA convinced themselves by arbitrarily tagging significant problems with labels such as *"sporadic results"* and *"not considered to be treatment related."* They've trivialized their own evidence and achieved acceptance from the scientific community by publishing the results in a peer-reviewed journal.

Juskevich & Guyer

Body weights of male rats given the high dose or rIGF-1 by oral gavage showed a statistically significant increase.

Juskevich and Guyer previously stated that the results of this study showed that there was no effect when rBST was taken orally. In the next line, they commented that body weights of male rats taking the drug orally increased. How will they explain this contradiction? Is it magic or is it incidental?

Juskevich & Guyer

However, this increase was considered incidental because it occurred in only half of the male rats, the body weight of the female rats in the HD gavage group did not increase, serum levels of IGF-1 were not increased in the HD animals as they were in the positive control groups, and there were no changes in hematology, clinical chemistry and urinalysis parameters, or organ weights that were consistent with the effects of GH or IGF-1, as observed in the positive control groups. Therefore, it was concluded that rIGF-1 is orally inactive at doses up to 2 mg/kg per day.

Residue Studies of IGF-I

Several companies conducted studies to determine the concentration of IGF-1 in the milk of rbGH-treated and untreated cows. The analytical methods used by the companies are exclusively RIA procedures that putatively measure free IGF-1 plus IGF-1 bound to carrier proteins. Bound IGF-1 is liberated by an acid-ethanol extraction step. Each company developed its own RIA and submitted the procedure to FDA for evaluation.

The survey of 100 raw bulk tank milk samples from a commercial processing plant was conducted to provide data on the naturally occurring range of IGF-1 concentrations in salable milk (68*). The mean IGF-1 concentration ($\pm$ SD) in these samples was 4.32 ng/ml $\pm$ 1.09 ng/ml with a range of 1.27 to 8.10 ng/ml (Fig.1).

A bulk tank truck of milk carries 50,000 pounds. Monsanto accessed samples from 100 bulk tank milk samples. Therefore, one must assume that 5 million pounds of milk containing pooled milk from thousands of different animals at different times of their lactations and energy balances and cycles would provide a UNIVERSAL NUMBER which could be accepted by everybody. Every combination and permutation is considered. One assumes that milk comes from

Guernsey, Jersey and Holstein cows. Cows in the beginning of their lactation cycle and cows at the end. Big cows, little cows, fat cows and skinny cows. Holy cow! I for once accept Monsanto's research on this subject.

There are 4.32 nanograms of IGF-I in each thousandth of a liter (milliliter) of milk. To convert milliliters to liters, multiply by 1000. Therefore, there are 4320 nanograms of IGF-I in a liter of milk. One liter of liquid milk is equal to 1.057 liquid quarts of milk. Therefore, there are 4566 nanograms of IGF-I in a quart of milk. A tall glass of milk, one pint, contains 2283 nanograms of IGF-I, approximately the same amount of free and unbound IGF-I contained in the average adult male's body. (21)

Juskevich & Guyer

The range of IGF-1 concentrations was also determined in salable milk from 408 untreated cows from five Missouri dairy herds (69*). The highest mean concentration of IGF-1 in milk was detected in early lactation (days 6 to 15 postpartum, 6.2 ng/ml), after which milk concentrations declined. Multiparous animals had significantly higher mean milk IGF-1 concentrations (2.83 ng/ml) than primiparous (first lactation) animals (2.15 ng/ml). Stage of lactation effects were detected in both parties, and the effect of parity was apparent at all stages of lactation. The survey studies determined that the concentration of IGF-1 in milk of untreated cows is quite variable, ranging from <0.7 to 8.2 ng/ml in 95% of the cows with a maximum of 30.5 ng/ml, depending on parity and stage of lactation of the cow.

What FDA is doing here is setting a range in which levels of IGF-I appear in normal milk. Despite the fact that Monsanto accessed 5 million pounds of milk from thousands of animals and determined a universal average standard, 4320 ng/L, FDA deliberately broadened the range so that the effects of rBST-treatment can be negated.

FDA, by this act, knows that different herds of cows yield different results. As a result of one cow having a sample reading of 30.5 nanograms per milliliter, FDA has now expanded the range to include 32,239 nanograms of IGF-I in a quart of milk to be well within the range. (There are 30,500 nanograms in one liter. We multiply that number by 1.057, the factor to convert liters into quarts. The resulting number, 32,239, is the number of nanograms of IGF-I in one quart.) Monsanto's average reading for a quart of milk was 4566 nanograms. The authors of this study have written that levels of IGF-I increase in milk from cows treated with rBST. If the amount of IGF-I increased by 7 times, 700 percent, FDA would say that it did not really increase because it was well within the normal range.

Juskevich & Guyer

Schams and Karg (70*) investigated the increase in IGF-1 concentrations in the milk of cows treated with rbGH. In the first experiment, eight cows (four controls and four treated) of different breeds were injected subcutaneously with 640 mg of rbGH in a prolonged release formulation every 28 days (approximately the proposed dose). Milk samples were collected in the morning before the third injection and after on days 1, 3, 6, 8, 10, 13, 15, 17, 20, 22, 24, and 27 and after the fourth injection of rbGH on days 1, 3, 6, 8, 10 and 13. Mean amounts of IGF-1 in the milk of treated cows were always higher than those found in the controls. The average IGF-1 milk concentration found in the control cows was 28.4 ng/ml, and the average IGF-1 milk concentrations in the rbGH-treated cows was 35.5 ng/ml, representing an increase of 25% of the mean.

In another study conducted for Elanco (71*), 36 cows that had completed at least one full lactation were given a single subcutaneous injection of 0, 320 or 640 mg of rbGH (12 cows per group). The concentration (mean $\pm$ SEM) of IGF-1 in milk was significantly higher by day 3 in cows treated with 320 mg of rbGH (13.9 $\pm$ 1.35 ng/ml) than in the control cows (9.5 $\pm$ 1.35 ng/ml) (P< 0.05, protected t test), but not in those cows treated with 640 mg of rbGH (12.6 $\pm$ 1.41 NG/ML) (P >0.05, protected t test). The values at 10, 17 and 24 days after treatment were also not significantly different for any of the groups (P > 0.05, protected t test).

White et al. (72*) conducted a study to provide additional data about the effect of exogenous administration of rbGH on concentrations of IGF-1 in milk. Eighteen lactating cows were administered subcutaneous injections of 500 mg of rbGH in a prolonged release formulation (approximately the proposed dose) or a sham injection at 14-day intervals (9 cows per group). IGF-1 concentrations in milk were significantly increased in rbGH-treated cows, although the increases were numerically small and occurred only in injection cycles 2 and 3 of treatment (Table 6).

There were only nine cows in this unpublished Monsanto study. The actual data are considered a trade secret and will not be released to the public.

Juskevich & Guyer

The overall range of concentrations was similar for both groups:
2.16 to 9.04 ng/ml for the control group and 1.56 to 8.83 ng/ml for the rbGH treatment group.

Miller et al. (73*) assessed the potential carryover of IGF-1 in processed milk. IGF-1 concentrations were measured in raw and pasteurized milk and in milk subjected to conditions similar to those used in preparation of infant formula.

Daily milk samples were obtained before and after pasteurization from a local commercial processing plant. The milk was pasteurized by standard procedures. Conditions used to process milk for infant formula (heating in a retort at 250 degrees Fahrenheit for 15 minutes) can be simulated in the laboratory. Raw (unpasteurized and pasteurized milk samples were autoclaved under conditions simulating retorting and then assayed for IGF-I content.

These results were then compared to IGF-I concentrations measured in a commercial infant formula. The mean ($\pm$ SEM) IGF-I concentrations in raw milk and pasteurized milk samples were 5.6 $\pm$ 0.56 and 8.2 $\pm$ 0.35 ng/ml, respectively. These same samples exposed to the heat treatment process for manufacturing infant formula contained concentrations of IGF-I of approximately 0.5 ng/ml and lower. The commercial infant formula also contained only trace amounts (approximately 0.7 ng/ml) of IGF-I. These results suggest that IGF-I is not destroyed by the pasteurization process, but the heating of milk for the preparation of infant formula denatures IGF-I, with only one-tenth of the concentration of the milk before heat treatment.

Although the pharmaceutical companies were not required to conduct studies with IGF-II, Monsanto conducted a study of milk residues to determine if IGF-II concentrations increased in rbGH-treated cows *(74*)*. Sixty-four lactating Holstein cows (21 primiparous and 43 multiparous) were used in the study; they received either 500 mg or rbGH in an oil-based prolonged-release formulation (approximately the proposed dose) or vehicle by intramuscular or subcutaneous injection at 14-day intervals. Treatments began at 60 $\pm$ 3 days postpartum and continued for at least 10 cycles. Composite milk samples from each cow were collected on day -7 of the pretreatment period and on day 7 of injection cycles 1 through 10. There was no significant increase in milk IGF-II concentrations in any of the sampling periods ($P > 0.05$). However, the concentration of IGF-I in milk from the rbGH-treated cows was significantly increased across the ten injection cycles. The average increase in IGF-I concentrations was 2.2 ng/ml in milk (Table 7).

This study was performed by Margaret Miller, Monsanto's most important bovine scientist. Miller was hired by the FDA, where she ended up reviewing her very own research. It is curious that when levels of IGF-I increase in milk only slightly, these FDA reviewers comment about the percentage. In the case of the Schams and Karg study *(70*)*, they wrote that levels of IGF-I increased by 25 percent. Schams and Karg only treated four cows. Miller's data, more reliable, were taken from 64 cows and readings were averaged over ten different cycles. Her data indicate that IGF-I levels in milk taken from primiparous animals (cows who had not previously birthed a calf) treated with rbGH increased by an average of 71 percent, and an average of 47 percent in multiparous animals (cows who had previously birthed at least one calf).

Juskevich & Guyer

It appears from these studies that IGF-I concentrations in the milk of rbGH-treated cows are increased above those concentrations of found naturally in untreated cows. However, the data indicate that stage of lactation and parity also significantly influence IGF-I concentrations in milk. IGF-II milk concentrations, on the other hand, are not affected by rbGH treatment.

Conclusions

The data evaluated by the FDA document the safety of food products from animals treated with rbGH. Bovine GH is biologically inactive in humans; therefore residues of bGH in food products would have no physiological effect even if absorbed intact from the gastrointestinal tract. The possibility that fragments of bGH produce metabolic effects in humans is not a basis for concern as it is unlikely that any active fragment could be produced in biologically significant amounts in the gastrointestinal tract. Very mild hydrolysis conditions are necessary to retain even the limited activity observed in test animals. No oral activity was found when rbGH was administered to rats at exaggerated doses. In addition, very limited residue studies suggest no significant increase in milk concentrations of bGH due to the treatment of dairy cows with rbGH. Furthermore, 90% of bGH in milk is destroyed upon pasteurization, and rbGH treatment appears to have no significant impact on the nutritional quality of milk.

The FDA concluded that an increase in growth factors secondary to rbGH treatment was unlikely to present any human food safety concerns. Nonetheless, the FDA felt it was important to establish the range of concentrations of growth factors after rbGH treatment and the potential for oral activity because of the widespread use of milk-based infant formula. IGF-I was chosen as the growth factor for study because it is the major factor that mediates the effects of GH.

The oral toxicity studies demonstrated that rIGH-I was not active at doses up to 2 mg/kg per day in rats. Additional information collected to resolve any concern for potential neonatal exposure to IGF-I, demonstrated that IGF-I is denatured by the process used to prepare infant formula, which eliminates any basis of concern for minor increases in IGF-I concentrations in milk. Although limited information is available about the concentration of IGF-I in human milk, the data indicate that the concentration of IGF-I found in milk from rbGH-treated cows is within the physiological range found in human breast milk. On the basis of this information, the FDA scientists concluded that the use of rbGH in dairy cattle presents no increased health risks to consumers.

In their summary, FDA made eight major errors:

1) *Bovine GH is biologically inactive in humans.*
   Actions of bovine GH are mediated by IGF-I and the IGF-I receptor. IGF-I is identical in humans and cows. FDA could also conclude that bovine GH is inactive in cows because there are no such receptors in the mammary tissues of cows.
2) *It is unlikely that fragments of bGH could reach the gastrointestinal tract.*
   Milk acts as an enzyme inhibitor. Milk buffers gastric pH from a normal 1.8 to a 6.0. At 6, growth hormones are not broken down.
3) *No oral activity was found when bGH was administered orally to rats.*

Here's What FDA Calls Evidence Contrary to Their Opinions:

A) INCIDENTAL FINDINGS
B) NO SIGNIFICANT INCREASE
C) BIOLOGICALLY INSIGNIFICANT
D) SPORADIC RESULTS
E) NOT TREATMENT RELATED

4) *No significant increase in milk concentrations of bGH occur after cows are treated with rbGH.*
   A 26 percent increase was reported!
5) *90% of bGH in milk is destroyed after milk is pasteurized.*
   Milk was heated for 30 minutes at a temperature reserved for a 15-second treatment and 82 percent of the bGH survived! Only 18 percent of the bGH was destroyed, yet this lie became the foundation of bGH approval.
6) *rbGH treatment appears to have no significant impact on the nutritional quality of milk.*
   The most powerful growth hormone in the human body, IGF-I, is the same as bovine IGF-I. Milk drinkers ingest enormous amounts of this hormone. Milk treated with the new genetically engineered hormone always contains increased levels of IGF-1.
7) *An increase in growth factors in rbGH-treated milk was unlikely to present any human food safety concerns.*
   These growth factors survive digestion.
8) *IGF-I is not orally active in rats.*
   Research indicates otherwise. Laboratory rats were fed IGF-I which was naturally destroyed by digestive processes. In milk, protected by casein and

the buffering effect which milk has upon stomach acid, IGF-I survived and has been shown to be active.

Judy Juskevich and Greg Guyer were selected to write the FDA paper that would end the controversy surrounding the genetically engineered bovine hormone. Scientific fraud has never passed inspection by so many members of a scientific community. If not for the many links in a long chain, Sam Epstein, Pete Hardin, Michael Hansen, William Von Meyer, Jane Heimlich, and, finally, this book, the American public would have no idea of the deception. Monsanto would have succeeded in their crime. That would have been a national tragedy. When Monsanto's rbST animal drug application was finally approved by FDA the agency cautioned that:

> Use of the product has also been associated with increased cystic ovaries and disorders of the uterus (in cows) during the treatment period. Treated cows are at an increased risk of clinical mastitis and subclinical mastitis. In some herds, use has been associated with increases in somatic cell counts in milk...Use may result in an increase in digestive disorders such as indigestion, bloat and diarrhea. Cows treated with this product may have increased numbers of enlarged hocks and lesions of the knee...and second lactation or older cows may have more disorders of the foot region. Use has been associated with reductions in hemoglobin and hematocrit values during treatment. (22)

"Behind every great fortune there is a crime."

Honore de Balzac

"What the scientists have in their briefcases is terrifying."

Nikita Khruschev

Chapter 4

Scientific Proof: Milk Hormones Are Hazardous to Your Health

The word *hormone* constitutes diversified meanings for different people. To teenagers with acne it's the cause of all pimples. To the husband of a pregnant woman desiring pickles and ice cream, experiencing mood swings, it's the foundation of her behavior patterns. To gang members who fight to defend a street corner as their turf, it's the chemical that brings about aggressive behavior. To a weight lifter or Olympic athlete, it's the way to illegally grow muscles quickly. To an animal psychologist studying wolf behavior, a hormone is a chemical messenger that causes a fixed action pattern in the brain eliciting the course of action in which a male will mark bushes and declare his territorial rights. Nobody instructs a male dog in how to mount a female and conduct himself in a manner as to reproduce his species. He does not read such advice in a book and he does not watch a movie. A chemical hormone called a pheromone creates an odor which when inhaled affects the male dog's brain in such a manner that he perform the same act done by generations of his ancestors. Chemical and physiological processes are so linked in the brains of all mammals.

Steroid hormones such as estrogen, progesterone and testosterone are responsible for a vast array of behaviors. Body organs secrete these chemical messengers at varied times for a multitude of purposes. There are other hormones which control miscellaneous body functions. One is called epinephrine, better known as adrenaline. Adrenaline is the powerful hormonal messenger that alerts humans to dangerous situations. When adrenaline is secreted into the bloodstream by the adrenal glands, animals, including humans, experience the "fight or flight" response. One other group of hormones works on cellular processes. Quite often the effects of these hormones are not readily observed.

The amino acid sequence of two such hormones, genetically engineered bovine growth hormone (rbGH, rbST) and insulin-like growth factor-I (IGF-I) are illustrated on the following pages:

Amino Acid Sequence of The Genetically Engineered Version of Bovine Growth Hormone (rBGH, rBST) *

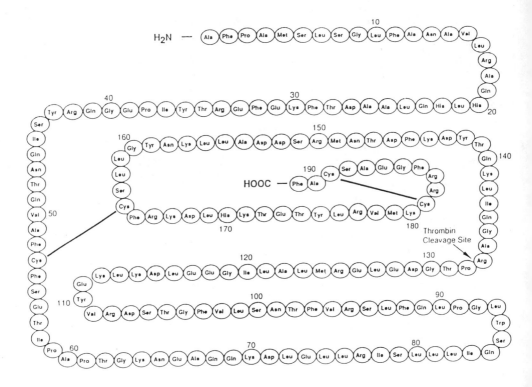

* From page 114 of the World Health Organization Monograph from the June, 1992 meeting in Geneva, Switzerland.

Amino Acid sequence of Insulin-Like Growth Factor-I (IGF-I), Identical to Bovines and Humans *

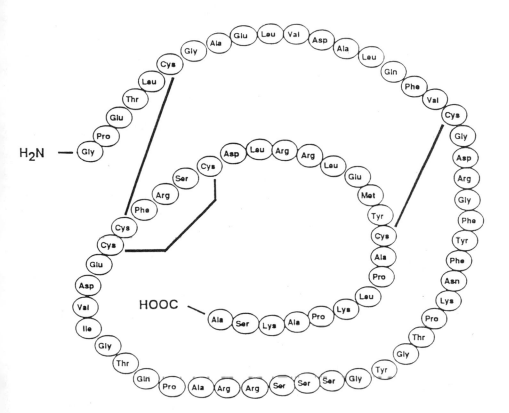

* From page 116 of the World Health Organization Monograph from the June, 1992 meeting in Geneva, Switzerland.

When a hormone doesn't function properly, an abnormal condition can often result. For example, diabetes can be an indication that the pancreas is not producing enough insulin to metabolize sugar. Less than 30 years ago, a powerful growth hormone was identified in the milk of cows. Subsequently, that same hormone has been identified in humans. Variations of that growth hormone have also been identified in hundreds of animal species. The actual date of discovery was never recorded. This hormone was similar to but not exactly like insulin. This hormone made cells grow. Since it resembled insulin and made cells grow it was called insulin-like growth factor. There are at least five different types of insulin-like growth factors. For this chapter and this book we concern ourselves primarily with insulin-like growth factor-I (IGF-I).

IGF-I works on an extremely tiny scale, a molecular level. It does not take a lot of IGF-I to exert cellular growth effects. Other chemicals work the same way. A similarly tiny amount of LSD would create powerful hallucinations for anybody experiencing an LSD "trip." Hormones are made up of amino acids. Amino acids are building blocks of proteins. There are approximately 28 amino acids that make up the hundreds of known proteins in the human body. Other species of animals have hormones that are similar to but not exact in structure to human hormones. There is one exception. IGF-I, the most powerful growth hormone in the human body, is identical between bovines and humans. IGF-I in both cows and people contains 70 amino acids in the same exact sequence. If somebody were to offer you a pill containing the most powerful growth hormone in the human body, would you take that pill? Every time you drink a glass of milk, you ingest the same amount of this growth hormone. Would you imagine that IGF-I works on a nursing calf? Of course it does! Why would you not assume that IGF-I in milk has the potential to exert a powerful influence on human cellular activity?

The Juskevich and Guyer journal article appearing in *Science* contained seven tables, each containing data from various experiments. For a table to appear, illustrating data, it is logical to assume that the experiment carried some weight. FDA relied upon these studies in reaching their determination.

Tables 1 and 2 contained data referenced in citation #42, an unpublished report prepared for Monsanto in 1989 by Searle (1). Tables 3, 4, 5, 6 and 7 also contained data from unpublished reports. It did not take a degree in genetic engineering to detect a pattern. Here was an article summarizing the research concerning the most controversial drug application in FDA history, appearing in a peer-review journal, and the actual data were not available for the peers to review.

Here's how FDA explained the data in their description of Table 1: *"Body weight changes (in grams) of control rats and rbGH-treated rats (means ± SD)."*

Note: Scientific data are analyzed by various standardized methods of statistical analyses. Without the raw data, these universally accepted tests of significance are impossible to perform. Terms such as mean (average amount) and SD, standard deviation, derive from all of the available data. Without a complete breakdown of all available figures, it is impossible to authenticate results and conclusions.

Table One - Caption

Charles River CD rats (one of the many different species of laboratory animal available for laboratory experimentation) were treated for 90 days with rbGH either by gavage or by subcutaneous administration. Groups of 30 rats per sex each were treated with rbGH orally by gavage; one group was treated with rbGH by subcutaneous injection; and one group of animals served as untreated controls. From (42) with permission, copyright, 1989, Monsanto Agricultural Company.

There were 360 laboratory animals in this study. There were 12 different groups. Six groups each of males and females. Of the six groups (for each sex) one group received no rbGH. One group of animals received an injection of the drug. Four groups received varying dosages of the drug orally, by gavage. A gavage is similar to a medicine dropper which delivers a carefully measured dose to the animal and insures that the entire dose of medication is swallowed by the subject.

The table is difficult to read and requires a guide. On the left-hand column are numbers, 8, 29, 50 and 85. These are the study days in which the animals were weighed. To the right of the words, *study date*, are numbers signifying the dosages or drug administered to each group. The dosages given to the six different groups were:

GROUP 1) Placebo, no drug
GROUP 2) 1.0 milligrams per 1000 grams of body weight
         (Group 2 received rbGH by injection under the skin)
GROUP 3) 0.1 milligrams per 1000 grams of body weight (oral)
GROUP 4) 0.5 milligrams per 1000 grams of body weight (oral)
GROUP 5) 5.0 milligrams per 1000 grams of body weight (oral)
GROUP 6) 50.0 milligrams per 1000 grams of body weight (oral)

The number 0 (zero) represents the control group.

Table 1
Body weight change (g) for dosage of rbGH (mg/kg per day)

Study day	Subcutaneous		Oral			
	0	1.0	0.1	0.5	5	50
			MALES			
8	58	72	61	62	62	59
29	170	207	174	178	181	176
50	239	294	240	241	239	243
85	324	432	327	318	325	328
			FEMALES			
8	24	33	21	25	25	25
29	81	101	69	80	81	83
50	110	150	99	116	112	114
85	148	217	140	152	147	152

When designing a study of this type the researcher must create the same conditions for the control animals and the animals receiving the drug. This study was poorly designed. There should have been two control groups because there were two methods of administering the drug. One group had the drug injected. There should have been a control group receiving "sham" injections containing a placebo. That way, possible effects resulting from the injection itself, or the suspension contained in the injection, could be discounted against control animals.

The same is true of the group receiving the rbGH by gavage. What effects, if any, were contributed by forcing a liquid down the throat of a laboratory animal? Would they eat properly? Would they eat more or less than the control animals receiving injections? Were their throats irritated? The group receiving the rbGH orally should also have had a control group receiving a placebo. Questions such as these could be answered and doubts eliminated by proper experimental design. Furthermore, who picked out the parameters? Day 8, 29, 50 and 85? Why not tabulate the weights once per week (i.e., day 7, 14, 21, 28) or once every 10 days (i.e., day 10, 20, 30, 40)? Analyses of data expose the reason and reveals how the data are manipulated. They picked these days after running the data so as to obtain results that did not reflect actual growth effects.

Additional data were listed after each weight. Those data, the means plus or minus standard deviation, were intentionally eliminated from this table. In order to determine the standard deviations, a simple statistical test, the actual weights of each animal must be available. Monsanto and FDA will not release those weights, citing trade protection and claiming that Monsanto will be irreparably harmed if such data are revealed.

FDA controls the "scientific game" by publishing only partial data. To a scientist, it is an unconscionable affront to the integrity of the scientific method to deny full access to all existing data. A review of the data indicates that oral ingestion of rbGH had no growth effects. This was to be expected, as any possible effects would be negated because rbGH would be destroyed by gastric enzymatic activity. Perhaps the experimental results would have been different had the rats ingested the hormones in fluid milk which has a buffering effect.

The results for the subcutaneous group were rather revealing. Even FDA admitted that "differences in mean body weights reached 16 percent in males and 20 percent in females by study week 13 (day 85), compared to the negative control group." What is actually learned by a careful review of the data is concealed by the presentation of this table. We are told that males injected with rbGH grew 16 percent more than untreated males and that rbGH-treated females grew 20 percent over control females. The data were carefully manipulated so that these relatively low results could be averaged out. First, notice that we are not told what the animals weighed at day 1 of the experiment.

Actual Weight Gains (Grams) From Table 1

TIME PERIOD	CONTROL GROUP	rBGH-TREATED	DIFFERENCE	% INCREASE
MALES				
DAYS 8-29	+ 112 Grams	+135 Grams	+23 Grams	+21%
DAYS 29-50	+ 69 Grams	+ 87 Grams	+18 Grams	+26%
DAYS 50-85	+ 85 Grams	+138 Grams	+53 Grams	+62%
FEMALES				
DAYS 8-29	+ 57 Grams	+ 68 Grams	+11 Grams	+19%
DAYS 29-50	+ 29 Grams	+ 49 Grams	+20 Grams	+69%
DAYS 50-85	+ 38 Grams	+ 67 Grams	+29 Grams	+76%

The actual weight gains demonstrate that there is a latency period accounting for the growth effects of subcutaneous injections of rbGH. FDA noted that rbGH-treated animals increased in size 16 percent (in males) and 20 percent (in females) over control animals. What actually happened was that the increases were in the 20 percent range during the first four weeks of the study. After that, there was a boomerang effect. The data are quite revealing, once they're broken down. During the last period, from day 50 to day 85, the male group experienced 62 percent greater growth than the control animals. The rbGH-treated females experienced a 76 percent increase over controls during that same period.

Something unusual was happening to these animals. Toward the end of the study the animals receiving rbGH experienced enormous growth spurts when compared to the control group animals receiving a placebo. FDA would have the reader believe that the study ended after day 90. That's what FDA wrote. It is clear that FDA never really examined these data. Had they, they would have discovered that the study continued until day 180.

Richard Teske, Associate Director for Policy at the Center for Veterinary Medicine (CVM) in Rockville, Maryland, oversees all pharmaceutical company applications for new drugs containing studies using animals for research. The August 10, 1995, letter from Teske to this author revealed:

> I should note that Dr. Condon did uncover some errors in the
> information as it was presented...in the *Science* paper. While
> the 90 day study did involve the use of 30 rats per sex per
> treatment group, only 15 rats per sex per treatment were
> sacrificed...(others) were scheduled for an effect reversal phase
> of the study. (2)

A reversal phase? That means that the study continued. It wasn't a 90 day study. It was a 180-day study! What will we find if and when the courts order Monsanto and FDA to release all of the raw data? In a world where deals are made behind closed doors and influence is exerted by multi-billion dollar corporations, is anybody naive enough to believe that Monsanto will ever be made to reveal the organ weights of these animals? Once an animal gets cancer, the secret must be carefully hidden away from public scrutiny. Especially if that cancer is caused by an additive now in our food supply!

This hormone should not be casually categorized along with thousands of chemicals which have been implicated in causing cancers. There is no evidence that this hormone causes cancer. This hormone merely increases the level of the most powerful growth hormone naturally contained in milk, and, coincidentally, the most powerful growth factor in the human body, IGF-I. Cancer is growth of an peculiar type of tissue. Growth hormones do not discriminate. They cause cells to reproduce. While you will not grow a larger nose or finger, there are no genetic reins on cancerous tumors. Growth hormones make already existing cancers grow.

Data contained in Table 2 are even more revealing:

Table 2

Absolute organ weight (g) for dosage of rbGH (mg/kg per day)

	Subcutaneous		Oral			
	MALES					
	0	1.0	0.1	0.5	5.0	50.0
Kidneys	3.677	4.188	3.178	3.695	3.540	3.544
Liver	16.549	20.364	15.164	15.740	15.993	15.098
Heart	1.726	1.941	1.645	1.608	1.618	1.640
Spleen	0.912	1.274	0.910	1.051	0.987	1.002
	FEMALES					
Kidneys	2.067	2.464	2.040	2.170	2.102	2.025
Liver	8.637	11.146	8.302	8.754	8.446	8.297
Heart	1.041	1.215	1.061	1.101	1.034	1.070
Spleen	0.585	0.855	0.601	0.663	0.630	0.608

In referencing this study, FDA revealed that 32 different tissue and organ weight samples were obtained from each laboratory rat. [3] Table 2 of the Juskevich and Guyer paper lists only weights from four organ samples. Freedom of Information Act requests for these original data for each animal (by this author) were denied by FDA and Monsanto. Here is how FDA explains the data in Table 2:

Absolute organ weights (in grams) in control rats and rbGH-treated rats (means ± SD). Charles River CD rats (n=30 rats per sex) were treated for 90 days with rbGH either by gavage or by subcutaneous administrations, and one group of animals served as untreated controls. From (42) with permission, Copyright, 1989, Monsanto Agricultural Company.

(As with Table 1, standard deviations are not reported)

FDA scientists noted significant changes in the weights of organs and in blood chemistry from animals that had received the rBGH by injection. However, the scientists and FDA reviewers concluded that there were no biological effects in the oral rbGH-treatment group. There were effects.

The average male rat receiving rbGH by injection developed a spleen 39.6 percent larger than the spleen of the control animals. The relative weight of the spleens from the female group averaged 46 percent greater weight than the spleens from the female control group. These are not normal reactions and signify an animal in distress. Similar growth of a spleen in a human would often result in a diagnosis of leukemia. These animals were "under attack" by a foreign invader, rbGH. Their spleens, the first line of defense in an animal's lymphatic system, began to grow, mounting a defense.

Spleens manufacture white and red blood cells. Spleens act as sentinels defending the body. The only ones who knew the spleen growth were the scientists performing autopsies, weighing tissue samples, compiling and analyzing data. Would it not have been appropriate for these scientists, who having noted the remarkable spleen growth from injections, to examine the spleen data from the animals orally ingesting rbGH?

FDA found no evidence of oral effects on these laboratory subjects. Data from Table 2 indicated that the average female treated orally with rbGH had gained 7 percent more weight in her spleen than animals from the control group. The average male orally ingesting rbGH gained spleen weight in excess of 8 percent! In addition, the average male lost in excess of 5 percent of his heart, liver and kidney weights when compared to the control group organs. During the first 90 days of treatment these male rats treated with oral rbGH had similar weights to the control group animals but their vital organs were completely out of whack.

The first thing I did was place a telephone call to Monsanto scientist, Robert Collier. (4) I told Collier that the data were disturbing. He listened as I told him of the data manipulation in Table 1. He listened as I reviewed effects of rbGH on the organs in Table 2. "The organ and tissue weights are not statistically significant," he responded. "You've gotta be kidding me," was my reaction. "If there was any evidence that this drug had oral effects it would never have been approved." "It's not significant," he repeated. "The drug has been approved after much debate and controversy. It's the most examined drug in FDA history. Anyway, that was just one of hundreds of studies. There are other studies which demonstrate no oral effects."

That was just one study, but it was the one study that FDA used to illustrate no oral effects and build two tables as evidence and publish their opinions in the most important scientific journal in the world. "Could I have the actual raw data and run my own statistical analyses?" I asked. Collier laughed. "Forget it! Those data are trade protected. We will not release the study." Then I'll get it myself, I thought, as I hung up the phone, then dialed the number for the Center For Veterinary Medicine (CVM), FDA's investigative branch. I reached Teske and was referred to Robert Condon, Ph.D., who was responsible for reviewing and performing statistical analyses on the data in question.

Condon commented that although my "averaging method" was mathematically correct, that was not the way proper statistical analyses were performed. I was handicapped by not having the actual raw data consisting of the tissue weights for 32 organs from 360 animals. I called back Teske and requested the original data from the Searle experiment (Richard, Odaglia and Deslex), the study from which the data in Tables 1 and 2 were taken. Teske informed me that FDA was not permitted to release that data. "The weights of those rats are a trade secret. If we release that information it would cause great financial harm to Monsanto," he said.

Out of frustration, I again called Collier of Monsanto. "Please, can I get access to just the weights of each animal in the study," I asked. "No. That information is a trade secret," was his answer. I then called CVM. "How can the animal weights be a secret?" I inquired of Teske. We're talking about human safety." "The data are not statistically significant," he responded, sternly.

Freedom of Information

On October 3, 1994, I filed a Freedom of Information Act (FOIA) request (5) for the actual data from this experiment. The Department of Health and Human Services oversees the FDA. According to a 1992 report issued by Richard P. Kusserow, the inspector general of the Department of Health and Human Services:

> [C]omplete disclosure of bST data will not occur unless
> and until FDA approves the drug for commercial use.

If the respected office of the inspector general can be relied upon, then data from Monsanto's application for drug approval should now be available to anybody who properly makes such a request. Formal approval for recombinant bovine somatotropin under the trade name of Posilac was given by FDA in November 1993, and actual marketing and sales by Monsanto began in February 1994.

In October 1994, I had indications that laboratory animals had contacted a vast array of illnesses from BST. In addition to "all gross lesions," which was cited as part of reference #45 in the landmark FDA publication in *Science*, 28 other organs and tissue samples cited as references in the Juskevich and Guyer article would reveal the scope of the activity of BST on these animals. In my gut I suspected that the data from the Richard, Odaglia and Deslex study (Searle report prepared for Monsanto in 1989) would confirm my suspicion that not only were there biological effects on laboratory animals from oral ingestion of BST but it would also prove that laboratory animals were developing cancers.

Monsanto and FDA in their joint publication had relied heavily upon that report to "prove" that there were no effects on laboratory animals. They had built Tables 1 and 2 around data from that experiment. Review of the actual data would allow me to conduct detailed statistical analyses. When Collier of Monsanto laughed at my request for the data from the experiment, his temperament represented the deed of throwing the gauntlet at my feet. Teske of FDA assured me that I would never review the actual data. Both men had to have known how incriminating those data were.

Again, my only recourse was to file a formal request under the Freedom of Information Act (FOIA), which I did on October 3, 1994. My original request was assigned Ref. #94-39274. There was no Freedom of Information Act officer at FDA, which was required by law. Billy Don Weaver, who previously held the position, had left his office. A vacancy remained; the void had not yet been filled. Certainly, I expected unbiased eyes to review my request and routinely release the article as a matter of law. The same people who reviewed the Monsanto drug application, writing comment and policy on BST use covered themselves by denying that these incriminating data be released. The ultimate decision of denial came from Mary Alice Miller, a press liaison. She should not be confused with Margaret Miller, the scientist who played a key role in researching this new drug for Monsanto, and then came to FDA to review her own research. Mary Alice Miller admitted to me that the final decision (which I suspected was made for her by Richard Teske) was her responsibility to make.

According to law, FOIA requests are decided in 10 days. Weeks and then months passed with no word. Finally, on December 24, 1994, I decided to call everybody I knew at FDA. Jerry Deighton, who works in FDA's FOIA branch, finally faxed a long-overdue decision, after repeated phone calls requesting a decision, that they were turning down my request for those unpublished data. By the time that I received this letter, I was ready to file my appeal. I knew that the decision would be negative because I understood that too many careers were based on the fraudulent approval process. Releasing the data would hurt too many reputations. What I didn't know was that my appeal would be heard by the same insiders who made the original denial.

I faxed my appeal to the Department of Health and Human Services on December 24, 1994. They responded immediately with a docket number which indicated to me that a separate "court, jury and process" would determine the FOIA request on the issues. Two letters came into my possession from a friend at FDA. One was a letter from Monsanto addressed to Billy Don Weaver, director of the Freedom of Information office. The other was from Eli Lilly Pharmaceutical Company. The letter from Eli Lilly slipped up and revealed the fraud which was being perpetrated. The March 6, 1995, letter stated:

> Mr. Howard Green of our company has been contacted
> by telephone by Ms. Linda Grassie (sic) of FDA concerning
> the request of Mr. Robert Cohen for information about
> studies cited as references in *Science*, 1990 related to bovine
> somatotropin.

This was the needed proof. Phillip Lee, Ph.D., assistant secretary for Health at the Department of Health and Human Services, was the one who was supposed to assign an independent group to investigate the issues relating to my appeal. Instead, Lee had returned my appeal to the same individuals who turned down the request in the first place. I do not hold anything against Grasse for her action. She has been at FDA for 20 years and I am totally convinced that she would do nothing that she believed was wrong. She is idealistic and believes that her colleagues place the health and safety of the American people above any other consideration. Linda Grasse had no business, as an employee of CVM, to be handling the matter of my administrative appeal. On April 4, 1995, Lee sent me a formal denial which said:

> Release of the information would cause substantial competitive
> and financial harm to the company (Monsanto).

All I wanted was the weights of thirty-two different tissues and organs. How could this benefit the competition? I wasn't asking for secret formulas. Financial harm? If the information proving animal sicknesses were released, Monsanto would lose an enormous investment. On June 7, 1995, the Freedom of Information Clearinghouse, a Ralph Nadir organization, sent a letter to Lee. The letter was written by two staff attorneys, Ann Begley and Robin Leibowitz. In addition to citing a number of legal precedents exposing the impropriety of the denial to the FOIA request, the letter stated:

> [T]here are serious questions as to the classification of the
> studies in question as *"confidential."* Accordingly we seek
> a reversal of the Department's previous decision and ask
> that the Department release the requested studies. If, after
> reconsideration, you decline to rule in favor of disclosure,
> we ask that you provide a more complete explanation of the
> applicability of Exemption Four to these studies. In accordance
> with FOIA, we expect a response within twenty working days.

The FDA finally responded on the Freedom of Information Clearinghouse request. They revealed that Margaret Miller had actually written parts of the landmark Juskevich and Guyer paper. Although the paper was published in August 1990 it was ready for publication in February of 1990. Miller had come to FDA in December 1989. She was prohibited from working on BST issues. The investigative agency of Congress, the Government Accounting Organization (GAO) assured the American people in their subsequent investigation into conflicts of interest that she had not broken the law by performing any task having to do with rbST analyses. GAO erred. The evidence clearly showed Miller admitting 5 years later that she wrote a key part of the paper. Journalistic fraud? Any author should have been so cited! Miller as author would have alerted investigators of an impropriety. Certainly, those at FDA had to know that she was writing this paper.

By law, I exercised the option to file an appeal of that first denial decision to the Department of Health and Human Services (HHS). After I lost that second request I still had an appeal open to me by filing a complaint in Superior Court, which I did in December of 1995. (7)

The complaint was filed in U.S. District Court in Newark, New Jersey. Judge William H. Walls was assigned the case. It was Robert Cohen, Pro Se (I acted as my own attorney, performing the legal research and writing my own briefs) versus FDA and HHS, represented by the U.S. Attorney's office. Monsanto joined the suit opposing my efforts to obtain the report held by FDA and they were represented by the legal firm of King & Spalding.

Freedom of Information Act Suit

In a noble universe there was no way that any judge with wisdom could ignore the evidence contained in my suit. The health and safety of every American citizen was imperiled by evidence indicating that laboratory animals got cancer from this new food additive.

The law allowed for the release of these data, or so I believed. I had the inspector general of the United States agreeing with my position. Here is the original complaint:

UNITED STATES DISTRICT COURT DISTRICT OF NEWARK, NEW JERSEY 07101-0419

Robert Cohen, Citizen of the	!	
United States of America, Plaintiff	!	
v.	!	
David Kessler in his official capacity	!	
as Commissioner, U.S. Food and Drug	!	Docket No. **95-6140**
Administration, and **Philip Lee** in his	!	
official capacity as Assistant Secretary	!	
of Health of the Department of Health	!	
and Human Services, Defendants	!	

COMPLAINT

Plaintiff, ROBERT COHEN, P.O. Box 36, Oradell, New Jersey, 07649 (201-599-0325), complaining of Defendants, DAVID KESSLER, Commissioner of the U.S. Food and Drug Administration, and PHILIP LEE, Assistant Secretary of the U.S. Department of Health and Human Services, respectfully alleges as follows:

Purpose of Action

1)   This action is for declaratory judgment, and for injunctive relief against the U.S. Food and Drug Administration (FDA) and the Department of Health and Human Services, who by their action of refusing to release research data which were submitted to FDA as part of a 53,000 page application by Monsanto Agricultural Company for approval of recombinant bovine somatotropin (rBST) continue to suppress the key evidence which will prove that laboratory animals ingesting rBST developed CANCER. This Action, filed on behalf of the health and safety of the American Public which now consumes milk and dairy products containing this new genetically engineered hormone, was filed because FDA denied a Freedom of Information Act request and the Department of Health and Human Services upheld that denial in a subsequent appeal. The actual request was for an unpublished paper that was cited as reference #42 and note #45 in an FDA paper published in the Journal, *Science* (August 24, 1990, Juskevich & Guyer, 875-883).

ANECDOTAL NOTE: A recent movie, *I Love Trouble* (Nick Nolte & Julia Roberts) had as the basic premise two reporters who attempted to "steal" the secret report that a genetically engineered cow hormone caused cancer and should not have been approved.

FDA possesses the **REAL LIFE** report authored by D. Richard, G. Odaglia and P. Deslex which will reveal the weights of 32 organs and tissue samples from rBST-treated laboratory animals.   These data, which were never properly reviewed by FDA, will result in a ban on rBST which has been implicated by numerous scientists and institutions as a key factor in human cancer. Americans have a right to know! FDA and Department of Health and Human Services incorrectly lends "TRADE PROTECTION" to Monsanto by not releasing these data in this one experiment. FDA and the Department of Health and Human Services correctly state that Monsanto will suffer financial harm if this paper is released. Monsanto hides behind this powerful protective legal veil which is being incorrectly applied and which violates FDA statues regarding "Trade Protection."

2)   The provisions of the Federal Food, Drug, and Cosmetic Act and regulations and actions thereunder pertaining to TRADE PROTECTION are

incorrectly being interpreted and implemented as policy and are short of statutory right.

Plaintiff

3) Plaintiff, Robert Cohen, resides in Oradell, New Jersey. He filed a Freedom of Information Act request with FDA on October 3, 1994 (94-39274) **(EXHIBIT #1)**, which was denied on December 23, 1994 **(EXHIBIT #2)** and then filed an appeal on December 24, 1994, with the Department of Health and Human Services **(EXHIBIT #3)** which was denied on April 4, 1995**(EXHIBIT #4).**

4) Cohen then FAXED a letter on July 17, 1995 to Linda Kahn, Esq., Chief Counsel for the Center for Veterinary Medicine. **(EXHIBIT #5)**. That letter contained specific provisions in the Administrative Code (Section 514.11) which allowed for the release of said data contained in the FOIA request of October 3, 1994.

5) Cohen received no response to that letter.

Defendants

6) Defendant David Kessler, M.D., J.D., is the commissioner of the U.S. Food and Drug Administration (FDA), and is responsible for its supervision.

7) Defendant Philip Lee, M.D., is the assistant secretary of the U.S. Department of Health and Human Services (HHS), and is the officer charged with the administration of Freedom of Information Act appeals which have been denied by FDA.

Subject Matter

8) The subject matter of this action is the necessity for public disclosure and independent review of data from newly approved pharmaceuticals in which adverse reaction problems are indicated. FDA correctly offers trade protection to drugs that are currently under review or drugs which have been turned down for commercial use. These trade secrets "protect" pharmaceutical companies from unfair competition and the validity of this protection is well founded. However, according to FDA, after an approval is published in the *Federal Register*, data must be made available for public disclosure. Cohen does not seek secret formulas or experimental techniques. Cohen seeks only raw data of organ and tissue samples of 360 laboratory rats which were treated with rBST. It is unfortunate that the American public can no longer trust FDA to impartially review data in a rigorous manner. Cohen will demonstrate under the section **BACKGROUND**

examples of how Monsanto and FDA manipulated data and committed scientific fraud which led to the approval of rBST.

Jurisdiction and Venue

9) The jurisdiction of this Court is invoked pursuant to Title 28 U.S.C. Sections 1331 and 1337. This action arises under the laws of the United States, namely the Federal Food, Drug and Cosmetic Act, Title 21, U.S. Code. The actions described herein are reviewable by this Court pursuant to Section 10(c) of the Administrative Procedure Act, 5 U.S.C. Section 704.

10) This action is authorized by 28 U.S.C. Sections 2201 and 2202. The Plaintiff is suffering legal wrong because of the agency actions of the FDA commissioner and assistant secretary of HSS hereinabove referred to, and is aggrieved by such actions. There is now existing between the parties hereto an actual, justiciable controversy in respect to which plaintiff is entitled to have a declaration of his right and further relief, of releasing the data requested in his FOIA request, because of the facts, conditions and circumstances herein set out.

11) Venue in this judicial district is proper by virtue of 28 U.S.C. Section 1391 (e).

Background

12) rBST is the most controversial drug application in FDA history. In order to answer some of the questions in that controversy, FDA (August 24, 1990) published an article in *Science* which was intended for "peer review" by an estimated weekly readership of 500,000 individuals in the scientific community. That article was written by Judy Juskevich and Greg Guyer, two FDA scientists. At the same time that article appeared, an article was published in the *Journal of the American Medical Association* (*JAMA*) written by two "independent" doctors. Both articles stressed the safety of rBST.

13) When Cohen first read these articles in July 1994 he noted some problems. The *JAMA* article, for example was not written by independent doctors at all. Both authors were on the Monsanto payroll. That information was revealed on page 1003 of the *JAMA* article (**EXHIBIT #6**) although that conflict was not revealed in subsequent FDA comments on that article.

14) When FDA wrote that wholesome milk and genetically engineered milk were exactly the same, indistinguishable, Cohen read the abstract of that Juskevich and Guyer FDA article which indicated otherwise. (**EXHIBIT #7**) That abstract indicated that a powerful growth hormone, insulin-like growth factor (IGF) increased in rBST-treated milk. Yet, FDA continued to misstate the facts. That misrepresentation was repeated by the national press and appeared in

newspapers and magazines. That lie became part of the public's basic understanding.

15) When Cohen applied simple math and observed that the spleens of laboratory animals grew enormously after rBST treatment (males spleens grew over 39 percent and female spleens grew 46 percent!) and FDA stated that there were no biological effects, Cohen requested in telephone conversations with Richard Teske, Ph.D., at FDA, and Robert Collier, Ph.D., at Monsanto, copies of the actual "raw data" so that he could perform actual statistical analyses of said data. Both parties refused this request.

16) When Cohen noted (**EXHIBIT #8**) in the Conclusion section of that article that FDA believed 90 percent of BST was destroyed when milk is pasteurized, Cohen searched for the reference. The FDA authors were quite sloppy and incorrectly cited J.A. Moore as the scientist who did this research. (They cited Moore, reference #47.) The work was actually performed by Groenewegen, reference # 49, who was not cited (**EXH. #8**)

17) When Cohen examined Groenewegen's work he discovered **SCIENTIFIC FRAUD.** Groenewegen, then an undergraduate student at the University of Guelph, Ontario, pasteurized milk at a high temperature for 30 minutes. The temperature used was normally reserved for a 15-second pasteurization process. No wonder the BST was destroyed. Or was it?

18) Cohen carefully reviewed Groenewegen's data. (**EXHIBIT #9**). Groenewegen's data revealed that only 19 percent of the BST was destroyed by this high heat! Somebody obviously lied. Somebody knew the lie and incorrectly cited the reference.

19) This was an important lie. FDA Commissioner Kessler, Director of Center for Veterinary Medicine Steven Sundlof, and Deputy Regulatory Commissioner Michael Taylor (Monsanto's ex-attorney who was appointed into this position of power) all testified before Congress as to the safety of rBST. These respected gentlemen repeated this pasteurization fraud which resulted in the following:

1) No further toxicology studies were required of Monsanto
2) A zero-day withdrawal period was determined for rBST
   making it safe for human consumption
3) No assay was required (identification tool) to measure
   the amounts of this genetically engineered hormone.

All of these things occurred because FDA investigators created this fraud.

20) On April 21, 1995, Cohen met with a group of FDA scientists at The Center for Veterinary Medicine in Rockville, Maryland. At that time it became clear that the original Richard, Deslex and Odaglia study was not rigorously

reviewed. Dr. Robert Condon agreed to "re-analyze" the data. This work was performed in late summer, 1995.

21) A number of contraindications surfaced as a result of that review. It became clear to Cohen that any conflicts of interest could best be eliminated by an independent review of said data. The actual reference (#45 in the Juskevich and Guyer paper) revealed that data existed for 32 organ and tissue samples. The last citation indicated that data existed for "all gross lesions." The scientific terminology "all gross lesions" indicates tumors and/or cancers.

22) Inspector General Richard Kusserow **(EXHIBIT 10)** in 1992 commented:

"Because FDA is constrained from fully disclosing data ***undergoing review*** (emphasis added), complete disclosure of bST data will not occur unless and until FDA approves the drug for commercial use." FDA has approved the drug for commercial use. The data should now be released.

23) Section 514.11 of the FDA administrative Code which allows for release of such data states (in section e):

After an approval has been published in the *Federal Register*, the following data and information in the NADA file are immediately available for disclosure unless extraordinary circumstances are shown.

Section 4 - "Adverse reaction reports, product experience reports, consumer complaints, and other similar data and information after deletion of..." (names, ingredients, methods)

24) In upholding the importance of releasing any adverse reaction report, FDA guidelines state in section f of 514:

All safety and effectiveness data and information not previously disclosed to the public are available for public disclosure at any time one of the following events occurs unless extraordinary circumstances are known:

#5 [A] final determination has been made that the animal drug may be marketed without submission of such safety and/or effectiveness data and information.

The pasteurization SCIENTIFIC FRAUD (described in paragraphs 16-19) indicate that an incorrect determination was made to not require additional safety documentation. Monsanto was relieved of its responsibility. The data indicating such problems existed must at this time be released. Every day that passes exposes Americans to increased levels of this new genetically engineered growth hormone which has replaced wholesome milk with a dangerous chemical. These data must be reviewed. By no stretch of the imagination can any lawyer or scientist argue that Monsanto will be compromised by exclusivity of trade secrets when Cohen has opportunity to review the actual weights of spleens, stomach, thymus, pancreas, testes, ovaries and brain tissues. Trade protection for these data is an unconscionable and wanton abuse of the legal system and provides a legal veil which has been incorrectly offered for Monsanto to hide behind.

25) The respected industry journal, *Food Chemical News,* (October 9, 1995, pp. #4-6) recently obtained evidence of errors in the Richard, Odaglia and Deslex report which Cohen has requested in the entirety. (**EXHIBIT #11**)

THE FOLLOWING PRINTED TEXT IS REPRODUCED EXACTLY AS IT APPEARS IN THE OCTOBER / 9/ 1995 ISSUE OF *FOOD CHEMICAL NEWS.*

According to this report, Dr. Condon of FDA "did uncover some errors in the information as it was presented in Table 2 of the Science paper." He noted that the heading of table 2 states that 30 rats per sex per treatment group were utilized in the study. "While the 90-day study did involve the use of 30 rats per sex per treatment group, only 15 rats per sex treatment were sacrificed to obtain organ weight data," Teske said, noting that 10 rats per sex per treatment were used for blood analyses and the remaining 5 animals per sex per treatment were scheduled for an effect reversal phase of the study. Noting that the weight of one heart in the negative control male rat was given as being almost 3.5 grams, Teske said no other heart weight was over two grams for this control group or any of the rBST oral groups. "In Dr. Condon's opinion, this heart weight is an impossible value." There is an unresolved issue regarding the average spleen weight for the female negative control group. Teske said, "The available data are not sufficient to determine the correct value. In either case, the effect on spleen weight is not considered to be biologically meaningful," he added. Cohen charged that Dr. Condon's reanalyses "demonstrates that the data from the study were never reviewed by FDA," saying FDA was guilty of blindly accepting data and conclusions from Monsanto. As Dr. Condon discovered error after error (including the grossly increased heart weight of 3.5 grams which you dismiss as 'an impossible value,') it becomes clear that independent review of these data is appropriate," Cohen wrote.

26) Plaintiff realleges and incorporates herein by reference the allegations contained in Paragraphs 1 through paragraphs 25.

27)   By not releasing the article referenced in the landmark Juskevich and Guyer FDA publication in the journal *Science,* FDA and HHS denies proper peer review to scientists and the American people. By not releasing the data from that experiment, FDA violates its own statute as written in Code 514.11.

COUNT I

28)   The illegal, improper, arbitrary and excessive actions by the defendant FDA commissioner and his subordinates, hereinabove set forth, have and will, unless corrected, interfere with the rights of all Americans to their physical well being, livelihoods, and quality of life, denying them right to review truthful accounts of cancer in laboratory animals from ingestion of rBST.

COUNT II

29)   The illegal and improper interpretation of a Congressional Act, the Delaney Amendment (1958) which has now become standard operating procedure at FDA as a result of Michael Taylor's (Monsanto's attorney turned FDA regulator) paper, "A De-Minimus interpretation of the Delaney Amendment," has allowed FDA procedural and operational jurisdiction, but not legal justification, in allowing a food additive to be approved which caused cancer in laboratory animals. Release of this paper will demonstrate the ontogeny of this scientific fraud. Release of this paper will demonstrate and invalidate an attempt at covering up this fraud. Release of this paper is consistent with applicable code and is in the best interests of the health and of the American people.

PRAYER FOR RELIEF

WHEREFORE, Plaintiff respectfully requests the following relief:
A.   As to Count I, that the Court instruct defendants and all persons acting on their behalf to release the scientific experiments and papers which were the basis of a Freedom of Information Act request (94-39274) filed on October 3, 1994.
B.   As to Count II, that the Court enter a judgment finding that FDA and HHS acted in an arbitrary manner, abusing their authority and discretion by offering trade protection to a pharmaceutical company at the expense of the health and safety of the American ɼublic.
C.   For such other further relief as this Honorable Court may deem proper.

Respectfully submitted,
Robert Cohen

FDA and HHS through the United States Attorney's Office, filed an answer to my complaint. They denied every allegation and cited many cases.

RESPONSE TO U.S. ATTORNEY'S ANSWER

1) As a Pro-Se attorney, one is not accustomed to writing briefs, arguing cases or reading phrases such as, **"Deny the allegations of paragraph 6."** When I wrote that in my complaint, dated December 4, 1995, **"David Kessler was the commissioner of FDA and responsible for overseeing FDA actions,"** I could not imagine any controversy. Yet, United States Attorney Robert Hannah felt it necessary to **"deny that allegation"** and in doing so he wrote that David Kessler was **"responsible for implementation of FDA's mission."** Gosh, he makes FDA sound like a church. As the U.S. Attorney continued his denials, his admissions substantiate and verify plaintiff's case.

2) Consequently, we have established, by the U. S. Attorney's answer that plaintiff has exhausted administrative remedies (paragraph 10), and is in the proper Court of jurisdiction (paragraph 11).

3) Furthermore, defendants admit that references in the landmark Juskevich and Guyer *Science* article were improperly cited, (paragraph 16) and that the *Science* article improperly used key terms (paragraph 17).

4) It is clear, by the answer in paragraph 18, that a careful review of, in fact a **"LITMUS TEST"** approach, be applied to Groenewegen's work, which was so heavily relied upon by FDA in both rBST approval and congressional testimony. Attorney for defendants does not **"deny the allegations..."**; rather, he mindfully **"denies knowledge the allegations"** while admitting that Groenewegen, et al., in their article **"state what they did and what their results were."** What they did was set out to commit fraud and succeeded, with the cooperation and creative interpretation of FDA reviewers!

5) By admission, in paragraph 21, **"FDA, in subsequent review in 1995 of Monsanto's rat study, found errors in the organ weight data."** FDA reviewed these data for the first time as a result of an April 21, 1995, meeting with this plaintiff. The errors were obtrusively overwhelming and this research, originally reported as a 90-day study, was actually an investigation lasting 180 days. These glaring irregularities would have been detected if the study was reviewed. However, the review process was flawed, the deck was stacked and the data ignored by Monsanto's personnel who conveniently found employment at FDA in key regulatory and review positions. These individuals included Margaret Miller, Ph.D., Susan Sechen, Ph.D., and Michael Taylor.

6) It is by proclivity and standard operating procedure, and not statute, that FDA continues to offer trade protection to Monsanto. Honorable Inspector General of the United States of America Richard Kusserow, wrote:

> **Because FDA is constrained from fully disclosing data**
> ***undergoing review* (emphasis added), complete *disclosure***
> ***of bST data will not occur unless and until FDA approves***
> ***the drug for commercial use* (emphasis added). Given**
> **that FDA continues to review data on bST, we agree that**
> **the Agency should not allow the public to have full access**
> **to data regarding a yet-to-be approved product.**

In 1992, when the above comment was written to James Mason, M.D., the assistant secretary for Health and Human Services, the data was still being reviewed, the drug was not yet approved, and Monsanto had valid justification for Trade Protection. The inspector general commented that after approval, trade protection would no longer be applied. Monsanto continued to hide behind FDA's protective veil.

      7)   When Section 514.11 is reviewed and rigorously adhered to, it will be clear that adverse data should be made available for review, if and only when that drug has been approved and said notice of approval published in the Federal Register. On November 12, 1993, FDA approved Monsanto's new drug   (58 FR 59946, 1993).

RESPONSE TO AFFIRMATIVE DEFENSES

      1.   Plaintiff has stated section 514.11 as regulatory statute which contradicts continued trade protection for these data. Plaintiff has submitted the written opinion of Honorable Inspector General Kusserow as it applied specifically to these data and these circumstances in 1992.

      2.   To state that the Court lacks jurisdiction, is to contradict paragraph 9 and add insult to the honorable inspector general and to this Court.

      3.   Records withheld from plaintiff were improperly withheld.

      4.   Both Defendants have been served in their official capacity in regulatory positions. The remedy made available to plaintiff by Dr. Phillip Lee, secretary of the Department of Health and Human Services **(EXHIBIT 4)** states:

Paragraph #1 **"I have now completed my review..."**
Paragraph #4 **"My review indicates..."**
Paragraph #5 **"My decision...**

Each time Phillip Lee speaks personally. His advice in paragraph six states:
> **[Y]ou may seek review in the District Court of**
> **The United States in the district in which you reside...**

I have done just that. It was his decision. I filed suit against Lee in his capacity.

     5.   In view of the above, plaintiff asserts such claims with proper legal standing.

     6.   Plaintiff wishes to avoid any disrespect to this Court by requesting a Jury trial. Three months prior to this brief, plaintiff predicted in a television interview the outbreak of Mad Cow disease in England because bovine proteins survive digestive processes. Plaintiff claims that the health and safety of all Americans are in perilous danger as a result of this new genetically engineered hormone. Admissions by FDA already confirm serious contraindications in these controversial data. It remains clear that independent review of these data is permissible by statute, and morally and ethically justifiable. If it is determined that plaintiff is not entitled to a trial by jury, plaintiff prays in the wisdom of Your Honor. Plaintiff also requests the opportunity to make oral argument.

     WHEREFORE, plaintiff respectfully prays that this action be determined by the merits so stated. A drug causing cancer in laboratory animals should never have been approved for America's food supply. Any such drugs should be immediately removed from our market place. Review of the Richard, Deslex and Odaglia unpublished report will ultimately lead to an rBST ban.

DATED: April 12, 1996   By: Robert Cohen - Pro-Se

There Just Ain't No Justice

     King & Spalding soon filed motions for summary judgment, requesting that the judge dismiss the case without the court considering arguments or even discovery. I opposed those motions for summary judgment.

The Honorable William H. Walls
United States Federal Judge
50 Walnut Street
Newark, NJ 07102

RE: Robert Cohen v. David Kessler, et al.
Civil Action No. 95-6140 (WHW)

Dear Judge Walls,

     Please accept this letter brief in lieu of a more formal brief. This is an answer to two motions for summary judgment in the above case. Since each contain the same argument and motion I will submit one response which should address all issues.

First, I recognize that there is some controversy regarding the issue of Mandamus. I originally served David Kessler and Philip Lee in their official capacities. It is my belief that each have made personal statements and accepted personal responsibility for their actions. However, any argument before this Court on the issue of Mandamus would only cloud the only important point of this suit. For this reason I filed a motion on July 25th to include the United States Food and Drug Administration (FDA) and HHS as either co-defendants or simply as defendants, the decision to be left to the discretion of this Court.

Another issue that is not in dispute is the lack of rights of the American people and the public interest. The public interest is not relevant in a Freedom of Information Act suit. Although the public's health interest might be compromised, the showing of need or public interest is absolutely irrelevant to the issue at hand.

The courts have considered Freedom of Information Act requests on numerous occasions. The U.S. attorney, in his motion for summary judgment, submitted a table of authorities citing 35 different cases.

King & Spalding, counsel for Intervenor, Monsanto, submitted citations for 25 cases. Although the evidence in those cases was not overwhelming, the effect on this Pro Se plaintiff was!

The only issue before this Court is whether or not Trade Protection applies to Monsanto for raw data from a study submitted as part of their NDA application to FDA for consideration of approval of their new genetically engineered bovine hormone, re-combinant bovine somatotropin (rBST).

The U.S. Attorney, in his brief, cited Public Citizen Health Research Group v. FDA, 704 f.2d. 1280 9D.C. Cir. 1983. Although Public Citizen sued for data in an ongoing study, which is clearly trade-protected, the Court made opportunity to define Trade Secret for the purpose of FOIA. The Court wrote:

TRADE SECRET FOR THE PURPOSE OF FOIA

TRADE SECRET is a secret, commercially viable plan, formula, process or device that is used for making, preparing, compounding or processing trade commodities and that can be said to be product of either innovation or substantial effort.

The Court went on further to state:

Records produced during ongoing clinical studies of safety and efficacy were not trade secrets and not protected as such under Freedom of Information Act exemption.

21CFR, section 514.11, clearly allows for the release of such data. This issue arose during 1992 and then-Inspector General Richard Kusserow wisely offered trade protection for the yet non-approved drug. This plaintiff applauds the concept of absolute trade protection for all data from drugs which have not yet been approved.

However, statute clearly defines the approval process and publication and notice of such approval. Once a drug is properly approved and notice published in the Federal Register, previously protected data becomes available for review. The Honorable Inspector General Richard Kusserow, in 1992, wrote:

> *Because FDA is constrained from fully disclosing data undergoing review, complete disclosure of bST data will not occur unless and until FDA approves the drug for commercial use.*

Section (e) of 514.11 of the Pure Food and Drug Act reads:

> *After an approval has been published in the Federal   Register, the following data and information in the NADA file are immediately available for public disclosure unless extraordinary circumstances are shown... Adverse reaction reports, product experience reports, consumer complaints, and other similar data and information after deletion of...(names, methods, ingredients, assays)...*

Section (f) of 514.11 states:

> *All safety and effectiveness data and information not previously disclosed to the public are available for public disclosure at any time any one of the following events occurs... A final determination has been made that the animal drug may be marketed without submission of such safety and/or effectiveness data and information.*

It is clear that FDA never reviewed this key study. Had they done so, they would not continue to cite this 90-day study which was actually a 180-day study. Curiously, affidavits supplied to this Court continue to insist that this study lasted for 90 days, despite evidence that it continued for 180 days. After day 90 the animals got cancer. It is also clear that Monsanto's attorney, Michael Taylor, left King & Spalding to assume a key regulatory position at FDA to assume a key role in the approval process of rBST.

Furthermore, it is clear that two key Monsanto scientists, Margaret Miller and Suzanne Sechen, were hired at a key time to direct and oversee the analyses of their own research data. This Plaintiff agrees with the U.S. attorney who writes on page 13 of his brief: "...disclosure is likely to cause substantial harm..."

The SYSTEM works! However, Monsanto clearly stacked the deck. The raw data of animals testes and ovaries, brains and stomachs...these were never reviewed. This was admitted by FDA scientists on April 21, 1995, when this Plaintiff met with a group of scientists at the Center for Veterinary Medicine, the investigative branch of FDA.

While the public has no rights in this matter, their rights being "irrelevant," the public continues to drink milk containing new genetically engineered hormones which caused cancer in laboratory animals.

King & Spalding, in a motion for summary judgment, admit that a suit of this type is unprecedented. On page 12, Laurence Senn, Esq., states:

> *[N]o Federal Court seems to have faced the issue of a*
> *FOIA request for information received as part of a NADA...*

Your Honor, never before has there been such a conspiracy (as detailed in the original complaint by this Plaintiff) of fraudulently reported data, miscited references, lies, deceit, bribery of Congress (12 members of the Dairy Sub-Committee receiving $711,000 directly from Dairy interests including Monsanto, which resulted in milk labeling bills stalling in committee).

Because this case is unique, both the U.S. Attorney and King & Spalding had to reference totally unrelated suits and concepts. Freedom of Information Act suits have been denied for various reasons. In one case, <u>Government of Virgin Islands v. Douglas</u>, 812 F. 2d 822 (3rd. Cir. 1979), a defendant was convicted of aggravated rape and possession of a deadly weapon used during the commission of a crime of violence. In another, an Iranian wanted to obtain the names of all CIA undercover operatives in the Mid-East <u>Ashfar v. Department of State</u> 702 F. 2.d 1125 (D.C. Cir 1983). There are groups seeking nuclear secrets, confidential FBI reports, personal financial statements. In all cases cited, FOIA requests were denied for reasons ranging from privacy to national security.

Although the amount of cases cited can be overwhelming, thousands of examples could have been provided by either side detailing how FOIA works and doesn't work. That is not the issue here nor the point of this suit. King & Spalding provided expert testimony in the affidavit of David F. Kowalczyk, V.V.D., Ph.D. This expert, in paragraph 17, continues THE BIG LIE, by stating that the study in question was a 90-day study. The study lasted for 180 days!

Your Honor, with all due respect, the "BST hit the fan" after day 90. In paragraph 13, the "expert" clouds the importance of this study by stating that 120 studies were analyzed for the FDA "peer-reviewed" Science publication.

Your Honor, this study was critical and table #1 and table #2 were constructed in the Science paper from data in this experiment. Results of four organs were published. This plaintiff seeks the raw data from 28 other organs. No techniques. No secret formulas. Peer review? Your Honor, I would have failed high school science for the amounts of mis-references and errors in this paper, ultimately admitted by U.S. Attorney in his original brief as a response to my original complaint. Peer review?

I appreciate the irony in the fact that Dr. Robert C. Livingston testified in an affidavit for the U.S. Attorney. When this Plaintiff met with FDA on April 21, 1995, it became clear that these data in question were never analyzed. It was Dr. Livingston who made the proposal that the data be formally reviewed by Dr. Robert Condon, who accepted. Four months later, the task was performed. A letter from Richard Teske, a copy of which is attached to this original complaint, admits to many disturbing discrepancies.

If the public interest was the only factor, then it would be clear that an independent review of these data be performed. Thankfully, statute 514.11 clearly supports the release of these data.

This plaintiff respectfully requests that Your Honor deny the motions for summary judgment and, furthermore, issue an order for the immediate release of these data. Your Honor, the average laboratory animal treated with rBST experienced a spleen increase of 46 percent! These animals were developing leukemias. It seems as if every time one picks up a newspaper, there's a story of another child needing a bone marrow donor. We are experiencing an epidemic because our national milk supply has been poisoned.

Having been armed with such data, it will be Monsanto's ultimate responsibility to explain to America why dollars were placed before public health. Having been armed with such data, it will be the burden of scientists and administrators at FDA to explain why career advancement was placed before public health concerns. Having one last remedy, this Court, I pray that your Honor has the wisdom to accept the words of the inspector general of the United States in 1992 and section 514.11 which clearly allow for the release of these data.

After completing my response to the motions for summary judgment, I received a copy of a letter (attached) which should be of critical importance in the determination of the trade protection issue. A letter, dated July 17, 1996, was sent by Victor F. Zonana, deputy assistant secretary of the Department of Health and Human Services. The letter was sent in response to Ms. Mullarkey's request for the same data which this Plaintiff requested, reference #42 in the Juskevich and Guyer joint FDA/Monsanto Science publication. Along with the letter were 250 pages of detailed data, trade secrets, methods and previously TRADE PROTECTED "secrets." The author of the letter in paragraph three states:

> *Pursuant to 21 CFR 514.11 (e), once an approval notice of an NADA has been published in the <u>Federal Register</u>, summaries of the drugs safety and effectiveness data are prepared and made available for public disclosure.*

However, the 1989 study cited as reference #42 of the Science *article was not included in the FOI summary_since it was not considered to be a pivotal study.*

Your Honor, I am stunned. FDA admits that they could have released this study. It was no longer a **TRADE SECRET***. It's just that they did not consider it pivotal. A review of EXHIBIT B included in the Motion by the U.S. Attorney reveals just how pivotal this study was. U.S. Attorney's Exhibit B is the landmark Juskevich and Guyer article. There are seven (7) tables in this article. Table number one (1), table number two (2) and table number five (5) were all built from data from this pivotal study.*

If this was not a pivotal study, the entire heart and body of this momentous article would not have utilized and relied upon its partial data. This study was THE STUDY!!! Your Honor, this evidence is in your hands. Trade protection no longer applies. The concept has been arbitrarily applied to protect guilty parties who are armed with damaging information at the expense of the American people.

> *Respectfully submitted,*
> *Robert Cohen DATED: July 29, 1996*

Judge Walls' decision was due on September 9, 1996. More than three months after the decision was due, I received a letter postmarked December 6, 1996, containing the Judge's decision.

The Judge's Decision

Dear Counsel and Litigant:

This matter comes before the Court upon the Governments' Motion to Dismiss or for Summary Judgment and Defendant Monsanto Co.'s ("Monsanto") Motion for Summary Judgment. Pursuant to Rule 78 of the Federal Rules of Civil Procedure, the Court decides these motions without oral argument.

The crucial part of that letter from the court stated:

[D]isclosure of the rat study's raw data would allow
competitors to develop or refine their products and avoid
the research and development costs because of the opportunity
to piggy-back upon Monsanto's development efforts.

What? In other words, release the data so other companies can develop a product which causes cancer in laboratory animals, too. Nice to know that the Judge decided the case this way.

I only requested the weights of organs and tissues from rbGH-treated animals. The judge makes clear his philosophy on the matter by writing:

Defendants have adequately demonstrated the likelihood
of competitive substantial harm (if released)...the Court finds
that the rat study's raw data is exempt...

Judge Walls so ordered that the Complaint be dismissed in its entirety. There are men of conscience who have possession of this study which will prove that all laboratory animals got cancer after treatment of this new genetically engineered hormone. This study, which contains only one secret, should be released.

Judge Walls is correct. If the study is released, who would ever drink milk? Milk contains hormones that caused cancer in every laboratory animal treated with rbGH. That hormone is now in our milk supply. It is also in the many dairy products that we consume.

"All truth goes through three stages. First it is ridiculed. Then it is violently opposed. Finally it is accepted as self evident."

Schoepenhouer

"The greatest blunders, like the thickest ropes, are often compounded of a multitude of strands. Take the rope apart, separate it into the small strands that compose it, and you can break them one by one. You think, 'That is all there was!' But twist them all together and you have something tremendous."

Victor Hugo

"To the rulers of the state then, if to any, it belongs of right to use falsehood, to deceive either enemies or their own citizens, for the good of the state; and no one else may meddle with this privilege."

Plato

Chapter 5

The Domino Effect: How FDA Misled America

The FDA reviewed Monsanto's research. Then the Government Accounting Office (GAO) reviewed FDA's review. After that the National Institutes of Health (NIH) reviewed FDA and GAO, and the Office of Technology Assessment (OTA) reviewed FDA, GAO and NIH. Of course, the *Journal of the American Medical Association* (*JAMA*) reviewed FDA, NIH, GAO, OTA, and, before this controversy became total alphabet soup, the World Health Organization (WHO) reviewed everybody else's work. How could so many intelligent scientific minds representing these most prestigious scientific organizations make the same exact mistakes? In order to clear the confusion and end the controversy, FDA published, for the first time in their history, a review of the research concerning rBST. Simultaneous to FDA's *Science* publication, two other scientific journals, *JAMA* and *Science News*, endorsed the new genetically engineered milk hormone. This endorsement was written and published before the publication of the *Science* article. The verdict, previously decided, was in. Each report contained innumerable contradictions and falsehoods. After formal approval on November 5, 1993, a three-month moratorium was placed on actual rBST use until the White House had the opportunity to issue their own report. That report, reviewed in this chapter proves that the best comedy writers in America are employed by the Executive Branch.

One individual challenging the FDA is a madman. So, why not do battle by tilting at windmills like Cervante's Quixote or hunt white whales like Melville's Ahab? I would stand shoulder to shoulder with some of the great monomaniacs of literature. Their stories were, however, works of fiction. A special cell in Bedlam has to be reserved for an individual taking on prestigious organizations like the Food and Drug Administration, National Institutes of Health, World Health Organization and American Medical Association. Right or wrong, who would take such an individual seriously? In concluding that the genetically engineered milk hormone was safe to drink, FDA also concluded that milk from hormonally treated cows was exactly the same as untreated milk.

And They Say There Was No Conspiracy?

FDA published their article on Friday, August 24, 1990, and on August 22, two days earlier, the *Journal of the American Medical Association (JAMA)* had jumped the gun and published their endorsement of FDA's conclusions. A third journal, *Science News* published news of the *JAMA* endorsement of the *Science* article just one day after the *Science* article appeared. (1) These *Science News* writers must have been working through Friday night, writing, editing and rolling the presses so that their story could be printed the following day.

JAMA raised their glass of milk and collectively said, "We'll drink to that!" The *JAMA* article and the *Science News* article appeared the same week as the *Science* article. Somebody was pulling the strings. *JAMA*, representing America's doctors, is respected for independent unbiased review of medical issues. Why then did they accept a paper authored by two doctors with economic ties to Monsanto? The *JAMA* article was dated 8/22, *Science News* 8/25 and *Science* was 8/24. All three journals need at least one week lead time for an article to appear.

Is There a Doctor in the House?

How did the doctors synchronize the publication of their informative BST article to appear two days earlier than the FDA paper was published? I am dazzled by the statistical improbability of such a random occurrence, and forced to recognize that only careful planning resulted in such timing. The AMA, recognizing that this most publicized controversy must be handled with surgical gloves, assigned the task to two independent doctors. One was David Barbano, hired by the Dairy Coalition to conduct a seminar on BST safety.

Ah, paper trails. Thank goodness for researchers who must see their names in print. These scientists document their relationships with other scientists by publishing articles with their colleagues. Names appearing together are smoking guns, testimony to the vain and the foolish. Dale Bauman, the scientist at Cornell who worked for Monsanto and published dozens of articles with their scientists (Miller for one), also published a paper with Barbano, the co-author of the so-called independent *JAMA* article. David Barbano was not an independent author writing for the *JAMA*. In 1988 Barbano and Bauman published an article on the influence of rbST on general milk composition! (2)

A Not-So-Independent Co-Author

Co-author, William Daughaday, M.D., had Monsanto ties. The actual words of the *JAMA* reviewer which were added as an addendum to the paper reveal:

> From 1984 to 1986, Dr. Daughaday was the recipient of a research
> contract from Monsanto Company, a small fraction of which was paid
> to Dr. Daughaday as a consulting fee. (3)

Monsanto's memo, *"Five Independent Authorities,"* had found rbST-treated milk to be indistinguishable from normal milk. (4) The *JAMA* authors downplay the significance of genetic engineering. Although Monsanto incorrectly translated the genetic code and created an entirely new hormone never before seen on the face of this planet with a bacterium amino acid in the #144 position, epsilon-N-acetyllysine replacing the normal lysine, the authors argue that genetic engineering is no big deal. They write in the *JAMA*:

> Bovine somatotropin is simply another milk production management
> tool that could be made available to the dairy farmer.

Right! And hydrogen bombs are simply another defensive management tool that could be made available to our armed forces. Examples of other management tools mentioned in the preceding paragraph of the *JAMA* article are enriched feeds, vitamins, improved sanitation, computerized ration balancing and record keeping and better milk cooling and handling systems. These authors compare genetic engineering to the other methods and state:

> This will help the dairy farmer produce milk at a lower cost, and
> lower milk production costs will ultimately benefit consumers.

Milk prices were increased 14 percent in California shortly after Monsanto's rbST was approved. The powerful Dairy Coalition is continuously lobbying Congress to increase milk prices. The consumer's interests are not a consideration of the coalition. As to BST-treated milk being indistinguishable from normal milk, the doctors write:

> The minor differences in milk composition shown between
> un-supplemented and bST-supplemented cows are well within
> normal biological variation in milk composition.

We trust doctors. We believe the *Journal of the American Medical Association*. When *Science* and *JAMA* ran their articles simultaneously, *JAMA* comments received more weight by the media. *Science* gave us their opinion and America's physicians gave us an unqualified second opinion, BST-treated milk is wholesome and reliably safe! Nobody was there to tell us that the "independent" *JAMA* investigators had received money from Monsanto. In the company of such overwhelming confirmation, the doctors had nothing to fear. Nobody would ever uncover the true facts. They nearly got that one right.

There were other medical opinions, not so well publicized, that tried to alert the public. Benjamin Spock, M.D., announced that cow's milk is inappropriate for children below the age of 1 because children react negatively to bovine hormones. (5) In the years preceding his death, Dr. Spock created quite a controversy by criticizing milk. After 50 years of telling parents that milk was a near perfect food, Spock made a 180-degree turn. After Spock's analyses, the American Academy of Pediatrics reexamined milk issues and withdrew their endorsement of whole cow's milk for infants on the basis that iron in milk cannot be properly absorbed. (6)

Neal D. Barnard, M.D., author of *Food For Life*, and director of Washington-based Physicians Committee for Responsible Medicine, made stronger statements. Barnard believes that consumption of cow's milk is totally inappropriate for humans. The scientific literature is filled with evidences of the inadequacy of cow's milk for human nutrition. According to Barnard:

> There is no nutritional requirement for dairy products, and there
> are serious problems that can result from the proteins, sugar, fat
> and contaminants in milk products. (7)

Harvey and Marilyn Diamond, authors of the best sellers, *Fit For Life* and *Living Health*, are strong opponents of milk consumption. They make a remarkable case against dairy products and their comments on the dairy industry are brilliantly presented. The Diamonds conclude that:

Dairy products are disease-producing. Pasteurization is a fraud because dead food cannot support life. Everything that you have been taught about calcium in milk is inaccurate and dishonest. Dairy products are a major cause of osteoporosis. (8)

Their books were on the *New York Times* best-seller list for two consecutive years. If all of the readers of the Diamonds' books had heeded the author's advice, we would have no dairy industry. Perhaps this book that you are reading will put a final nail in the dairy industry coffin.

The *Journal of the American Medical Association* once had an immaculate reputation. Then they started to play politics. A review made by this author of PAC donations reveal that in 1994 the AMA gave nearly $3 million dollars to various members of Congress. The AMA will not publicly comment on their political donations, records of which are kept on file by the Federal Election Commission.

In the same year Monsanto published their revealing article admitting a gene error in producing BST, *JAMA* said that they were baffled by an explosion of increased cancer rates. (9) *JAMA* suggested that unknown carcinogens, perhaps environmental, yet to be identified, have been introduced over the past 50 years. The *JAMA* report was particularly concerned about an increase in tumors among farmers. Farmers, according to the report, are exposed to increased levels of insecticides, fungicides, chemical solvents and animal viruses. Some studies referred to an increased level of leukemia among dairy farmers.

Medical school. A place where doctors learn that when they drop the scalpel, they are not supposed to say "oops." A place where a class called Malpractice 401 is more important to a practitioner's education then Nutrition 101. Doctors learn to diagnose and prescribe. They do not understand the words of the great twentieth century philosopher, Tiny Tim, who informed his adoring public that "you are what you eat." If you consume the same daily level of dairy products eaten by the average American, you eat the equivalent fat of 11 slices of bacon, the equivalent cholesterol contained in 53 slices of bacon, and enough hormones to "ignite" the processes which break the tight genetic control which your immune system has most likely placed on an existing cancer. Ready to light the fuse? Drink that glass of milk!

The World Health Organization (WHO) is a respected agency of the United Nations. Certainly their review would be independent. Same for the National Institutes of Health (NIH). These agencies endorsed the new hormone. These agencies had strong ties to Monsanto. Even the White House got in on the act.

The Executive Branch - A letter from the White House

Dear Mr. Cohen,   *October 20, 1994*

Thank you so much for your letter. President Clinton greatly appreciates the trust and confidence you have shown in him by writing.

To ensure that your concerns are addressed, I am forwarding your letter to the Department of Agriculture for review and any appropriate action. Please bear in mind that it may take some time to look thoroughly into the issues you have raised. Should you wish to contact the Department of Agriculture directly, you may write to: Department of Agriculture, 14th and Independence Avenue, S.W., Washington, D.C. 20250. Many thanks for your patience,

James A. Dorskind
(Special Assistant to the President, Director of Correspondence)

A few weeks later I received the following response from the Department of Agriculture. At the same time, Michael Taylor, Monsanto attorney turned FDA employee, was filling a new position as USDA's under secretary for food safety.

Dear Mr. Cohen,   *November 7, 1994*

This is in response to your letter to President Clinton of September 7, 1994, on the subject of bovine somatotropin (bST) administration to dairy cows. The Food and Drug Administration (FDA) approved a bST product developed by the Monsanto Company on November 5, 1993. The approved use of this product is to increase the volume and efficiency of milk production by dairy cows. Commercial marketing of this product was subjected to a 90 day moratorium during which time the administration prepared a report for Congress on the economic impact of bST on the dairy industry and the Federal Budget. That report was released on January 10, 1994, and the commercial sale of the Monsanto product began February 4, 1994.

FDA addressed the issues of human safety of meat and milk from cows treated with bST early in their evaluation process. The information to which you make reference in your letter was a part of that evaluation process. The conclusion made by FDA that the use of bST is safe for humans has been reaffirmed by a National Institutes of Health Panel of Experts asked to review all of the information on the topic in December of 1990, by an Office of Technology Assessment report requested by Congress and published in May of 1991, by the World Health Organization Joint Expert Committee on Food Additives in 1992, by the American Medical Association, by the drug <u>regulatory bodies of the</u>

European Union, (emphasis added), *and by a number of other scientific organizations both within the United States and around the world. Among the reasons for this conclusion is the fact that bST is normally present in cow's milk and the <u>milk from treated cows cannot be distinguished from the milk of untreated cows.</u>* (emphasis added)

      The position of the Department of Agriculture is to support the <u>objective</u> (emphasis added) *and <u>scientific evaluation</u>* (emphasis added) *of the safety and efficacy of bST. The Department of Agriculture has no legal authority to reverse the decision of FDA to approve the use of bST. However, if the Department were to become aware of new information relative to the safety or efficacy of bST use, this information would be brought to their attention immediately.*

      <u>Virtually</u> (emphasis added) *all of data FDA used to arrive at their conclusion are a matter of public record and have been published and discussed in the scientific and popular press. If I can be of any further assistance, please do not hesitate to ask.*

           Sincerely,   *Betty Lou Guilliland*
           (for William Carlson, Acting Administrator)

      Here is what was happening at the United States Department of Agriculture (USDA) at the time this letter was written. Michael Espy, ex-secretary of the USDA, had recently resigned his post in disgrace for having accepted gifts from a poultry producer. In addition to accepting gifts, Espy solicited tickets to Chicago Bulls basketball playoff games. Espy took advantage of "freebies," including lavish parties, dining and trips sponsored by private industry. USDA was in a turmoil. A new director had not been named. An individual was needed to stabilize Agriculture. Taylor, ex-Monsanto attorney, was chosen to be the president's man. Taylor was appointed to the important position of under-secretary of agriculture. This USDA form letter gave the same standard answers to questions that I had not even raised, while my specific questions were not addressed. The words that I have underlined in the preceding letter are quite revealing. In order of my highlighting:

1) The "**regulatory bodies of the European Union**" have placed a new seven year moratorium on the use of BST on dairy cows in Europe. If the Department of Agriculture is proud of listing the Old World continent as proof that BST is heartily accepted and endorsed by the rest of the world, they should recognize that BST has been banned in Europe.

2) "**Milk from (rbST) treated cows cannot be distinguished from the milk of untreated cows.**" Even FDA Commissioner Kessler is now carefully wording his comments to include the words, "virtually no difference." All of the assumptions leading to approval were based upon the fact that all of the experts accepted the fact that the two milks were indistinguishable.

3) "**Objective...evaluation**?" In this milk controversy there is only one oxymoron more absurdly applied than objective evaluation, and that is the term *wholesome milk.*

4) "**Virtually**" When this catchall phrase, "virtually all data from scientific studies," is applied, I recall the experiment by Richard, Odaglia and Deslex prepared by Searle for Monsanto in 1989. (10)

Previous to the letter written to me, the White House issued a report in January 1994 titled "Use of Bovine Somatotropin (BST) in the United States: Its Potential Effects."

The basic premise of the report invalidated all which was to follow. The executive summary states:

> There is no evidence that BST poses a health threat to
> humans or animals. It has been studied more than any
> other animal drug, and been found safe by FDA and
> many other scientific bodies in the U.S., Europe, and
> around the world. FDA also concludes there is no
> legal basis requiring the labeling of BST milk, since the
> milk is indistinguishable from non-BST milk. Voluntary
> labeling is permitted. (11)

You're probably tired of reading all of the prestigious scientific agencies and government offices that repeat the same lie, particularly after you have read contradiction after contradiction from these same authorities. This was science/industry/government's way of teaching you. In 1994, this is the method in which you were repeatedly "bombarded" with information extolling the virtues of milk. Television was filled with not so subtle advertisements of actresses and athletes with milk mustaches invading your prime time viewing pleasures. Full page ads in every major magazine displayed those cute milk mustaches on the lips of beautiful models. Repeated radio and newspaper exposure told you that genetically engineered milk and normal wholesome milk were indistinguishable.

This is the same way that Hitler's "Minister of Popular Enlightenment" (translate that as "propagandist"), Goebbels, brainwashed the residents of Berlin into believing that their capitol city was not under siege when Allied forces were dropping bombs on their heads. Well, we are under siege too. With bombs, we can hide in the basement. Sometimes explosives miss their mark. Milk is a different matter. Drink rbGH-milk and the hormones will find a way to hit their target. The White House report summary included 11 points. The first is included in a special category underlined with the heading "Safety."

Point #1 "**BST-treated milk is safe** (emphasis added) **because it is indistinguishable from normal milk**." We know that BST-treated milk and untreated milk are different. That must logically change the conclusion of Point

#1. If we assume that BST milk is <u>safe</u> because it is indistinguishable from non-BST milk, then the converse must be true. BST-milk is (fill in the blank) _____ because it is different from non-BST milk.

Point #2 "**Income for individual farmers who use BST is likely to increase because BST favors good herd management**." Not for the 500 farms and 9500 animals reported with mastitis. (Mastitis is a condition of ulcerations and sores to the udders of cows. This condition results in pus entering the milk which increases the bacterial cell count in milk.) Many animals had to be destroyed. Many more farmers experienced no problems. Those that were successful produced more milk. The government (using your tax dollars) purchases milk surpluses. We had a large milk surplus before BST came on the market. We will have an even larger milk surplus now. Income for most farmers will increase. They will be receiving subsidies for their extra milk which will be converted into butter and cheese and shipped off as donations to countries needing our overabundance.

Point #3 "**BST will lead to lower milk prices**." Milk prices are "fixed" and controlled. Milk producers are under a microscope and cannot lower or raise their prices. However, the dairy industry had their lobbyist working to release those controls so that prices would be free to increase, simultaneous to rbST approval and their carefully constructed media blitz.

Point #4 "**Lower milk prices would result in decreased Federal costs for food stamps and other supplemental food programs**." I do not know who wrote this report, but, as it comes from the White House, I must assume President Clinton had to be aware of it. Doesn't the "buck" stop on his desk? Hey, Mr. President, you're pushing it here. You've lost credibility, yet you're sinking even deeper. In other words, public welfare costs will decrease because we allow Monsanto the right to distribute a genetically engineered hormone that causes cancer to laboratory animals and makes the milk different? You're pulling my leg, aren't you? Milk prices have increased since rbST approval. This has added costs to all of the above programs. Guess who is paying the price?

Point #5 "**Federal dairy price-support program would increase by approximately $150 million per year and decline in later years**." The first part contradicts points #2, #3, and #4. The second part suggests costs will decline in later years. We've heard things like this before from politicians promising tax hikes for next year and then adding, "Don't worry, taxes will decrease in later years."

Point #6 "**Savings in the costs of Federal feeding programs will completely offset the cumulative costs of the Federal dairy price-support system over 10 years**." Federal feeding program? You mean to tell me that you guys feed their cows? The government subsidizes the milk, buys the surplus, gives tax breaks to companies doing research designing chemicals to poison us, and feeds their animals. What's the point? Why not just pay the dairy farmers to come to Washington, D.C., and sit at a desk like the rest of you bureaucrats and do nothing? It would probably save us money, and we'd be a heck of a lot healthier, too.

Point #7 "**Consumers will benefit over the next six years with BST use because of lower prices**." If you believe that one, I've got a bridge to sell to you. I'd like each American consumer to give me one penny saved from a quart of milk. That would be 250,000,000 people times one cent equals $2,500,000. Give me two-and-one-half-million dollars and I'll sell you the Brooklyn Bridge.

Point #8 "**No significant reduction of demand is expected to result from BST use. Some consumer surveys reveal resistance to BST milk**." There appears to be a need for nutrition education on rbST's effects. Oh, oh. Here comes "Big Brother." We need re-education? It's obvious who needs re-education, isn't it? If every American realizes that the "new milk" contains increased levels of hormones, will milk consumption increase or decrease? Point number nine is worthy of nomination for a very special classification by itself. The category is "The Environment." This rates as one of the silliest things I have ever read.

Point #9 "**BST is expected to have a minor, but beneficial net impact on the environment. It should lead to a slightly smaller U.S. dairy herd, and therefore less pollution through decreased use of fertilizers for feed production, and less cow manure and methane production**."

This kind of manure is appropriate for something coming out of the Executive Office. Are fertilizers for feed production bad? Do they cause pollution? If we decrease the amount of fertilizers can we save the environment? Is cow manure bad? I certainly don't want to step in it, but I buy a couple of bags every year for my small tomato garden. Does cow manure cause pollution? As for methane, now they're finally beginning to make sense. After all, cows fart. Farts smell bad. I wouldn't want to be in a closed room with friends and a dairy cow or two, with everybody suddenly turning to point at me. That could be embarrassing. Methane gas. Sure. That certainly affects me when cows in Wisconsin participate in communal "fartathons." Why, you could light up Hackensack, New Jersey, with all the methane gas produced from those bovines "breaking wind."

Thank goodness our government scientist realizes that fewer cows will mean fewer farts. I wonder just how many federal dollars they spent to come up with the data for this brilliant deduction. However, consider that rbST-treated cows will eat more food to produce 20 percent more milk. If they do not eat more food, then they will have to dissolve their own bones and melt their own proteins to produce that 20 percent more milk product. So, if they eat more, and you've got to assume that they will, then they're going to fart more, stupid. Perhaps we can get the author of this study a job on *Saturday Night Live* or Leno or Letterman.

Point #10 **"BST should have little, if any effect on U.S. dairy exports. Nearly half of U.S. dairy exports go to countries that have approved the use of BST, and more countries are expected to do so."**

The European Community placed a seven year moratorium on the use of rbST in their markets until the year 2002. This ban occurred sometime after the publication of this Executive Report. This not only invalidates point #10, but helps to invalidate points 1 through 9 as well. This ban was done for safety reasons.

Point #11 **"U.S. leadership in biotechnology, as well as private-sector investment for research and development in the biotechnology industry, would be enhanced by proceeding with BST, and would be impeded if there were new government obstacles to such bio-tech products following their approval for use by FDA and other regulatory agencies."**

In other words, if we determine that BST is not safe, we will hurt the prospects of the new genetic engineering technology. It has not yet been perfected. In Steven Spielberg's movie, *Jurassic Park*, we became witness to a scenario where errors in genetic engineering caused horrible consequences. When just one amino acid in a hormone or protein differs from the normal genetic code there can be dire consequences. Sickle cell anemia is just one example. Another example occurs in Alzheimer's disease. The substitution of just one amino acid, phenlylalanine, appears to be the basis for one type of hereditary Alzheimer disease. With rbST, improper research developed a product with a resulting gene transcription error. That error surfaced long after all of the research on rbST had been performed and submitted to FDA. (Amino acid number 144 should have been lysine; it was manufactured as epsilon-N-acetyllysine, a bacterium amino acid).

In our rush and excitement to get rbST to market, sloppy research was tolerated. When laboratory animals became sick, the incriminating data were hidden. When people like myself requested specific data proving laboratory animals get cancer from rbST, the government, in its great display of bureaucratic strength, did not allow such data to be released. "BST-treated milk is indistinguishable from normal milk." Approval was based on this assumption. On page 22 of the 64-page Executive Report we are treated to the following:

"There are slight variations in milkfat and milk-protein content immediately after BST treatment."

"The meat from BST-treated cows tends to have a lower fat content."

"A slight shift in the Kjeldahl nitrogen factions (casein, whey protein, and nonprotein nitrogen) has been observed."

These have been clues to a puzzle not yet solved. Combined with the irrefutable fact that levels of IGF in milk increase after cows are treated with rBST, it is a shame and a crime for any government employee or public figure to attempt to convince us that the milks are indistinguishable.

The National Institutes of Health

The National Institutes of Health (NIH) conducted a Technology Assessment Conference in December 1990. A Conference Statement entitled "Bovine Somatotropin" was published as a result of a two-day conference in which 37 individuals were given the opportunity to present their arguments, both pro and con. Among the speakers were FDA employees, Monsanto scientists and vocal critics of rBST including Sam Epstein, M.D., and David Kronfeld, Ph.D. A panel of thirteen doctors were assigned the task of assessing and evaluating the available scientific information and resolving the safety and efficacy issues as they related to biomedical technology.

In all fairness to the panel, significant research was not available for their review at the time of their assessment. They could not have possibly imagined what research in 1993 and 1994 would reveal about the biochemical activities of IGF. At the time, these doctors possessed Monsanto's research data. None of the doctors had opportunity to review the most critical piece of research, the report by Richard, Odaglia and Deslex which indicated that laboratory animals experienced increased spleen growth, decreased heart, kidney and liver growth as a result of oral ingestion of BST.

That report, which indicated that laboratory animals got cancer, was kept from review of these esteemed doctors. They did the best they could in analyzing the limited evidence which they had opportunity to examine. Monsanto and FDA will not release the key evidence which would have helped these panelists. The NIH group answered six questions in their conference statement. The questions were:

1. What is the role of milk in human nutrition, and how is its safety for human consumption monitored?
2. What is the comparative biology of human and bovine lactation and milk composition?
3. What is the effect of administration of rBST on milk production of cows and on the nutritional quality and hormonal content of their meat and milk?
4. What are the health effects on cows resulting from administration of BST?
5. What are the health effects on humans resulting from consumption of meat or milk from cows given rBST?
6. What further animal and human research is needed on use of rBST?

Question #1 - *What is the role of milk in human nutrition and how is its safety monitored? Their answer was that "Milk is an important food throughout the life cycle, especially in the diets of infants, children, pregnant and lactating women, and the elderly. Recent research emphasizes the importance of milk* *products in providing calcium throughout life to promote bone density and to prevent or delay osteoporosis."*

Cows do not drink milk. There is enough calcium in the normal diet of a cow or human to remain healthy. Nations with low milk intake also have low levels of osteoporosis. In countries where milk is consumed there are much higher rates of bone disease including arthritis and osteoporosis. Adult animals do not need milk for their bones to remain strong. That applies to elephants and whales, too.

As far as safety monitoring goes, when industry adds more pollutants to our food supply, the FDA changes the monitoring levels and safety criteria. They monitor the milk. A group of anonymous FDA employees wrote a letter to Congress complaining that Miller "arbitrarily" increased the level of accepted antibiotics in milk to include many different antibiotics. This change occurred because cows were getting mastitis as a result of being treated with rBST. More antibiotics were needed for sick cows. Additional antibiotics were needed to insure that healthy cows would not become sick cows. A Monsanto employee ends up at FDA to write labeling laws on this hormone. This same employee makes sure to write new levels of acceptance standards for antibiotic levels in milk. Other FDA employees (the letter writers), criticizing rBST, are harassed by the Director of the Center for Veterinary Medicine who happens to have become, in the words of a confidential letter to GAO, an "extremely close friend" with this female ex-Monsanto employee, Miller.

Question #2 - *What is the comparative biology of human and bovine lactation and milk composition?*

"The content of hormones, growth factors, and hormone-like peptides, where they are known, appear to be similar in both milks. Because these hormones are digested in the gastrointestinal tract and are not absorbed intact into the bloodstream, they are not believed to have biological significance when ingested, at least after the newborn period." Contrary evidence exists that milk hormones survive digestion and are absorbed intact through the lining of the intestinal. NIH could not have known this because this revealing research was performed in the years after this conference. We now have reason to believe that milk is an enzyme inhibitor. Gastric acidity is approximately a "2." Milk raises the pH to a level of a "6."

Question #3 - *What is the effect of administration of rBST on milk production of cows and on the nutritional quality and hormonal content of their meat and milk?*

"Pasteurization of milk destroys most BST but has little effect on IGF-I. Levels of IGF increase in milk after cows are treated with BST."

The NIH admitted that levels of IGF increase after rBST treatment. Why did the *JAMA*, WHO, Executive Branch report, newspapers and magazines quote the NIH as stating that the two milks are indistinguishable?

Question #4 - *What are the health effects on cows resulting from administration of rBST?*

"The panel was appraised of the fact that a large body of data has been submitted to the FDA that is not yet available either to the public or to the committee. The panel was informed that an evaluation and analyses of this data will be forthcoming. If there is an increase in mastitis in rBST-treated cows, there might be a concomitant increase in antibiotic therapy."

Monsanto reported only a handful of complaints by dairy farmers. FDA reported that there was a low level of mastitis complaints. Rifkin's Pure Food successful Freedom of Information Act request revealed that Monsanto and FDA participated in the identical cover-up. They both had to be aware that thousands of animals were getting mastitis. In fact, 9500 got mastitis. Nobody measured the amounts of pus finding its way into milk and then into a bowl of cereal. Nobody measured the increased levels of antibiotics which people consumed with that milk. Miller had arbitrarily increased the tolerable levels of antibiotics which she (and Monsanto) believed would safely enter your body. What will be the cumulative effects of the increased levels of these disease battling drugs on people's immune systems? How will their tolerance of antibiotics be affected if they ever get sick enough to actually need them?

Question #5 - *What are the health effects on humans resulting from consumption of meat or milk from cows given rBST?*

"Even if BST is absorbed intact, the growth hormone receptors in the human do not recognize BST, and therefore, BST cannot produce effects in humans. Similarly, there is no evidence that proteolytic fragments of IGF-I are biologically active in man, nor is there evidence of systemic biological effects in man from any IGF-I absorbed intact, because the amounts of IGF-I that might potentially be ingested are orders of magnitude less than those required to produce such effects."

Receptors. Cow mammary glands do not contain receptors for their own BST. Nobody really knows how "it" works. There are no binding sites when we examine the cells of udders in test tubes outside of a cow's body. (Scientists call that in vitro.) One must examine delicate tissues in vivo, in the body while they are alive. Hammond and Collier published a paper (see page 39) for Monsanto in 1990 in which they wrote:

> Bovine milk has been reported to contain trace levels of BST although it is not clear how it enters the milk, since no BST receptors have been identified on the surface of mammary glands.

Furthermore, Hammond and Collier said:

> While the lactating mammary glands of dairy cows do not appear to have receptors for somatotropin (BST), receptors for IGF-I and II have been identified in the mammary tissue of pregnant cows. Since somatotropin does not appear to have a direct effect on mammary secretory tissue, it is conceivable that the galactopoietic effect of somatotropin may be mediated, at least in part, through IGF-I, since this somatomedin has a stimulatory effect on mammary growth.

Translation: BST works in cows, even though there is no way that it possibly can. There are no receptors. In spite of that, it works. However, it cannot work on people because people have no receptors. Why not accept the work of Monsanto and assume that IGF has an effect in assisting BST to properly function? There are no BST binding sites in humans. Monsanto scientists themselves yield the clue as to how IGF can react with BST to make both active in the human body. While BST is different than the normal human growth hormone, IGF in humans is identical to IGF from cows. The human body will receive the IGF molecule from a cow and treat it as its own.

As for the orders of magnitude issue (the actual level of IGF already present in the human body), IGF and BST contained in meat will not be orally active. This is because strong digestive enzymes break down the hormones. Milk, on the other hand, was designed so that it would inhibit enzymatic breakdown. Factors such as casein, decreased size of fat globules (as a result of homogenization) increasing cellular permeability, and lowering of gastric pH all contribute to hormonal survival and activity. We also produce and swallow large quantities of IGF in our saliva. This IGF is broken down into their basic protein components in our stomachs. The liver and spleen and kidneys and other organs produce IGF. Unprotected by casein and other factors which keep it intact and safe in milk, this IGF is quickly bound to other receptors.

Miller of FDA told me that a typical human has 500,000 nanograms of IGF in his or her blood system. However, those IGF molecules are already bound to other material, just as the glue in your house has been bound inside of wood and sheetrock and carpeting. The glue is present in these items and can be measured. However, it can never regain its original character and essence to bind and perform like glue again. Levels of "free and unbound IGF" are relatively quite low. They were measured and the results published by Frystyk in Denmark on July 11, 1994. This occurred four years after the NIH assessment panel had even a clue as to the relatively low levels of "free" IGF present in the body.

If NIH panelists had known, they would have never used the phrase "orders of magnitude" when referring to the relative quantities of IGF and the insignificant quantities contained in one glass of milk. If you drink one glass of normal untreated milk you nearly double the levels of IGF in your body! When you drink a glass of rBST-treated milk the level of the IGF hormone always increases. There are scientists (Sam Epstein is one) who claim that the increase is as much as nine-fold!

Question #6 - *What further animal and human research is needed on use of rBST?*

The panel identified several areas of research that would help to gain further understanding of BST effects. It was the opinion of the NIH doctors that none of these studies were critical enough to delay decisions on the commercial use of rBST. NIH had made their minds up early on in this process that rBST was safe. However, they were cautious enough in each of their carefully worded conclusions to first include the following proviso:

"Based upon the data reviewed by the committee..."

The one determination that I absolutely upon agree with the NIH panel on is their first conclusion:

"In the unanimous judgment of the panel, rBST treatment increases milk production of cows."

The NIH review committee recommended that further studies be performed. None ever were.

Inspector General's Report

DATE: 2/ 21/ 92 FROM: Richard P. Kusserow Inspector General

TO: James O. Mason, M.D., Assistant Secretary For Health

*SUBJECT: **Audit of Issues Related to the Food and Drug Administration review of Bovine Somatotropin (A-15-90-00046)***

This final report provides you the results of our audit of issues related to the Food and Drug Administration's (FDA) review of the yet-to-be approved new animal drug bovine somatotropin (bST). This audit was requested in May 1990 by Congressman John D. Conyers, Jr., Chairman, House Committee on Government Operations, who was concerned that:

-- little actual research exists on the human safety aspects of bST;

-- industry files indicate high levels of bST are found in the milk of bST-treated cows;

-- critical research information regarding health effects of bST on animals and humans has been withheld from public scrutiny by FDA and the Monsanto Agricultural Company (Monsanto), one of the firms developing bST; and

-- Monsanto and FDA have manipulated and suppressed animal health test data showing that bST-injected cows suffer low fertility rates, mastitis (inflammation of the udder), and other chronic defects.

It was not possible for this audit to determine the adequacy of FDA's review at the time of publication because the approval process had not yet been completed. However, the audit was quite critical of public statements made by FDA officials regarding the safety of rBST and the likelihood of its approval. This audit concluded that while the FDA did not violate any Federal law or regulation by making such statements, the appearance that FDA gave was that they were prematurely predicting the outcome of the BST process. As a result of FDA comments, Monsanto improperly acted by disseminating pre-approval promotional materials which claimed, without supporting scientific data, that rBST was safe and effective prior to actual FDA approval of the drug.

Pre-approval promotion is contrary to Federal regulations. Monsanto received a verbal slap on the wrist, but took full advantage of this head start. The CVM actually completed the review of Monsanto's rBST human safety data in 1986, determining that food from rBST-treated cows posed no threat to human health.

Congressman John Conyers (D-MI), chairman of the House Committee on Government Operations, in requesting the inspector general's audit, was concerned that there was so little research actually performed on the human safety aspects of rBST use. The FDA had relied on data from experiments performed in the 1950s showing that BST does not produce growth when injected into human dwarf children. FDA became increasingly concerned with IGF in 1988 after learning that bovine and human IGF-I were identical. CVM requested data from Monsanto on IGF oral activity which Monsanto supplied. The rat studies (Chapter 9) were the primary determining factor for "lack of biological activity from oral ingestion of bST." Yet, laboratory animals did demonstrate biological effects.

Congressman Conyers was concerned that critical research was withheld from public scrutiny. The inspector general's report confirmed that these data were withheld. However, FDA was prohibited by Federal regulations from releasing any information from its investigational and new animal drug application files without Monsanto's permission if that information had not been previously and lawfully disclosed to the public. Despite the fact that Monsanto submitted part of the data for peer review to a committee of scientists at the prestigious journal *Science*, the bulk of data have not yet been released despite Freedom of Information Act requests and appeals to the Department of Health and Human Services by this author.

FDA is prohibited by Federal regulations contained in FDA statute 21 CFR 514.11 and 514.12 of the statutes under which FDA operates from releasing any information regarding Monsanto's investigational new animal drug file or new animal drug application. According to the FDA, the reason for this protective shield was to safeguard Monsanto from unfair competition. If the data were disclosed they could be used by competitors to obtain approval for their drugs.

If the data are released, not only would no competitor want to develop a similar product because that evidence revealed that animals were developing a wide spectrum of serious illnesses, but that competitors would be prohibited from doing so by the agency chosen to protect the health and safety concerns of American citizens.

One paper. One experiment performed on 360 rats. This paper will reveal the different organ weights of animals tested with varying doses of rBST. The Inspector General found no evidence that data were manipulated. That's because they didn't know where or how to look (more in Chapter 9). Tables in the *Science* article were presented in a biased manner.

Monsanto released data on spleen, liver, heart and kidney weights. They withheld data on twenty-eight additional organ and tissue samples which are cited as reference 42 of that *Science* article. The last referenced sample is "and all gross lesions." FDA Commissioner David Kessler, as well as Inspector General Richard Kusserow missed this. Everybody missed this! All gross lesions? Does that sound like a normal organ condition? Hope I don't grow one of those on my arm or leg. The drug has been approved for commercial use. It was approved in November 1993. The concluding comment in the inspector general's report regarding proprietary interest and disclosure of data to the public is:

> Our review found that FDA and Monsanto have acted appropriately in their decisions as to what data may be disclosed regarding the human and animal safety of bST. Because FDA is constrained from fully disclosing data undergoing review, complete disclosure of bST data will not occur unless and until FDA approves the drug for commercial use.

World Health Organization

The World Health Organization (WHO) held a 10-day meeting in Geneva, Switzerland in June 1992. The purpose of the meeting was a technical assessment of the residues of the hormones created from the new genetic engineering technology. Although the official title of the meeting was "Residues of Some Veterinary Drugs in Animals and Foods," the meeting was convened to study and analyze the published research, effects and implications of bovine somatotropin. The meeting resulted in a publication of the studies, or monographs - abstracts of those studies. One can get an indication of the spirit of the meeting by reviewing the papers presented and references on pages 137-142 of that report. There are 58 references. Monsanto employees, scientists and researchers produced 36 (62 percent) of the papers which were presented to the WHO. This document is informative. The studies are presented in a clear and scientific manner.

Although this example was illustrated previously, it's appropriate to repeat how scientists examine data. For example, the standard for expressing the presence or quantity of a drug in a liquid, be it milk or human blood, is to reveal the levels of that drug in a milliliter. Now, I don't know about you, but I have trouble imagining what a milliliter looks like. Open up my refrigerator and I challenge you to find a milliliter of anything. Open my cupboards and you will not find a milliliter container to hold a milliliter of milk or orange juice or whiskey. Perhaps my bird would drink a milliliter of water at one sitting. I would not. Therefore, I translate, when applicable, milliliters to liters. That's easy. I multiply by 1000. A liter is more or less one quart (1 liter = 1.0567 quarts). We all know what one quart looks like. This understanding will become critically important later on.

When scientists present data to politicians they know that politicians will understand only what the scientist wants them to understand. So, if the presence of a drug in milk is 4 nanograms per milliliter (ng/ml) and rBST treatment increases that presence to 50 ng/ml, the increase seems insignificant. However, if I translate milliliters to liters, then 4000 nanograms/liter (ng/L) would become 50,000 ng after rBST-treatment. Now the difference becomes substantial. We drink liters or quarts, not milliliters. Would you laugh if I reported the levels of a powerful growth hormone as milliquarts. You drink only 3 ng of IGF-I, a most powerful growth hormone in every milliquart of milk? However, you drink 3000 ng of this same hormone in a quart.

"Mom, can I have some milk with my chocolate cake?" "Sorry, honey. I only have a milliquart left in the refrigerator." Milliquart? I'd barely get a crackle out of one Rice Krispie from a milliquart of milk. However, my cells would probably experience the "snap" and "pop."

As for nanograms, a nanogram is one-billionth of a gram. There are approximately 28 grams (gr) in one ounce and 454 gr in a pound. There are one trillion nanograms in two pounds. Anyway, various hormones and drugs work on a very tiny scale. Sometimes only one molecule can trigger a biological response. The word which explains this submicroscopic level of biological activity is "nanomolecular." LSD works on a nanomolecular scale. So does BST, and so does IGF. When scientists note the small quantities of a drug which are sometimes present in a sample, they are usually aware that large quantities of that drug are not necessary to exert strong effects. One dot of the powerful hallucinogenic chemical acid (LSD) on a blot of paper applied to your tongue could send you on a "Magical Mystery Tour."

We begin on page 114 of the WHO report which displays a long necklace-type structure made up of an amino acid chain representing the configuration of bovine somatotropin. (see page 68) With this chart one would know, for example, that amino acid #10 should be leucine and #26 should be alanine and #144 should be lysine. This is Monsanto's version of BST. Any change in this sequence would create a new chemical with new characteristics. In the movie, *Jurassic Park*, there's a cartoon used to explain how genetic engineering works. When one company tampered with the genetic code and made some tiny changes in that code things began to go seriously wrong. The scientists reviewing this monograph and the chart on page 114 had no idea that a mistake had been made in manufacturing this hormone. Monsanto wouldn't learn of this mistake for some while. While it is unclear just when Monsanto learned that they had created a gene transcription error which resulted in a mutation, it is clear that Monsanto never told the FDA of that error. A publication in the British journal, *Protein Science*, in July 1994, revealed that amino acid #144, which should have been lysine, became an unusual amino acid called epsilon-N-acetyllysine. Anybody drinking milk containing this hormone had potentially assimilated a genetically created bacterium amino acid into their system. I drank milk during those years, 1988-1994.

The most important part of this monograph of studies begins on page 120. Here we learn that Monsanto conducted several studies to determine the average baseline levels of insulin-like growth factor (IGF) in untreated natural milk. Monsanto took 100 raw bulk tanks of milk and analyzed the levels of IGF. When Monsanto analyzed these milk samples they came up with an average reading of 4.32 nanograms per milliliter (ng/ml) which translate to 4,320 nanograms per liter (ng/L). However, Monsanto scientists added a range of between 1.27 and 8.10 which translates to 1270 - 8100 ng/L. That was an artificially created and enormous range. That is not necessarily an indication of the average or typical reading. However, this critical range allowed FDA to apply the following comment when levels of IGF nearly doubled in milk after BST treatment:

"Any increase is well within the normal range."

By testing 100 tanks of milk they are mixing the milk from thousands of cows at different stages of their lactations and combining every combination and permutation of IGF content that can be imagined. The level of IGF-I in milk, expressed as 4.32 ng/ml or 4,320 ng/L, is now an industry standard and should be the number that all other milk samples are based upon. To add a range is a trick of science allowing hormones to exert abnormal effects which can be designated as "normal range."

On the bottom of page 120 is one of my two favorite sentences of this study. The other is on page 128. These two quotes cannot be erased. Once printed they are evidence that this conspiracy and fraud exists. (They are also an indication that scientists do not proofread their own reports.) Taken together, these two sentences reveal the truth about rBST's effect on milk, and the lie which a small group of Monsanto scientists, with assistance from a small group of FDA "insiders," fooled the scientific community of the entire world.

Page 120 reveals:

AFTER SOMIDOBOVE (rbST) INJECTION, MEAN IGF-I LEVELS IN THE TREATED ANIMALS ARE ALWAYS HIGHER THAN THOSE FOUND IN THE CONTROLS.

Page 128 reveals:

THE MOST DEFINITIVE AND COMPREHENSIVE STUDIES DEMONSTRATE THAT IGF-I CONCENTRATIONS ARE NOT ALTERED AFTER rbST TREATMENT.

These two statements contradict each other. They came to Switzerland to get their act together. Like Swiss cheese, their credibility had been shot full of holes. If only somebody had bothered to carefully review this report, the contradictions might have been exposed and truths disclosed. I received one of my two copies of this report from Linda Grasse, editor of numerous FDA publications and spokeswoman for the Center for Veterinary Medicine, an investigative branch of FDA. Her name is written (photocopied) on the front cover. I received another copy from Robert Collier of Monsanto. Both copies remarkably begin with page 116. I have not had the opportunity to get the rest of the report. Perhaps neither has FDA.

The studies in this monograph were published without accompanying complete data. In study after study, no significant increase in IGF levels is reported because the relative increases fall within "the normal range." The experiments were designed by Monsanto scientists. They intentionally omitted the first 30 days of lactation in some studies and 60 days in others. This was done with knowledge that a cow's level of IGF is highest after giving birth to her calf. This study design is an example of scientific bias and fraud. The data were controlled even before the experiment started.

When Eli Lilly made application for their BST product called Optiflex 640, they represented that their product would not create IGF-I levels greater than 50,000 ng/L. Compare that with a baseline of 4,320! However, the way they put it, it was 50 ng/ml vs. 4.32 ng/ml. This doesn't seem like much when they present the data this way. Consider that one tall glass (1 pint) of natural milk contains 2,044 ng of IGF. The equivalent glass of Eli Lilly's milk would not contain more than 23,657 ng of IGF. The level of "free" (unbound) IGF in a 60-year-old male is 450 ng/L. The average male has 5-6 quarts of blood in his body. That would mean that one glass of natural milk would nearly equal the entire level of "free" IGF hormone in his body. One glass of Eli Lilly's rBST-treated milk could bathe an adult's system with up to nine and one-half times the level of IGF --- this is one powerful growth hormone.

Office of Technology Assessment

The Senate Committee on Agriculture, Nutrition and Forestry along with the House Committee on Agriculture requested the Office of Technology Assessment (OTA) to examine the emerging technology of genetic engineering and how the dairy industry might be affected by approving rBST for use on dairy cows. Although the final 118-page report was published in May 1991 before much of the rBST research was available to FDA reviewers, the OTA had this to say:

> The report concludes that, based on today's research findings,
> bST poses no additional risk to consumers and does not produce
> adverse health effects to cows. However, if approved by FDA,
> bST will accelerate trends that already put additional economic
> stress on dairy farm operators in many areas of the country.

It is interesting that this summary pessimistically identifies that rbST will exacerbate economic pressures that dairy farmers would feel as a result of increasing the milk supply which already produces a large surplus. The Executive Branch of our government painted an optimistic scenario suggesting how farmers and consumers would benefit from this new technology. In addition to five thoroughly researched chapters overviewing the dairy industry and emerging technology of rBST, the report projects detailed national and regional analyses of scenarios in which rBST use is adopted.

The OTA raised interesting points about the escalating rBST controversy. OTA raised a need for increased dissemination of research information before new technologies receive formal approval. It was noted that there is no agency able to develop information on the risks of new drugs and no formal agency which provides input to and from farmers to researchers and consumers. OTA notes that had such an agency existed a decade ago, much of the bST controversy could have been avoided. OTA warns:

> If demand for milk declines sharply with the introduction of bST,
> supply-management programs such as production quotas or
> termination programs may be required.

OTA recognized the risk assessments from implementing this new technology. OTA suspects that dairy farms would shut down as a result of rBST technology. Did they suspect that rBST had a potential to destroy an entire industry? We have learned that rBST-treated milk contains increased levels of IGF. However, milk naturally contains IGF. The natural levels of IGF are bad news for adults. We might never have come to this realization if Monsanto had not increased IGF levels in milk through their genetic engineering errors. Monsanto, in genetically engineering milk, might have created a hormone powerful enough to destroy the dairy industry. Now that's a hormone with a negative growth effect!

When the OTA report was written, the latest dairy industry figures (1989) accounted for an industry with total cash receipts of $19.4 billion dollars. Many geographic regions of the United States had operated negative cash flows, existing only because of government subsidies. The new emerging technology put enough fear into two states which placed moratoriums on rBST use even before approval. Four states wrote labeling laws fearing consumer reaction. The federal government did not hear this message from farmers and congressmen representing citizens concerns. Why do we need this new technology, wondered farmers who were just scraping by, fearing total loss of assets with the new technology? OTA lends credence to claims of activists like David Kronfeld, Jeremy Rifkin and Sam Epstein by stating:

> Although these individuals offer no specific documentation
> of scientific fraud, such claims are not to be taken lightly. Current
> events demonstrate that research fraud is possible. However,
> a distinguishing feature of science is that research results are
> examined and repeated by others.

Not only was research deceit possible, misrepresentations became the standard operating procedure regarding rBST information released by FDA and Monsanto. Would OTA describe the FDA and Monsanto representation that few cows got mastitis to be a lie? FDA repeatedly issued statements verifying only a handful of sick cows from rBST treatment. When a FOIA act request revealed that 9,500 animals had ulcerated udders as a result of rBST use, Monsanto and FDA were exposed in that lie. Not only did the February 1995 FOIA request reveal this damaging information but it also revealed the fact that ten people were injected in various incidents by rBST. One of those people was a female who experienced an enlarged breast thirty days after she was injected. If FDA and Monsanto had simply said, "No comment," when asked about mastitis incidents, we would have been annoyed and frustrated. However, they both lied to the American people by stating that there were only a handful of mastitis complaints from dairy farmers. Now that is fraud! OTA continues:

> The claims of Kronfeld, Rifkin, and Epstein imply a world-wide conspiracy involving at least 1,000 animal scientists in academia, government, and industry and hundreds of dairy farmers involved in the bST experiments. The possibility of such a conspiracy seems remote.

We accept on good faith the fact that scientists conducted honest and unbiased research. We accept on good faith the fact FDA will scrupulously review the data in drug applications. We accept on good faith that it is impossible for a pharmaceutical company like Monsanto to have the power to place their own scientists (Miller and Sechen) and attorneys (Taylor at FDA, and Michael Burros, the son of a *New York Times* food writer who had mysteriously changed her opinion about rbST, at GAO) in key FDA research and regulatory positions of power. We accept on good faith that our elected congressmen would not openly solicit and accept bribes in the name of PAC money from companies like Monsanto and trade organizations doing business with Monsanto. We accept on good faith that data on animal research would openly be available for review. We accept on good faith that when the proof is found that laboratory animals got cancer from rBST that proof would be reviewed by FDA and that we will be protected. We accept on good faith the representation made to us by FDA Commissioner Kessler that BST-treated milk is indistinguishable from normal wholesome milk.

The Executive Branch Report Concluded:

> BST has been examined, found safe, and approved for use by numerous foreign government regulatory agencies. **In fact, no professionally recognized scientific group has concluded, on the basis of current knowledge, that there is doubt about the safety of BST in milk production.** (*emphasis added*)

European Community

Europe banned rBST on December 15, 1994.

In February 1993, the Commission of the European Communities (EC) issued their final scientific report for their own Committee for Veterinary Medicinal Products (CVMP) for SOMATECH, Monsanto's European version of rBST, and OPTIFLEX-640, from the Eli Lilly company. France had received an application from Monsanto in 1987 for approval of the rBST hormone. Subsequently, Great Britain and Italy received applications as well. A committee had been formed in November 1987 to study biotechnology issues and that committee noted differences in the Monsanto documentation between the French and British applications. The committee prepared a comprehensive series of questions which were transmitted to Monsanto.

In July 1989, Monsanto responded to those questions with 22,000+ pages of documentation to all member states of the European Community (EC). However, instead of being overwhelmed (the way FDA was by Monsanto's 53,000-page application), EC deemed that the original submission was unacceptable for the purposes of assessment. An amended submission, eliminating the contradictions contained in the first, was received by EC in December 1989. In May 1990, the committee concluded that several answers relating to the quality and biotechnological aspects of rBST and safety of the product in "target species" remained unsatisfactory.

In the February 1993 report, EC took into consideration the human food safety evaluation of bovine somatotropin by the American FDA published in *Science* in August 1990. They also were influenced by the NIH conference and the WHO monograph of studies. Presented with all of the available data, including the FDA, NIH, and WHO policy statements, EC concluded that rBST was safe and should be approved for use. An assessment report was prepared for the CVMP by the French Laboratory for Medical Research. One curious comment (page 16) reports a study on rats carried out in the United States in 1950:

> Studies carried out in rats in 1950 showed an increase in the
> incidence of tumors after administration of raw bovine pituitary
> abstracts.

Every American agency citing the 1950 studies reported that there was no reaction in rats from injections of bovine pituitary extracts. On page 16 of the final assessment report, Eli Lilly comments on increased levels of IGF:

> The amount of IGF-I in milk may be increased in cows
> treated with (BST) somidobove. However, the increase

is small in comparison with the variation between cows
and some studies have been unable to detect a significant
difference. Total IGF-I in the milk of treated cows is
unlikely to exceed 50 ng/ml.

Lilly lived to regret that statement. Translate ml (milliters) into liters. 50 ng/ml (fifty ng/ml read as nanograms per milliliter) is the same way of saying 50,000 ng/L. Monsanto's baseline average of IGF in normal milk is 4,320 ng/L. When one divides 50,000 by 4,320 the subsequent result is that IGF levels in milk increase eleven and one-half times! Is that within the "normal range?" The European Community placed a moratorium on rBST use until the year 2002 which allowed continued rBST testing on cows in Europe. In addition, they took this opportunity to observe the enormous laboratory study being conducted on the American public by Monsanto.

Recognizing that Monsanto and Eli Lilly had an enormous investment in rBST, and that biotechnology might one day improve humanity's lot, the EC allowed rBST treatment on selected herds to continue for five years of additional studies. Monsanto and FDA both reacted promptly to the EC decision, which was painful to one and embarrassing to the other. One "partner" reacted in anger, the other party rationalized the news to be "good news."

TO: David Kessler, Director of FDA   *December 7, 1994*
FROM: Friedrich-Wilhelm Graefe zu Baringdorf
     Vice-President of the Agriculture Committee, EC

Dear Dr. Kessler,

Consumers in the European Community and their representatives in the European Parliament are apparently much more concerned about the unresolved human health issues related to recombinant Bovine Somatotropin than your agency was when it authorized the product. That is why the European Parliament unanimously adopted an amendment to the European Commission's proposal for a 7-year moratorium on rBST which would extend the prohibition to the import of dairy and meat products from animals which have been treated with the drug (Official Journal No. C 20, 24.01.94 enclosed for your information). Such a ban might necessitate convening the GATT Panel; however, we feel fairly confident in being able to demonstrate that the safety of European citizens who consume rBST-products cannot be guaranteed. More and more scientific evidence, such as the recent pieces in the British medical journal Lancet, *is accumulating to support this position.*

But rather than ban ALL meat and dairy products from the United States (and other countries where the drug is currently in use), a less contentious approach would simply be to label the meat and dairy products which are

<u>exported to the EU</u>. *Of course, the implementation of an export labeling requirement would depend upon the availability of an effective test to determine whether synthetic BST had been used in the production process. We understand from numerous reports in the US press and occasional statements from representatives of your agency that such a test is currently available in the United States. Could you please inform us as to the status and nature of this test and provide information about where it may be obtained? Obviously, the EU would also have to have such a test in order to enforce import labeling requirements for rBST products, and we would like to contact the supplier. Thank you for your assistance.*

Yours sincerely,
Friedrich-Wilhelm Graefe zu Baringdorf

Two lovers, Monsanto and FDA, coitus interruptus, were shocked by this letter. Their reactions revealed their personalities. Monsanto's said, "It's all right honey, we'll make the best of this. We're here to stay." FDA's reaction was angry, defensive and accusatory, protecting its partner, Monsanto. Kara Pharmaceuticals in New Jersey is developing an assay (test) to detect the presence of genetically engineered rBST in milk. That assay was paid for by a group of New York State farmers. In their letter, FDA commented that such a test, while theoretically possible, would be inconclusive. The FDA letter and Monsanto response to the EU ban follow.

NEWS RELEASE FROM MONSANTO
CONTACT: Ken Baker - (Brussels) Tom McDermott - (St. Louis)

EU MODIFIES MORATORIUM TO PERMIT LIMITED USE OF BST

BRUSSELS, 15 December 1994- Today's EU Agricultural Council decision which allows farmers to use supplemental BST was welcomed by the Monsanto Company. The decision permits member states to authorize limited use of the company's supplemental BST product over a five year period.

This is consistent with the company's intentions for the product in the EU, where a milk quota system is in effect until the year 2000. Monsanto is sensitive to the differences in the economics of milk production between the United States and the EU, and limited utilization will enable the company and farmers to learn how BST can best be used in the context of a quota system. The company will work with European farm and dairy industry groups to ensure that questions or concerns they have are addressed.

Monsanto's supplemental BST product was approved in 1993 by the EU's Committee for Veterinary Medicinal Products (CVMP), which determined that the product is both safe for humans and animals.

It has also been approved in 15 countries around the world, including the United States, where it continues to be a resounding success with dairy farmers. In the first six months of sales, more than 10,000 American dairy farmers have administered the product to more than 800,000 cows.

Despite concerns prior to approval, U.S. consumer patterns for fluid milk and other dairy foods remain steady. During the first nine months of 1994, consumption of all milk in the U.S. increased by 4.2 pecent over 1993, the largest increase in several years.

The EU Agricultural Council calls for the collection of data to evaluate the effects of the utilization of BST on cow health and safety. Monsanto has already committed to the CVMP that it will conduct a BST "pharmocovigilance" program in the EU. Monsanto has voluntarily initiated a similar post-approval monitoring program in the United States under the direction of the U.S. Food and Drug Administration."

In a public statement released following the first six months of the program, the FDA said the "number and severity of the reported conditions are no greater than the expected" and "are no different from the types normally occurring in cattle not treated with rBST." The agency concluded: "Based on reports submitted to date, FDA does not find any cause for concern."

Monsanto markets its supplemental rBST product as POSILAC in the United States and has received approval for the product as SOMATECH in the European Union.

FDA took 47 days to answer the letter from the European Community Agriculture Department. The letter was sent by Stephen F. Sundlof, director of the Center for Veterinary Medicine.

TO: *Frederich-Wilhelm Graefe zu Baringdorf - January 23, 1995 Vice-President of the Agriculture Committee, European Parliament*
FROM: *Dr. Stephen F. Sundlof, Director of CVM at FDA*

Dear Mr. Graefe zu Baringdorf,
This is in response to your letter of December 7, 1994, addressed to Dr. David A. Kessler, Commissioner of Food and Drugs in the United States.
We thank you for your interest but found your letter somewhat confusing, both in its depiction of European Union (EU) actions concerning recombinant bovine somatotropin (rbST), and in its allegations about unresolved safety questions concerning rbST.

Regarding the depiction of EU actions, we wonder why you chose not to inform us about an amendment offered by the European Parliament (EP) a year ago that was never adopted by the European Union. In an interesting coincidence of timing, just a week after the date of your letter, the EU Council of Ministers announced its extension of the rbST moratorium for another 5 years (not the 7 years cited in your letter), without expanding the moratorium to cover the import of products of animals treated with rbST, as was proposed by the parliament. Thus, the need you posited for a method to distinguish between products from rbST-treated and from non-treated animals, so as to avoid undue trade difficulties, would appear not to exist.

Regarding your statement about unspecified "unresolved human health issues" pertaining to rbST, I must take issue with your claim that "more and more scientific evidence" is raising questions about the safety of rbST, and with your apparent implication that FDA approved rbST prematurely. I can assure you that FDA's human food safety experts have been diligent and thorough in their review of all aspects of the human food safety of milk from cows receiving supplemental rbST. FDA activities in this regard have been extensively reviewed and investigated by Congressional oversight committees and other institutions of the U.S. Government. They have upheld the rigor of FDA's review process.

Further, the WHO/FAO Joint Expert Committee on Food Additives, the U.S. Congress Office of Technology Assessment, and a panel of experts convened by the U.S. National Institutes of Health all concluded that milk from cows receiving rbST is safe.

With respect to your reference to the report by Mepham and colleagues published in The Lancet, I would refer you to the reports by Collier and colleagues (Monsanto Company), and by Wilkinson (Lilly Industries) also published in The Lancet (VOL. 344, September 17, 1994) which point out "several inaccuracies and inconsistencies" and errors contained in the Mepham report. Of particular interest is the error contained in the Mepham report quoting Lilly as indicating in a submission to the CEC Committee of Veterinary Medicinal Products, that milk from cows receiving supplemental rbST might contain IGF-I at levels tenfold above the bulk tank average IGF-I level of 4 ng/ml referred to by Juskevich and Guyer in their report published in Science (Vol. 249; page 875; 1990). However, Lilly was referring (in a submission to the U.K. Veterinary Products Committee and Medicines Commission) to a study conducted in hypophysectomized rats, in which the milk from the rats had a hypothetical maximal level of 50 ng IGF-I/ml. In that study, the rats, which were highly sensitive to parenteral IGF-I, showed no adverse health effects from the daily administration of rbST at 1000 micrograms/kg body weight.

You also indicated that it is your understanding that there is "an effective test to determine whether synthetic BST" has been used in the production of milk. There have been reports on work done to measure recombinant human somatotropin in the blood of humans (where circulating HST levels are high compared to levels in milk). However, competent scientists maintain that while theoretically possible, a test to identify milk from rbST-supplemented cows by measuring rbST in milk would not only be extremely difficult, but would also be inconclusive and useless for any regulatory purposes. Furthermore since human food safety experts from the U.S. FDA, the EU, the WHO/FAO JECFA, and other official regulatory bodies have concluded that milk from cows treated with rbST is safe for human consumption, there is no basis for developing and implementing such a difficult and costly analytical test, which in the end would provide inclusive results.

Sincerely yours,
Stephen F. Sundlof, Director of CVM

The study which Sundlof refers to (50 ng/ml) was an unpublished Lilly study cited as reference #66 in the Juskevich and Guyer paper. Eli Lilly and Monsanto have demonstrated that they will not release the data in their unpublished reports. Furthermore, a review of Eli Lilly's application specifically referred to cow's milk, not rat's milk. Eli Lilly never mentioned the rat study when they stated that cow's milk would not contain IGF levels greater than 50 ng/ml.

Representations from FDA and the Monsanto Agricultural Company demonstrated how data and statistics are easily manipulated.

"There's many a mistake made on purpose."

Thomas C. Haliburton

"If science produces no better faults than tyranny, murder, rapine and destruction of national morality, I would rather wish our country to be ignorant, honest and estimable as our neighboring savages are."

Thomas Jefferson

"Suppose you were an idiot. And suppose you were a member of Congress. But I repeat myself."

Mark Twain

Chapter 6

The Plot Thickens: Collusion Between Monsanto, FDA & Congress

---

The investigation of the genetically engineered milk hormone was an enormous puzzle and each individual factor contributing to its approval was but a single clue which, when added together, revealed the solution to a far greater puzzle.   There were three critical questions to be answered, each one relating to the other. The first question was, After cows are treated with rBST does their milk contain increased levels of IGF-I? The answer to that first question was *yes*. The second question was, Is IGF-1 in milk bioactive and does it exert growth effects? The answer to that second question was also *yes*. The third question was one that nobody wanted to ask. Not FDA, not the *Journal of the American Medical Association*. Not even the anti-rBST activists. Certainly not the dairy farmers. The third question was, Does normal "wholesome" milk contain powerful growth hormones? The answer to this question is a Pandora's box which might never have been opened had not Monsanto genetically engineered the bovine hormone, beginning this controversy.

Monsanto learned many of the answers to these questions. Perhaps that is why they had to have their scientists, Miller and Sechen, and attorney, Taylor, hired by FDA to carefully review and write the regulations and approval of their own research. Perhaps that, too, is why so many members of Congress became wealthy from PAC money. The most important study considered by the FDA reviewers in their *Science* publication was never reviewed by FDA scientists and investigators. Although two of the seven tables of the Juskevich and Guyer paper presented data from an unpublished study by Richard, Odaglia and Deslex, FDA did not refer to that study as "pivotal." Had FDA called that study "pivotal," the data would have been released to the public for review after final approval. Despite Freedom of Information Act lawsuits, those data still remain secret. Monsanto continues to receive trade protected status from FDA for the weights of 32 organs and tissue samples from 360 laboratory animals. Monsanto claims that the release of these data will cause them financial harm. Monsanto's $600 million dollar investment remains safe, thanks to FDA's protective shield.

Simultaneous to FDA's review of Monsanto's scientific data, a different type of campaign was being conducted on Capitol Hill. Monsanto's lobbyists were purchasing influence from our elected officials. One group of recipients of Monsanto's generosity was the Congressional Committee considering a bill intended to label milk and dairy products produced from cows treated with the genetically engineered hormone.

Those Crooks on the Hill

BRIBERY - The act or practice of giving or accepting money or some other payment with the object of influencing the action or judgment; the application of influence to gain votes at a parliamentary hearing or other election.

Secretary of Agriculture Resigns

Michael Espy, agriculture secretary, abruptly resigned from his Cabinet position on October 3, 1994, in the midst of a controversial hearing into allegations that he received gifts from and gave favors to friends in the agriculture business. Espy had been a congressman for 6 years and had served as a member of the House Agriculture Committee. Ethical behavior for a Congressman should not differ from unethical behavior for a Secretary. The same act of taking gifts or bribes for influence should applied to all government officials. In a statement accepting Espy's resignation, President Clinton commented that Espy's timely resignation was appropriate because of his improper acceptance of gifts from Tyson Chicken, Quaker Oats and Sun Diamond.

In addition to accepting sports tickets and requesting Chicago Bulls playoff tickets, Espy received special lodging, the use of private industry jets, lavish parties and the lease of a Jeep Cherokee which was charged to the U.S. government. If Espy had not resigned, Congress was poised to investigate election law violations which might have led to the Oval Office. Espy's prompt resignation saved President Clinton enormous embarrassment. An investigation might have revealed the pattern of abuses which Clinton the candidate had pledged to end when he became president. A confidential informant had originally triggered an investigation into a 1992 PAC (Political Action Committee donating dollars to congressmen while seeking influence and access) called the Farmer's and Rancher's PAC. Espy's appointment, politically motivated, resulted in substantial donations to Clinton's presidential war chest. Espy was gone, but business continued as usual on Capitol Hill.

The Crooked Ones

The Center for Responsive Politics and the Federal Election Commission reported 1994 PAC donations given to all members of Congress including those congressmen serving on the Dairy Committee of Agriculture from companies having direct interest in bills which they considered in committee:

Congressman	State	Total PAC $	Agri. $	AMA $
John Boehner	(OH)	$ 216,076	$ 59,306	$ 3,200
Wes Cooley	(OR)	$ 131,890	$ 26,300	$ 5,000
Cal Dooley	(CA)	$ 219,475	$ 97,857	$ 3,000
Robert Goodlatte	(VA)	$ 150,069	$ 39,400	$ 2,606
Steve Gunderson	(WI)	$ 278,710	$ 21,750	$ 10,000
Earl Hilliard	(AL)	$ 257,424	$ 42,600	$ 1,350
Tim Holden	(PA)	$ 361,586	$ 47,300	$ 7,350
Frank Lucas	(OK)	$ 195,924	$ 36,550	$ 5,000
Collin Peterson	(MN)	$ 363,530	$ 59,880	$ 5,000
Richard Pombo	(CA)	$ 252,600	$ 84,385	$ 5,900
Pat Roberts	(KS)	$ 220,637	$113,456	$ 5,000
Nick Smith	(MI)	$ 0	$ 0	$ 0
Harold Volkmer	(MO)	$ 326,320	$ 82,969	$ 5,000

Total Bribes (PAC): $2,647,921
Total Agriculture-Related PAC Bribes: $711,753

In January 1995, I sent letters to the aides of each of these Dairy Committee members. The letters addressed rBST issues. In addition, I sent certified letters, return receipt requested, to each congressman on the above list. I detailed problems in the FDA and Monsanto research and expressed concerns for human safety issues. Not one congressman responded to my letters or phone calls.

On this list I have included total PAC donations and total donations from companies that are related to the agriculture business. While there are dozens of different types of categories for donations and literally thousands of different

PACS, each congressman (with the exception of Smith) received money from the American Medical Association (AMA).

While one can hardly understand the motives of individuals or groups, nor witness what goes on behind closed doors, one wonders what the AMA is doing handing thousands of dollars to individuals on the Dairy, Livestock and Poultry Committee. Then I made the connection. Why did AMA heartily approve BST in the August 20, 1990, issue of the *Journal of the American Medical Association* simultaneous to the August 24, 1990 article in *Science*? **BECAUSE MONSANTO GAVE THE AMA MONEY.** Monsanto donated money to the AMA. In their journal the AMA endorsed the new genetically engineered milk hormone. Money also found its way to congressmen voting in committee on BST issues. While the AMA donated a total of $53,406 to the congressmen on this committee willing to accept money, Monsanto gave only to a select few.

Four congressmen accepted these bribes directly from Monsanto: Volkmer, $2000; Dooley, $1000; Gunderson, $1000; Pombo, $500. They were voting on labeling issues impacting on Monsanto, yet they accepted money.

Who Can We Trust?

In the fall of 1993, the Physicians Committee for Responsible Medicine, an organization consisting of more than 6,000 medical doctors, asked the question:

Why would the American Medical Association (AMA) get
involved in dairy politics? [1]

In answering that question, the physician's organization links the American Dietetic Association (ADA) and the AMA to Monsanto. Monsanto gave $30,000 to the AMA to fund a television program "educating" consumers (brainwashing them) into believing that milk treated with hormones is as healthy an untreated milk. Monsanto also gave $100,000 to the ADA to run an education hotline with positive information about the bovine hormone.

On January 23, 1997, a study reported by the Associated Press revealed that members of Congress vote on specific issues according to the amount of money they receive from "interest groups" in various industries affected by pending legislation. This study performed by the Center for Responsive Politics revealed how decisions are made on Capitol Hill. Among the examples given are the following:

Industry/ Product	Average $ Given to Those Voting *YES*	Average $ Given to Those Voting *NO*
Peanuts	$ 1,542	$ 152
Timber	$ 19,503	$ 2,675
Oil	$ 64,460	$ 12,000
Cable TV	$ 5,994	$ 853

Do uneducated consumers really stand a chance? Is there anybody in a position of authority, power or influence immune from the dollars?

One American Hero

Conspicuous by his absence from the PAC money recipients is Congressman Nick Smith, Republican from the state of Michigan, who made PAC reform a campaign issue in his successful election bid. The "buying of congressional influence" is one of the greatest evils in this country, responsible for the enormous debt which America has accumulated by the deal making on Capitol Hill. The influence exerted by PAC groups and the hundreds of millions of dollars in legal bribes that they pay our representatives have taken America away from the goals and philosophy which made it a once great nation.

In July 1995, I asked Ann Begley, an attorney working for the Freedom of Information Clearing House, a Ralph Nader organization, to help me to obtain the unpublished secret study in which all laboratory animals either developed, or were developing, cancer from the new genetically engineered milk hormone. In turning me down, she explained in a letter that she had spoken to Jerry Deighton of FDA who had spoken to Margaret Miller, Ph.D. In referring to the Juskevich and Guyer *Science* paper, Deighton told Begley:

> Ms. Miller states that she wrote the parts of the article referring to
> the Eli Lilly studies and that she did not share the information she
> relied upon with Monsanto. (2)

FDA admits that Margaret Miller wrote the "Eli Lilly" portion of the Juskevich and Guyer paper. Margaret Miller, prohibited by law from anything to do with the rbGH investigation, was quietly behind the scenes "running the show."

At the very least, Miller should have been named as one of the authors of this article. After all, she wrote part of it. To give her credit would be to admit that she broke the law. Miller, having just come to FDA from Monsanto, was prohibited in any way from working on or reviewing her own research. Yet, it was clear that nobody in the world knew more about the subject of cows, IGF-I and the bovine hormone than Miller. By not citing Miller for her work, the authors of this study and FDA committed scientific fraud. In the case of scientific journal articles, scientists and their lab assistants usually are given credit as co-authors for studies and are so named. Credit is usually given to secretaries, proofreaders and sometimes clerical assistants. Reference # 75 thanks Suzanne Sechen for her contributions, yet Margaret Miller was not cited as an author or contributor.

Rotten to the Core

There are three groups of individuals who, armed with the truth about rbST and the power to change things, could have acted in the best interests of the American people. Instead, these three groups acted only in the best interests of the Monsanto Agricultural Company. Each individual or group of individuals acted with knowledge of the statements and positions of the other groups. Taken individually, their acts should be considered criminal. Taken together, their actions represent an American tragedy. These three groups include members of Congress, individuals employed by Monsanto, and a small group of people at FDA.

The co-conspirators were:

1) David Kessler, FDA commissioner
2) Monsanto Agricultural Company
3) C. Everett Koop, ex-surgeon general, Monsanto lobbyist
4) Michael Taylor, Monsanto attorney, hired by FDA
5) Margaret Miller, Monsanto scientist, hired by FDA
6) Suzanne Sechen, Monsanto scientist, hired by FDA
7) 12 congressmen who served on the House Agriculture Committee

Who's in Charge Here?

Who was in charge of the FDA? It all boils down to the former FDA Commissioner David Kessler. Doctor Kessler is an attorney and a physician. President George Bush appointed Kessler to head the FDA in 1990. Kessler, top man at FDA, must accept responsibility for FDA's "mission," which he oversaw during the period from 1990 until his resignation in January 1997. *The Wall Street Journal* published an editorial in 1994, titled, "First Step To an FDA Cure: Dump Kessler." In that editorial, James Bovard wrote:

Freedom is a difficult concept for the doctor to grasp.
In 1992, Dr. Kessler declared: "If members of our
society were empowered to make their own decisions...

then the whole rationale for the (FDA) would cease to exist." He has derided "freedom of choice" as an illusion unless people are presented with only government-approved choices. (3)

Monsanto

National Geographic, September, 1980. A Monsanto advertisement displays a perfectly manicured hand holding an unblemished orange and long register tape listing the ingredients of the natural orange. The ad reads:

> All foods, even natural ones, are made up of chemicals. But natural foods don't have to list their ingredients. So it's often assumed they're chemical-free. In fact, the ordinary orange is a miniature chemical factory. And the good old potato contains arsenic among its more than 150 ingredients.
>
> This doesn't mean natural foods are dangerous. If they were, they wouldn't be on the market. The same is true of man-made foods. All man-made foods are tested for safety. And they often provide more nutrition, at a lower cost, than natural foods. They even use many of the same chemical ingredients.
>
> So you see, there really isn't much difference between foods made by Mother Nature and those made by man. What's artificial is the line drawn between them. (4)

The Monsanto Pledge

In 1990, the chairman of Monsanto, Richard J. Mahoney, unveiled a seven-point corporate promise (5) at a meeting of the National Wildlife Foundation. Monsanto's actual pledge can be found on the INTERNET at:

www.monsanto.com/MonPub/EnvironmentPledge.html

Permission to print this pledge has been denied! Apparently Monsanto does not wish to have anyone remember their pledge and to be held to the promise of reducing toxic chemicals in our food supply. Not after a corporate history of manufacturing cance-causing agents such as PCBs, dioxins, Agent Orange, aspartame and rbST. One day Monsanto, through genetic engineering, could influence every food product in our supermarkets.

Monsanto on Ethics

Meet Monsanto Agricultural Company of St. Louis, Missouri. Thomas McDermott, Director of Biotechnology Communications for Monsanto, wrote an editorial on the subject of Biotechnology and Ethics:

> Although it is true that ethics or moral philosophy does have some important things to say about these and other questions (How are we to act?, What should we value? Where do our moral obligations lie?), I am afraid that those of you who think that hard and fast answers can be found are going to be disappointed.
>
> Common arguments, such as those that contend that biotechnology is too risky and may have unintended consequences, are either not ethical arguments at all-owing to the simple fact that higher-risk activities are not automatically less ethical than less-risky ones-or else they contend, from a utilitarian perspective, that we have not properly assessed the outcomes. The latter charge seems to me to be more of an empirical question, and one that our regulatory agencies should be equipped to handle. (6)

This is Monsanto's official position. They rationalize the death chemicals which they manufacture. McDermott speaks of the FDA when he mentions regulatory agencies. If the FDA says our chemicals are safe, then the ethical and moral responsibility is on their shoulders, not Monsanto's. Here's how this same philosophy has been historically applied by other pharmaceutical companies. A company manufactures a product like diethyl stilbesterol (DES). Their research indicates problems. Many years later second generation cancers and genetic deformities occur. Is this the fault of the FDA? Or the manufacturer, who suspected the truth? Funny how one can warp reality and lecture on ethics and morality.

In 1985, Monsanto acquired G.D. Searle Pharmaceutical Company. In doing so, Monsanto purchased all of the licensing rights to manufacture and distribute NutraSweet, an artificial sweetener. In doing so, Monsanto also accepted all liability for all lawsuits involving Searle's intrauterine copper coil birth control device. For Monsanto, the coil and the artificial sweetener represented tactical war games. Monsanto was able to accumulate legal expertise and political connections which allowed a new chapter to be written in the "empirical" game of ethics and morality. Lisa Watson, a Monsanto spokeswoman, appeared on a Canadian television show called "The Fifth Estate." In that September 9, 1994, broadcast she said, "Out of those 10,000 dairy farmers and 800,000 cows we had only received 95 complaints from dairy farmers." (7) At that time the FDA had actually received complaints concerning nearly 9,500 BST-treated cows contracting mastitis.

This Canadian TV program also reported that Canadian government officials, while debating legalization of BST, received multimillion dollar bribes from Monsanto officials. If Monsanto bribed officials in Canada, is it possible that they did the same in the United States? The Congressional Record of May 7, 1985, published a condemnation of the research techniques which result in severely flawed experiments. Investigators found that such biased research experiments performed by pharmaceutical companies were the rule and not the exception. (8)

One example comes from another Monsanto product, Aspartame, originally developed by Searle Pharmaceutical Company. Shocking testimony reveals that thousands of volunteered complaints have been received by the FDA from aspartame users, use of which has been associated with hundreds of ailments. They include migraines, seizures, vision problems, depression and memory loss. He who has the most dollars is the most ethical and moral. That should be the title of McDermott's next article.

STATEMENT OF C. EVERETT KOOP ON THE INTRODUCTION OF SUPPLEMENTAL BST - February 6, 1994

"Milk from cows given supplemental bovine somatotropin is the same as any other milk. So, there should be no doubt in the minds of consumers that the milk they drink is just as safe, nutritious and wholesome as it has always been. Every issue and every question about BST has been thoroughly and carefully studied by the federal government and several independent scientific institutions. Consumers can continue to enjoy milk and dairy foods with complete confidence.

"Unfortunately, a few fringe groups are using misleading statements and blatant falsehoods as part of a long-running campaign to scare consumers about a perfectly safe food. Their long-range goal is to prevent the benefits of biotechnology from reaching the public. Because dairy foods are an important, widely consumed source of nutrition, it is necessary to condemn these attacks on the safety of milk for what they are; baseless, manipulative and completely irresponsible.

"Even worse are attempts by some persons to use school children as pawns in their opposition to BST. Any suggestion that milk from BST-supplemented cows is unsafe for children to consume at school, or at home, is a potential threat to their health and well being. We should be reinforcing the message that all dairy foods, when consumed as part of a varied and balanced diet, are healthful - and not burden our children with unwarranted fears about food safety.

"Supermarkets and dairy processors can play an important role by assuring consumers of the safety of the milk supply, by providing the facts on BST to interested customers, or by referring them to credible health and nutrition authorities."

How Monsanto Plays "Politics"

After leaving government service, C. Everett Koop, M.D., the respected ex-surgeon general, issued a well-publicized and strongly worded statement in favor of Monsanto's genetically engineered hormone. Koop relied upon statements made previously by Monsanto in attacking critics of the new hormone. It was clear which side he had chosen. I called and wrote to Koop. I faxed a letter to him on April 3, 1995. He did not return telephone calls, letters or my fax.

Did Monsanto make direct payment to Koop so that this letter would be written to influence regulators and members of Congress? America had a love affair with the respected ex-surgeon general and his assertion carried great weight. That affirmation was reproduced in newspapers and magazines and marketed to benefit Monsanto's agenda. The first line of Koop's statement reads, "Milk from cows given supplemental bovine somatotropin is the same as any other milk."

When we review Juskevich and Guyer's abstract in their landmark *Science* paper we find that the authors state, "Recombinant bGH treatment produces an increase in the concentration of insulin-like growth factor-I (IGF-I) in cow's milk." What appeared to be "the same as any other milk" to Koop was significantly different to FDA scientists.

It appears that Koop never read Juskevich and Guyer's paper. Had he done so he could not have said that wholesome milk "is the same as" genetically engineered milk. Ethics and morality are directly proportional to and measured by dollars invested to shape perception, which becomes the one and only reality. Koop was part of the problem. Did he review Monsanto's BST data? Why doesn't he demand that they release the unpublished article cited as reference #42 in the August 24, 1994, *Science* article? Is Koop an ethical man and do you really believe that "a few fringe groups are using misleading statements and blatant falsehoods?" How much money did Monsanto pay him to pen those words? Will he stand up for truth and demand that Monsanto release the documents which will ultimately prove to the world that laboratory animals were developing cancer from BST?

Congress Acts to Prevent Cancer

In 1958, Congress added a revision to the Pure Food and Drug Act. That legislative addition was called the Food Additives Amendment, and has been known ever since as the Delaney clause, named after Congressman Jim Delaney (D-NY), who wrote and sponsored the clause. The Delaney clause established the requirement that food additives be approved by FDA before they were added to foods. Manufacturers of these additives and companies using these additives had to first present scientific data demonstrating the safety of these additives before FDA would issue approval. The Delaney clause stipulated that no food additive would be deemed safe by FDA if it was shown to be the cause of cancer in laboratory animals.

Food manufacturers and pharmaceutical companies have long been uncomfortable with the Delaney clause. People should be free to buy products that cause cancer if they so choose. The Constitution of the United States guarantees that right. That's the thinking of those who are aware that food additives cause cancer. On the other hand, Congress, in passing the Delaney amendment, believed strongly that the average person cannot always know everything and therefore gave the power to FDA to review research intending to prove such additives safe. In 1988, Monsanto was beginning to learn that laboratory animals were getting cancer from its new genetically engineered cow hormone. The approval of this hormone represented a new technology, genetic engineering, that would propel Monsanto into a leading role in the biotech industry.

Monsanto's Attorney Negates the Delaney Clause

Taylor tackled the Delaney Clause before coming to FDA. He wrote a paper called, "The De Minimus Interpretation of the Delaney Clause: Legal and Policy Rationale." (9) Michael Taylor's paper was published in the *Journal of the American College of Toxicology*. Attorneys who write papers usually publish those papers in law journals. There are hundreds of law review journals. Taylor is an attorney, not a toxicologist. He easily got his paper published in a peer-reviewed scientific journal. Scientists with credentials have difficulty having their papers published in a journal, and yet this attorney had no such problem. Interesting. What favors were called in and what creative deals fashioned in private corridors?

Cancer is a "Trivial Matter"

Taylor wrote:

The term *de Minimus* is a legal one embodying the concept
that, even when the literal language of the law would permit,
the reach of a regulatory statute need not be extended to
truly trivial matters.

In other words, cancer is sometimes a "truly trivial matter." Taylor continued:

> The decision if an animal carcinogen is safe for human consumption is not solely scientific, policy or legal, but, like all safety decisions, is a combination of these.

Politics plays a role in determining the seriousness of cancer. Michael Taylor's brilliant paper received top billing at FDA. Attorney Taylor was hired shortly after this paper was written. One of his roles at FDA was to help to institute a "De Minimus" interpretation of the Delaney Amendment. Another role of Taylor's was to oversee a De Minimus interpretation of cancers in laboratory animals ingesting the new genetically engineered milk hormone. As Deputy Commissioner for Policy at FDA, Taylor was responsible for all FDA rule making and policy development activities. Taylor then led a major overhaul of the USDA food safety program.

Conflicts of Interest: FDA Employees "Confidential" Letter

On March 16, 1994, a letter signed "concerned CVM employees" was circulated to members of Congress, GAO, Dr. David Kessler - Commissioner of FDA, the Inspector General of the United States, Richard P. Kusserow, and Michael Hansen of Consumer's Union.

To whom it may concern:
·   *We are a group of CVM/FDA employees who are very concerned about the FDA's recent decision not to label milk treated with BST. We are afraid to speak openly about the situation because of retribution from our director, Dr. Robert Livingston. Dr. Livingston openly harasses anyone who states an opinion in opposition to his.*
    The basis of our concern is that Dr. Margaret Miller, Dr. Livingston's assistant and, from all indications, extremely "close friend," wrote the FDA's opinion on why milk from BST-treated cows should not be labeled. However, before coming to FDA, Dr. Margaret Miller was working for the Monsanto company as a researcher on BST. At the time she wrote the FDA opinion on labeling, she was still publishing papers with Monsanto scientists on BST. It appears to us that this is a direct conflict of interest to have in any way Dr. Miller working on BST. As you know, if milk is labeled as being from BST-treated cows, consumers will not buy it and Monsanto stands to lose a great deal of money. Several of Dr. Miller's former colleagues would lose their jobs.
    To add to this, Dr. Livingston had Dr. Miller write a policy on use of antimicrobials in milk. She picked an arbitrary and scientifically unsupported

number of 1 ppm as being the allowable amount of antimicrobial in milk permitted without any consumer safety testing. This is for any antimicrobial. A cow could be treated with several antibiotics and each one would be permitted to be in milk at a level of 1ppm without additional consumer safety testing. Effects of the different antibiotics could be additive and this is not taken into account.

As you know, one big concern for BST is that it leads to increased antibiotic use. Monsanto has said this is not a concern. This issue held up the approval of BST for a long time. Dr. Miller's policy was used as the basis for approval of BST despite increased antibiotic usage. This also is a direct conflict of interest to have Dr. Miller working on this issue.

This is not the first time that CVM employees have charged Dr. Livingston with fraud and abuse leading to an endangerment of the public safety. However, it seems if anyone speaks out, they, not Dr. Livingston, end up in trouble. We as government employees cannot understand why it is allowed to continue.

We would appreciate a full investigation of the charges. We have sent letters to GAO, Consumer's Union, Dr. Kessler, and the Inspector General.

Thank You,

Concerned CVM Employees

On April 15, 1994, a timely letter was sent to Charles Bowsher, the comptroller general of the U.S. General Accounting Office. The letter was signed by three members of Congress: California Democrat George E. Brown, Jr., who at the time was the chairman of the Science, Space and Technology Committee, Vermont Independent Bernard Sanders, and Wisconsin Democrat David Obey.

Congress Calls for an Investigation

Dear Mr. Bowsher,

We are writing to request a targeted investigation and prompt letter report (within 30 days) concerning potential conflicts of interest involving the Food and Drug Administration's (FDA) review of recombinant bovine somatotropin (rBGH/BST) and FDA's decision not to require national labeling of milk products produced with the synthetic hormone.

Your agency has worked with us and other members of Congress in the past on a different dimension of the rBGH/BST controversy and the GAO staff, specifically Boris Kachura and Kwai-Cheung Chan were very helpful to us. Accordingly, we hope you will detail GAO professional staff to assist us in validating or debunking very troubling information we have received about alleged past and on-going conflicts of interest on the part of several key officials who have been or continue to make critical decisions about the safety and marketing of this synthetic hormone.

Specifically, we want GAO to conduct a focused investigation on an expedited basis to examine:

1) Potential conflicts of interest regarding individuals involved in the FDA's review of rBGH, and very serious concerns raised in the letter sent last month to GAO, and others, by anonymous "Concerned CVM Employees" (Center for Veterinary Medicine), copy attached. The individuals include:

- Margaret Miller, Deputy Director of the FDA's Office of New Animal Drugs and a former Monsanto Company employee. According to the letter from "Concerned CVM Employees," Miller wrote the FDA's opinion on why milk from BST-treated cows should not be labeled, while, "she was still publishing papers with Monsanto scientists on BST." Miller also developed the FDA policy rationale on antibiotics that provided the basis for FDA's approval for BST. This occurred in spite of the fact that rBGH treatments result in an increased use of antibiotics and a likely increase in antibiotic residues in the milk supply. The CVM letter claims Miller's policy is arbitrary and does not account for the cumulative effects of different antibiotics. Because of Miller's relationship with Monsanto, and the importance of the antibiotic issue to rBGH approval, the letter calls it 'a direct conflict of interest to have Dr. Miller working on this issue.'

GAO's own report, "BGH: Approval Should Be Withheld Until the Mastitis Issue is Resolved", challenged FDA's failure to adequately consider the human health effects of increased antibiotic use in cows treated with rBGH. Also, GAO investigators had to abandon their investigation of rBGH effects that was undertaken at the University of Vermont because of the Monsanto Company's refusal to make available to them all pertinent clinical and related data.

Dismissing GAO's concerns, and ignoring Monsanto's lack of cooperation with GAO investigators, FDA went ahead and approved rBGH based on their position, presumably supported by Dr. Miller's policy, that increased antibiotic use was not an issue worthy of further review. FDA subsequently and unilaterally declared that rBGH was a "manageable risk."

- Michael Taylor, Deputy Commissioner of FDA for Policy was previously with the law firm of King & Spalding where Monsanto was his personal client regarding food labeling and regulatory issues. Taylor approved and signed the FDA's labeling guidance thereby justifying the FDA's policy prohibiting the labeling of milk produced with rBGH. His former law firm, King & Spalding, is now representing Monsanto in suits against companies who are choosing to label milk "rBGH free." They rely heavily on the guidelines approved by Mr. Taylor and have even enclosed them when threatening companies with lawsuits.

- Susan Sechen, an rBGH data reviewer at FDA previously worked with Cornell University researcher Dale Bauman, a consultant to Monsanto (and other rBGH sponsors), who conducted Monsanto-sponsored research and has played a key role in defending Monsanto's rBGH product. Ms. Sechen appears to have *done rBGH work for FDA, while still involved with the Monsanto-sponsored work at Cornell.*

Thus, there is strong evidence that all three of these employees may have violated at least two ethical regulations applicable to them pursuant to the Code of Federal Regulations (43 CFR s.7373b-201 and 5 CFR s2635.502). Furthermore, the current FDA approval of the use of rBGH appears to be a direct product of these violations. This requires further investigation.

2) Reports of employee intimidation and endangerment of the public health as alleged in the "Concerned CVM Employees" letter. According to that letter, Dr. Robert Livingston, Director of the Office of New Animal Drug Evaluation, "openly harasses anyone who states an opinion in opposition to his," and, "this is not the first time that CVM employees have charged Dr. Livingston with fraud and abuse leading to an endangerment of the public safety." The validity of these charges should be reviewed.

This review should also investigate the case of Dr. Richard Burroughs. Burroughs involvement does not appear to be a conflict of interest controversy, but may be a case of retaliation against employees who challenge the CVM's review of animal drugs. Burroughs supervised the rBGH target animal safety studies before being fired by FDA. He maintains that his problems with CVM stemmed from his insistence on stringent animal health standards in rBGH research.

3) Identities of other FDA employees who are former employees of Monsanto or who maintain an on-going direct or indirect relationship with that company which may raise potential conflicts of interest.

While we have not sought to identify by name those who initiated the CVM Employees letter, their concerns certainly warrant further investigation, especially when added to questions raised previously inside and outside the Congress about potential conflicts of interest in FDA's rBGH review.

The entire FDA review of rBGH seemingly has been characterized by misinformation and questionable actions on the part of both FDA and the Monsanto Company officials. This includes the Monsanto Company's apparent repeated violations of the laws prohibiting pre-approval promotion of a drug under FDA review, as well as continuing questions about the credibility of the FDA's scientific review.

Finally, taking all of this new information into account, we also want you to undertake a technical review of the FDA decision to approve commercial usage of rBGH, including but not limited to the March, 1993 discussion of the risks posed by increased antibiotics usage and the subsequent recommendation of the Veterinary Advisory Committee of the Center for Veterinary Medicine to approve rBGH usage.

Thank you for your prompt attention and follow up action in this matter. Time is of the essence for probing this troubling new information. Accordingly, we respectfully request that we quickly agree on an approach to initiate this limited investigation immediately with a view to GAO providing us with your first batch of findings within a month. This will enable us to consider any appropriate oversight or legislative follow-up action in a timely fashion during this session of Congress.

Sincerely,

George E. Brown, Jr., Bernard Sanders, David Obey

An FDA Employee with Integrity

"FDA has become an extension of the drug industry. I don't think that FDA is doing good, honest reviews," Richard Burroughs, Ph.D., told the *Village Voice* in 1995. (10)   Burroughs, a veterinarian, was fired from the FDA in November 1989 after working closely on the review of Monsanto's data in their rBST application.   While working at FDA during the mid-1980s at the height of review of Monsanto's drug application (originally filed in 1981), Burroughs would later testify that he was often frustrated that Monsanto would not comply with his suggestions.   He had noted a large number of udder infections to dairy cows treated with rBST.   Burroughs noted biased research and wanted Monsanto to design experiments that would closely parallel effects of rBST if the drug was approved.

For example, on a dairy farm, after the birth of a calf, the cow must be "put back into service" as soon as possible.   Cash flow and proper management are necessary for a dairy farmer's financial survival.   Do you believe that a dairy farmer "dumps" milk from that cow early in the lactation period because there are more hormones in that milk?   He is required to!   In spite of the fact that FDA does not believe that hormones in milk work, it is against the law for a farmer to sell the early milk because people must be protected from drinking milk containing large amounts of hormones, hormones that they claim do not work.   What logic!

Bad Science

One prime example of bad science is a study listed as reference #49 in the landmark Juskevich and Guyer paper, authored by Paul Groenewegen, in which only three cows were treated with rBST.   The study began at twenty-eight days postpartum.   The design of the experiment was unscientific.   Three animals for a statistical study!   Imagine if they did Nielsen television ratings that way or determined presidential elections by polling the opinions of three people?   The FDA reviewer commenting on this study wrote:

The need to pursue more definitive studies has already

been stated as unnecessary because bGH (rBST) is
biologically inactive in humans and orally inactive.

Orally inactive? Tell that to the lab animals developing cancer in reference
#42 of the Juskevich and Guyer paper. Imagine the pressure on this idealistic
veterinarian, Burroughs. He was in a political environment. He was witnessing
sick cows as result of rBST treatment. The data that he reviewed were biased and
manipulated. He could not go the press. Monsanto would not cooperate. His
boss, the director of new animal drug studies at the CVM, would harass him each
time that Burroughs noted a problem. Burroughs knew that the health and safety
of the American people would be in jeopardy if this drug were approved. What
was in greater jeopardy was Burroughs' job security at FDA.

What was Richard Burroughs' reward? A close family friend recently said
that on his last day at FDA Burroughs was slammed against a wall by a security
guard injuring his nose. A member of Burroughs' family confirmed this story. His
arm was twisted and his thumb bent into an awkward position which ripped
tendons. Burroughs was handcuffed and arrested and an ambulance had to take
him to a hospital under police guard. All of this while his wife and two children
waited outside for him in the family car. Charges were later filed against him for
animal cruelty in attempts to destroy his veterinary practice. Thousands of dollars
in legal fees were included in the severance package to this public servant. The
letter which three congressmen sent to GAO included a reference to this treatment
of Burroughs. That letter asked for an investigation of what appeared to be:

> [A] case of retaliation against employees who
> challenge the CVM's review of animal drugs.

Burroughs is living proof that pharmaceutical companies are not as evil as
Hollywood would make them out to be. In the movie, *I Love Trouble*, a man like
Burroughs would have met an untimely accident. Getting fired was a gift, and
Burroughs can maintain his sanity and regain his dignity. People like Burroughs
are the real American heroes. It is a shame that more individuals like this are not
in positions of power. They have never learned the complicated art of combining
science and politics.

Margaret Miller, Ph.D.

My FOIA request made on July 17, 1995, revealed that Miller began work
at FDA on December 3, 1989. Who, possessing all of their faculties, leaves a
company a few weeks before Christmas bonuses are due? Miller had as much to
do in having researched rbST as anybody still employed by Monsanto. She now
would be working for the key agency, FDA, which would insure approval for her

previous employer, Monsanto. On her job application Miller indicated that she was a senior research specialist at Monsanto and that she had averaged 50 hour work weeks. In describing her tasks at Monsanto, Miller wrote on her federal employment application:

> Currently I supervise the residue and metabolism and clinical
> chemistry, endocrinology Laboratory. This laboratory develops,
> validates, and performs analyses on blood, milk, and meat;
> required to demonstrate the safety and efficacy of recombinant
> bovine and porcine somatotropin and other biotechnology
> products. This position requires understanding of FDA and
> EEC regulations, development and validation of assays to fulfill
> these requirements, writing reports and documentation for
> submission to regulatory agencies. I am responsible for having
> developed and validated several immunoassays for analyzing
> proteins and steroids in complex biological matrices,
> implemented a microwave-based laboratory automation system,
> validated a ⟨WORD BLACKENED OUT⟩ clinical chemistry
> analyzer to perform blood chemistries on animal samples and
> supervise five to eight technicians. All laboratory procedures
> are performed under Good Laboratory Practices Guidelines; and
> data is submitted to FDA. (11)

Miller, by her own admission, was an important member of Monsanto's biotechnology "team." Monsanto placed this important employee directly within FDA to review, analyze and help gain the approval of their new technology. FDA never required Monsanto to develop a test to detect the levels of genetically engineered bovine proteins in blood and milk. It is curious that Miller, in her questionnaire, found it necessary to blacken out a key word that might have revealed the secret that such a test had already been developed. Dr. Miller had left Monsanto in 1989. She was the instrumental researcher on BST safety studies. When she joined the FDA she was careful to impose a self-moratorium so as not to work on any BST-related issues. The letter from the three congressmen to GAO specifically cited the statutes violated by Miller (and others):

> Thus, there is strong evidence that all three employees
> may have violated at least two ethical regulations
> applicable to them pursuant to the Code of Federal
> Regulations (43 CFR s.7373b-201 and 5CFR s2365.502).

In spite of Miller's caution, she was the expert, and the bulk of BST research and review crossed her desk. She knew that there was a direct conflict of interest each time she made a suggestion or determination on any BST issue. Yet, Miller wrote the FDA labeling opinion which guaranteed that consumers would be kept in the dark when they purchased milk that was genetically engineered. To label or not to label? That was just one of the many BST questions facing FDA. Would consumers purchase milk that had been treated with genetically engineered hormones? FDA reasoned that they would not. The policy of proving that genetically engineered milk was indistinguishable from normal wholesome milk became FDA's primary directive. Monsanto had to enjoy FDA's help. This was just the first of many genetically engineered food products Monsanto wished to control. After BST came tomatoes. Monsanto purchased Calgene, a biotechnology company owning the patents to the new tomato gene. In 1996 Monsanto Agricultural Company would spin off from all other Monsanto enterprises to position themselves for the new millennium. In late 1996 and early 1997, Monsanto's genetically engineered soybeans, corn and wheat began to find their way into America's foods. Thanks to precedents set with BST, the labeling of these new foods became a moot point. Miller and Taylor, two ex-Monsanto employees, had a mission at FDA. They paved the way for a nonlabeling policy. Americans have a right to know. Thanks to FDA, they do not. During this controversy David Kessler acted as FDA commissioner, overseeing FDA's mission from 1990 through 1996.

Miller joined FDA in December 1989. Why then, did she submit a paper with Collier of Monsanto to a peer-reviewed scientific journal after she began working at the FDA? The note on the paper reads:

" The article was written by MAM (Miller) in her private capacity?" (12)

In other words, this was perhaps her hobby, along with knitting and needlepoint. The note further insults the reader's intelligence by continuing:

"No official support or endorsement by the agency (FDA)
is, or should be, inferred."

The title of the paper was "Nutrient Balance and Stage of Lactation Affect Response of Insulin, Insulin-Like Growth Factors I and II, and Insulin-Like Growth Factor-Binding Protein 2 to Somatotropin Administration in Dairy Cows." She must have done this work with Monsanto on her own personal time. A more appropriate title might have been, "How I Spent My Summer Vacation." The paper was presented at the 82nd Annual Meeting of the American Society of Animal Science in Ames, Iowa, and also presented at the American Dairy Science Association Meeting in Lexington, Kentucky, and published in the *Journal of Animal Science*. Did Margaret Miller travel to these conventions to present her paper? If so, did she pay for her plane tickets, or did Monsanto, or FDA? Did she travel on company time? Conflict of interests? Maybe this was just her hobby.

Miller also had another paper presented at meetings in 1990 while she was working at FDA. This second paper was "Response of Somatomedins (IGF-I and IGF-II) in Lactating Cows to Variations in Dietary Energy and Protein and Treatment with Recombinant n-Methionyl Bovine Somatotropin." (13) This project was conducted with Dale Bauman, Ph.D., who was on Monsanto's payroll performing research at Cornell University Agricultural Station. Miller is quite expert on BST and IGF matters, but having left Monsanto in 1989, perhaps she felt that she had no obligation to keep up with current IGF research. Our conversations in 1994 confirmed her ignorance of current research performed by hospitals and universities outside of Monsanto's influence.

Miller admitted to me that she drank milk and consumed dairy products. She researched levels of IGF more than ten different lactations and found them to increase by an across the board average of 78 percent. Miller believes that IGF does not increase after rBST treatment, in spite of her own research. Miller worked under the impression that 500,000 ng of IGF were present in the adult body. How could drinking a glass of milk which contained 2000 ng have any significant effect, she wondered? There is the reference and the author of a study in which total levels of free and unbound IGF were measured to be equal to the same amount of IGF contained in one glass of normal untreated milk. (Frystyk, Institute of Research, University Hospital, Aarhus, Denmark, published on July 11, 1994). This research contradicted Miller's previous assumptions, proving that her conclusions were incorrectly applied.

Miller should never have been judge, jury, and prosecutor on the rBST drug application. If one individual were to have that awesome power, that individual should not have arrived in Washington, D.C., with Monsanto stickers on her baggage.

Miller "pulled the strings" behind the scenes at FDA. She did not sign into policy the actual milk labeling order. She simply wrote it and Taylor signed it. When opinions were published in FDA papers or newsletters, Miller was the expert, the one behind those opinions. She was careful not to leave a paper trail. Her name did not appear in the articles. Judy Juskevich revealed that Margaret Miller reviewed the research in the IGF-I discussion and presented data for her to write. Linda Grasse, who edits FDA newsletters, told me that it was Miller who instructed her to write:

> There is no absolutely no possibility that the consumption of milk from rbST-treated cows could increase the risk of breast cancer. (14)

Margaret Miller's Crime Against America: The Mastitis Controversy

While performing her research at Monsanto, Miller observed that cows treated with rbGH developed ulcers on their udders. A group of FDA employees wrote that confidential letter to numerous members of the House of Representatives and the Senate complaining that Miller "...arbitrarily changed the acceptable level of antibiotics in milk."   While Miller worked at Monsanto, before leaving the pharmaceutical company for her new job as an FDA employee, the allowable limit, by law, of antibiotic residues in milk was one part per hundred-million. After Miller arrived at FDA she changed that number to one part per million. She increased by 100 times the amounts of antibiotics Americans could drink. The CDC has issued memorandums alerting America that antibiotics no longer seem to work.

Suzanne Sechen, Ph.D.

Suzanne Sechen's name sticks out in reference #75 of the Juskevich and Guyer paper which says, "We thank S. Sechen for her contributions to the manuscript." A second individual investigated by the GAO was Suzanne Sechen, Ph.D., who had been a student at Cornell University.   Sechen worked with Dale Bauman, who published numerous papers with Margaret Miller. The scientific community performing bovine research was a small one. All of the "players" knew each other and had close working relationships with Monsanto. Sechen reviewed rBST data for the agency in 1988 after performing research for Monsanto. FDA began writing the landmark paper authored by Juskevich and Guyer in 1988. Sechen worked with Margaret Miller who wrote part of that report while working for Monsanto. Why wasn't Miller thanked for her contributions to the manuscript? Sechen was no minor participant in this "game" although her involvement has been downplayed by FDA, Monsanto and the GAO.

Miller was cleared by the GAO investigation. So was Sechen. GAO found that there was no evidence that Miller participated in the approval process for rBST. However, Miller has recently admitted writing part of the Juskevich and Guyer paper. She made this admission to two investigators from the Freedom of Information Clearing House who included this information in a July 11, 1995, letter to me which said:

> He (Deighton, a Freedom of Information Act FDA employee)
> spoke with the chief researcher on the *Science* article, Ms.
> Margaret Miller who states that she wrote the parts of the article
> referring to the Eli Lilly studies and that she did not share the
> information she relied upon with Monsanto. (15)

Here's the evidence that GAO never investigated. Miller was not supposed to be working on this subject. This was a conflict of interest. Furthermore, if she was one of the authors of this scientific article her name should have been listed as an author. This demonstrates a lack of scientific and journalistic integrity. Miller's role could be compared with the actions of a virus. Lurking where she was unobserved, she invaded the host and exerted her influence. Better analogy. Margaret Miller was no virus. She was a powerful growth factor. Miller was the human insulin-like growth factor. She did not initiate this firestorm of controversy. She was simply the "gasoline added to the fire."

Nobody will ever know (except the participants) the actual duties performed by Sechen. Nobody will know the conversations she had with her colleagues or with Monsanto personnel during the approval process. One seemingly random event after another occurred involving researchers from colleges and universities, independent labs and pharmaceutical firms, and key government officials. Was it conspiracy, coincidence or a conspiracy of ignorance? Either way, Monsanto was the beneficiary.

Michael Taylor, Esq.

Michael Taylor, Esq., was a partner at King & Spalding, Monsanto's Washington law firm. Taylor's hiring preceded FDA Commissioner Kessler's tenure. Kessler had to be aware of Taylor's Monsanto connections. Kessler, the attorney, had to know that he was "protected." Why did Taylor go to FDA from a powerful firm where Monsanto was his special client? He could not have continued to draw his share of partnership profits from his firm, could he? That angle was never investigated by GAO, and if it had occurred it would be the same type of conflict of interest that has placed lesser men in jail, from Watergate through the Iran-Contra Affair to Whitewater. If, at the FDA, he received his share of partnership money from his law firm while Monsanto was still a client, Taylor would have to be held accountable for his action.

Maybe he was not compensated for his move from a high-paying partner in a prestigious law firm to that of a public servant at FDA. What was Taylor promised? How was he recruited? By whom? Did Taylor take orders from Kessler or vice versa? Who instructed Kessler? In 1991, while he worked at FDA, Taylor officially recused himself from participating in any policy decisions regarding Monsanto. He recognized that it would be a conflict for him to be involved in any activity in which Monsanto received benefit by regulatory actions. Yet, Taylor, deputy FDA commissioner for policy, signed the memorandum in which FDA published its approval of Monsanto's rBST application. Furthermore, amid great controversy, Taylor reviewed and signed the labeling law regulations which did not require rBST-treated milk or dairy products to be so identified.

Taylor performed a role that was even more important for Monsanto (and the entire pharmaceutical industry). Taylor's interpretation of Congressional cancer laws alleviated the responsibility of companies like Monsanto in this and future drug studies and applications. While working as an attorney for King & Spalding, Taylor wrote a legal opinion which was submitted to and published in the *Journal of the American College of Toxicology*. Taylor worked closely with other King & Spalding attorneys who performed different tasks for Monsanto. King & Spalding lawyers have a history of being rewarded by our government for such service. Michael Taylor followed another lawyer from his firm into serving his nation. That other Monsanto attorney? Clarence Thomas, now a Supreme Court Justice. As of September, 1997, King & Spalding's Food and Drug Practice group consisted of twelve attorneys who together have worked for a collective period of 45 years in FDA's Chief Counsel's Office.

Michael Taylor, FDA, under-secretary at USDA, and Clarence Thomas, Supreme Court Justice. Both King & Spalding attorneys who represented Monsanto. Donald Rumsfeld, ex-G.D. Searle President (G.D. Searle was purchased by Monsanto in 1989) and Bob Dole's campaign chief. America? The land of opportunity and opportunists! Taylor gave clue to his future performance by inserting a quote on the title page of his Delaney Amendment article:

> One of the most delicate tasks a court faces is the application
> of the legislative mandate of a prior generation to novel
> circumstances created by a culture grown more complex.

> Judge Irving R. Kaufman

Many have made similar arguments as they apply to the Constitution of the United States. The founding fathers never imagined that we would genetically engineer milk. The Supreme Court has intermittently dealt with similar premises over the years and had repeatedly struck down such arguments. Taylor attempted to supersede this important act of Congress by writing "The De Minimus Interpretation of the Delaney Clause: Legal and Policy Rationale." Many people believe that Taylor's move to FDA was a Monsanto set-up. They believe that he was moved there to determine rBST policy. These people are wrong. Miller had already accomplished the task. Taylor signed Miller's work into policy and law. Taylor came to FDA to rewrite policy as it was affected by the Delaney Clause.

The Delaney Clause. People are terrified of cancer. Four decades ago Americans lived in fear of two major cataclysms. One was nuclear war with the Soviet Union. Another was receiving a diagnosis of cancer, which was most often an incurable and painful death sentence. In the late 1950s, one of the goals of Congress was to enact a Food Additives Act. People were becoming more aware of the factors that were known to induce cancer. Although only a few substances were actually identifiable as carcinogenic, scientists were developing new techniques including analytical methods which were implicating chemicals in our food supply to be carcinogens.

As a result of much debate, Congress passed the Food Additive Amendment to the Federal Food, Drug and Cosmetic Act in 1958. The goal of this amendment was to insure that the safety of Americans would be safeguarded from the consumption of any food product containing a chemical additive. The Delaney Clause was actually a safety standard which stated that no food additive would be deemed safe if it was found to induce cancer when eaten by people or laboratory animals. Taylor's interpretation of this clause would set new policy at FDA. This amendment is one of the reasons that pharmaceutical companies conduct short term studies, such as the 90/180-day study which was so heavily relied upon by Monsanto. If rats got cancer, poof, good-bye investment. Monsanto could hardly justify $600 million dollars for researching one drug application. When rbST-treated laboratory animals experienced enormous spleen growth and developed cancers in the 1988 Searle experiment (reference #42 in the Juskevich and Guyer paper), they had to protect their investment in the new genetic engineering technology. BST represented the future of genetic engineering. Bad publicity at this point in time could set back Monsanto's plans.

Taylor's incipient assignment? Attack the 1958 Delaney Clause. Just what is a "reasonable certainty?" FDA now ignores the original intent of the Delaney Clause. According to Taylor:

FDA now interprets the Delaney Clause as simply not operating
to prohibit substances that, although found to induce cancer in animals,
can be judged to pose extremely low or essentially non-existent risks
under anticipated conditions of human exposure.

Taylor argues that FDA should have leeway in determining just how trivial those risks might be. Taylor goes in, writes policy, uses his capabilities to remove all obstacles, and then is promoted to under-secretary of Agriculture. What will Taylor do next? Secretary of Agriculture? Newly appointed director of FDA? Still to be determined is who actually put him there and why. As of the fall of 1996, Taylor was back at King & Spalding. If you believe that Monsanto will get a return on their investment, first, buy plenty of their stock. This newly designed milk hormone is only the tip of the iceberg. Second, buy a couple of acres and start growing your own fruits and vegetables. That's the only way you will know what goes into your own body. Monsanto, FDA, Congress - they all have other interests, and those interests do not include your safety. Michael Taylor laid the groundwork for the repeal of the Delaney Amendment. At FDA he set into motion a new set of standard operating procedures which ignored the law and intent of Congress. In

August 1996, a bipartisan Congress enacted HR 1627, the Food Policy Protection Act, which once and for all invalidated the Delaney Act.

The GAO Investigation: Conflicts of Interest

The United States General Accounting Office (GAO) is an agency that audits issues rather then financial records. The GAO exists as the investigative branch of Congress. At the formal bequest of a congressman, GAO will assign staff to investigate any problem that exists in our government. GAO was involved in two rBST investigations. The first study reviewed health concerns, particularly mastitis issues. GAO can only make recommendations in response to congressional requests. GAO recommended a delay in rBST approval. Congress did not act on GAO's analyses.

The second study was a conflict of interest hearing which ended with release of GAO's report on October 30, 1994. FDA's Commissioner Kessler announced that "GAO conducted a thorough and exhaustive review of the actions of these employees (Taylor, Sechen and Miller). This report clears them and they have the full support of this agency." Bernard Sanders, Independent congressman from Vermont, commented:

> The FDA allowed corporate influence to run rampant in its approval
> of the drug. The report showed problems with FDA leadership.

Sander's aide, Anthony Pollina, added, "When you read it carefully as we have, you see at least eleven violations of the rules that are clearly there." Jeremy Rifkin of the Pure Foods Campaign, said the report was "devastating." GAO called the eleven violations minor because no financial conflicts of interest were found.

Margaret Miller violated FDA ethics rules at least eight times, the report concluded. She illegally published eight articles for Monsanto while writing the labeling laws which Taylor "drafted, refined, and signed off on." Suzanne Sechen, as a graduate student, researched rBST studies for Monsanto. She was assigned the role of reviewing her own studies. She also reviewed what GAO calls a "pivotal study" which was presented by her co-author (and professor at Cornell) Bauman. Pollina's final comment on the matter reflected the feelings of many rBST critics:

> I honestly don't know why GAO played this down. We were frankly
> quite surprised at their resistance in pursuing it. But one must
> remember that Monsanto has an immense amount of political and
> financial power. And this goes beyond rBGH, calling into question
> the larger issue of biotechnology.

On August 6, 1992, GAO finished its first rBST investigation. In a report addressed to five United States senators, including Al Gore, and four members of the House of Representatives, the GAO recommended that FDA approval of rBST should be withheld. The title of the GAO report was "RECOMBINANT BOVINE GROWTH HORMONE FDA Approval Should Be Withheld Until the Mastitis Issue Is Resolved." At the time of this report FDA had approved rBST for research only. Actual approval for Monsanto to market their rbST drug, "Posilac," would come in November 1994. GAO was particularly concerned that evaluation of indirect human food safety risks were never investigated. According to GAO, the increased milk production in cows would trigger an increase in the incidence of mastitis, which would often be treated with antibiotics. As a consequence, higher levels of antibiotics would enter the milk supply. FDA's innovative solution to the mastitis issue was to have Miller determine new specifications for acceptable levels of antibiotics found in milk.

GAO also was critical of the entire process of research. They discovered that a gap existed in the data given to FDA and in FDA's ability to review such data. The FDA guidelines failed to include a potentially critical area for human food safety. No research has examined this area. The reason FDA did not require additional tests was because they accepted Monsanto's representation that the milk hormones were not orally active. FDA's conclusions were made despite the fact that research from all over the world from dozens of colleges, laboratories and hospitals implicated these hormones as exerting powerful effects. These data were not part of Monsanto's application and were not considered.

It would have been the responsibility of FDA scientists to abstract these articles taking into consideration not only biased Monsanto research but unbiased research as well. Being the "experts," they should have acted in a professional manner. FDA experts, who had been assigned the task of reviewing data in an unbiased and impartial manner, turned out to be ex-Monsanto employees carefully chosen and placed into positions of power. GAO recommended that FDA study the feasibility of labeling milk and dairy products derived from cows treated with rBST.

GAO found that insulin-like growth factor does increase in milk treated with rBST, but they went on to comment that these increases may not pose a risk because IGF is not toxic and is already present in the human system. GAO did not review specific data from Monsanto's research. If they had they would have discovered that rBST was orally active. GAO conclusion accepted FDA statement of no evidence of oral activity. Boris Kachura, senior investigator at GAO, made possible my meeting with FDA scientists. Kachura smelled a laboratory rat at work but never had the opportunity to trap that rat. Rats are careful not to leave crumbs. "Crumbs" (rotten people) are careful not to leave paper trails. Yet, one trail exists. That secret report which FDA possesses and Monsanto refuses to release will prove that laboratory animals got cancer from oral ingestion of rBST.

There is only one reason for keeping it secret, and that is to protect all of the guilty parties in this conspiracy.

The Food and Drug Administration

      I was thirty minutes early for my appointment at the Center For Veterinary Medicine (CVM) in Rockville, Maryland. The date was April 21, 1995. I had been invited to discuss rBST issues with a team of scientists within the branch of FDA that investigates new drug applications. This meeting with scientists was also scheduled to include Robert Sauer, who would be discussing my concerns regarding the FDA's procedure in dealing with my Freedom of Information Act requests. Also in attendance were Richard Teske, Ph.D., Robert Condon, Ph.D., John Leighton, Ph.D., and William Marnane, Ph.D. Margaret Miller, Ph.D., was also scheduled to attend our session. I was disappointed when she did not make the meeting. No individual who I had spoken to had more knowledge about IGF.

      Teske explained that she had other commitments. Although this meeting was a "commitment," one of the group later commented that her anticipation of the meeting had caused such anxiety that she had simply called in sick. Every time that a decision of comment or conclusion was made about rBST, Miller was attributed as the source. Miller was quietly controlling people and events at the CVM. Regarding her rBST actions, she was clearly the one, behind the scenes, who was in charge.

      Security at this building was tight, offering peace of mind to visitors of any federal building one week after the horrible bombing in Oklahoma City. The building was of modern design, with exquisite marble floors adding an air of out of place elegance to an edifice housing government scientists.

      I had attained a great deal of knowledge of FDA personnel and their personalities in the months preceding my meeting, and understood that these were no ordinary scientists. These were men and women of science who had to be on the alert to every political implication in each statement, both written and orally made. The pressure to stay true to one's scientific philosophy and objectives had to be enormous. Rockville, Maryland, is a lovely community located in the shadow of Washington, D.C. The main road contained mall after mall of upscale shops which my wife, who accompanied me, referred to as "shopping mall heaven." Because of Rockville's proximity to Washington, FDA employees refer to the nation's capitol as "downtown." The pressures of politics trickle down and play key roles in FDA decision making.

      I was invited to this meeting by Stephen Sundlof, Ph.D., the director of CVM. Sundlof was at a meeting "downtown." The actual agenda of the meeting was conducted by Teske, who is the "hands on" director of animal research and the drug approval process. The meeting occurred because Boris Kachura, a senior investigator at the GAO called Linda Suydam (who was second in command of the entire FDA under Commissioner Kessler). After filing my citizen petition which called for the removal of rBST from the market more than six months earlier, I had continued learning and researching the rBST and IGF issues and I presented my theories and evidence at this meeting.

Cohen Paper Submitted to FDA

TITLE

Recombinant bovine somatotropin (rBST) increases levels of insulin-like growth factor (IGF) in milk; IGF in milk is orally active; IGF is a key factor in the growth and survival of cancer in animals and humans.

INTRODUCTION

The Food and Drug Administration (FDA) approved the use of a genetically engineered version of bovine somatotropin (rBST) after a process which represented the most researched and controversial drug application in history. This paper will explore three major topics:

1

The data presented to FDA was not rigorously reviewed, was presented in a biased manner, and the actual product which was approved by FDA was significantly different than the actual product in use today.

2

Numerous tests including toxicology studies were not performed because it was predetermined that there could be no biological effects upon animals or humans from oral ingestion of rBST or IGF. This conclusion was made because of a belief that strong digestive enzymes would destroy milk hormones. This paper will demonstrate that milk is an enzyme inhibitor and that hormones survive digestion.

3

IGF is a key factor in the growth and survival of tumors in humans. IGF is a proliferative growth hormone which increases after cows are treated with BST.

Milk and dairy products are staples in the American diet and represent the largest food industry in the United States. To increase milk output of cows, scientists have genetically engineered bovine growth hormone through DNA technology and have developed a substance which was meant to be similar to a cow's normally occurring somatotropic hormone. Through the use of genetic engineering technology the bacterium, E. coli, received the gene that enabled it to produce a synthetic version of the natural bovine growth hormone.

A GENE TRANSCRIPTION ERROR

Monsanto (1*) has admitted that an unusual amino acid was created by their new technology. Amino acid #144 which should have been lysine has been replaced on the normal chain with epsilon-N-acetyllysine. Monsanto's publication did not indicate how long (after rBST was introduced into milk in 1990) this unusual amino acid has been consumed by the American milk drinking public.

DATA WERE NEVER PROPERLY REVIEWED

The FDA and Monsanto, manufacturer of rBST, collaborated on a paper (2*) which was published in *Science*. This article was intended to end the controversy surrounding rBST. As a result of this article, the *Journal of the American Medical Association* and the National Institutes of Health endorsed rBST use. Evidence exists that the data in that article were not reviewed by the NIH or *JAMA*. Unpublished reports were cited but never made available for peer review. By not making available actual data for tissue and organ weights of subjects treated with genetically engineered hormones, peer review was compromised. References were requested through the Freedom of Information Act office but Monsanto cites "trade protection" and hides behind a protective veil.

ACTUAL REFERENCES NEVER PEER REVIEWED

(From the Juskevich and Guyer paper:)

Ref. # 40 is an unpublished Upjohn report.
Ref. # 41 is an unpublished Hazleton Lab report.
Reef. # 42 is an unpublished Searle report.
Ref. # 43 is an unpublished American Cyanamid report.
Ref. # 44 is an unpublished Eli Lilly report.
Ref. # 70 is an unpublished Elanco report.

It is clear that these reports are shared by Monsanto competition. Trade protection should not be reason to deny a researcher access to reports cited as references.

BST-TREATED MILK DIFFERS FROM UNTREATED MILK

The Juskevich and Guyer paper contradicts the conclusion reached by FDA, NIH and the World Health Organization. All agree that milk from rBST-treated cows is indistinguishable from the milk of nontreated cows. Their conclusion contradicts the actual data presented. The authors state:

Recombinant bGH treatment produces an increase in the concentration of insulin-like growth factor-I (IGF-I) in cow's milk.

BIOLOGICAL EFFECTS

Data in the Juskevich paper suggest that there are indeed biological effects from oral ingestion of rBGH on laboratory animals. Animals reacting to subcutaneous injections demonstrated significantly large and abnormal spleen growth rates (as compared to the control group). From table #2 on page 878 we note that the typical male spleen increased in size 39.6 percent while the female spleen grew 46 percent. Those doing the research had to note these dramatic numbers and had to have observed the spleen effects from oral ingestion.

Reprinted from *Science* - August, 1990, Page 878

Table 2 Absolute organ weights (in grams) in control rats and rbGH rats. Charles River CD rats (*n*=30 rats per sex) were treated for 90 days with rbGH either by gavage or by subcutaneous administrations, and one group of animals served as untreated controls. From (42) @ 1989 Monsanto Agricultural Company.

Organ		Subcutaneous	Oral			
	0	1.0	0.1	0.5	5.0	50.0
MALES						
Kidneys	3.677	4.188	3.178	3.695	3.540	3.544
Liver	16.549	20.364	15.614	15.740	15.993	15.098
Heart	1.726	1.941	1.645	1.608	1.618	1.640
Spleen	0.912	1.274	0.910	1.051	0.987	1.002
FEMALES						
Kidneys	2.067	2.464	2.040	2.170	2.102	2.025
Liver	8.637	11.146	8.302	8.754	8.446	8.297
Heart	1.041	1.215	1.061	1.101	1.034	1.070
Spleen	0.585	0.855	0.601	0.663	0.630	0.608

Let us examine what occurs to the animals (mean averages):

1) subcutaneous males gained 39.69 percent spleen weight
2) subcutaneous females gained 46.15 percent spleen weight
3) oral males gained 8.33 percent spleen weight
4) oral females gained 6.92 percent spleen weight

The subject animals in this study were sacrificed after 90 days. Scientists at the Albert Einstein College of Medicine found that mice treated with IGF-II developed a diverse spectrum of tumors at a higher frequency than controls after 18 months of age. This long latent period before tumors arise and the wide spectrum of tumor types suggest that IGF may function primarily as a tumor progression factor in mice via autocrine and endocrine mechanisms of action. **(3*)**

There is evidence of such latent effects in Juskevich. Data is presented in a remarkably biased manner:

Table #1 (Page 877) Body weight changes (in grams) of control rats and rbGH-treated rats. Charles River rats were treated for 90 days with rbGH either by gavage or by subcutaneous injection; and one group of animals served as untreated controls. From (42) @ 1989 Monsanto Agricultural Company

Only The Control Group And Subcutaneous Group Weights Appear To Illustrate The Point Of Data Manipulation By The Monsanto/FDA Publication.

STUDY DAY	Control		Subcutaneous
		MALES	
8	58		72
29	170		207
50	239		294
85	324		432
		FEMALES	
8	24		33
29	81		101
50	110		150
85	148		217

The average weight gains for subcutaneous animals (per time period) are 20-30 percent greater than the control group. Look closely at the parameters. Is this a standard chart? Day 8, day 29, day 50, and day 85? Did the data simply fit neatly into these designated time slots?

Let's examine what occurs to the animals between days 50 and 85. The average male gains 62 percent more weight than the control male during that period. The average female gains 76 percent more than the average control female.

This is a very clever nonpresentation of data. There is indeed a dramatic latency growth spurt that occurs at some time two months after initial introduction of the hormone.

It would be interesting to do statistical analyses on all of the subjects cited in the Juskevich article, but alas, FDA and MONSANTO will not release such data, citing the privilege of protection from exclusivity of "trade secrets."

No oral effects? In addition to the average male (Table 2) gaining (from oral ingestion) 8.33 percent in his spleen weight, the average female gains 6.92 percent. The average male also loses 5.10 percent kidney weight, loses 5.6675 percent liver weight, and loses 5.692 percent heart weight (when compared with the control group). These are biological effects! Are they statistically significant? We may never know because freedom of information requests are not enough to induce FDA or Monsanto into releasing data necessary to perform such analyses. (Requests by this author have been denied.)

IGF - CELL PROLIFERATION AND CANCER

Should IGF (insulin growth factor) be such a concern? Hammond and Collier, writing for Monsanto Agricultural Company state:

> Based upon the no oral effect levels determined in rat
> gavage studies (oral ingestion of rBGH), it is possible to
> approximate safety factors for ingestion of these two
> proteins (sometribove and IGF-I). However, estimation of
> safety factors for sometribove (BST, rBGH) consumption
> is not necessary, since it would not be orally active in
> humans even if it could be absorbed. IGF-I is not
> orally active in laboratory animals supporting a large
> margin of safety for their consumption. **(4*)**

The most recent research would tend to support the dramatic role that IGF plays in cellular growth. Kleinman reports that IGF-I is found to be involved in the growth regulation of endometrial tumor cells and is 30 times more potent than insulin suggesting that the effects of these growth factors are mediated by the IGF-I receptor. **(5*)** D'Errico notes that results obtained using molecular biology techniques suggest a possible role for insulin-like growth factor II (IGF-II) in the pathogenesis of hepatocellular carcinoma (HCC). **(6*)** Kwok has found that the biological effects of IGF-I are initiated by its binding to the IGF-I receptor, which is able to transduce mitogenic and metabolic signals, supporting the hypothesis that the IGF-I receptor is involved in the development of diabetic vascular complications. **(7*)** Wimalasena found IGF-I to increase cell growth, and a maximal effect of three-to-five-fold increase in cell number was observed. **(8*)**

There is evidence that IGF functions on a nanomolecular level. MCF-7 cancer cells proliferate in response to nanomolar concentrations of IGF-I and IGF-II. De-Leon reported that the actions of both peptides are mediated through the IGF-I receptor concluding that IGF-I and IGF-II are potent mitogens in MCF-7 cells and can stimulate cell proliferation through all three receptors. **(9*)** Martin reports that IGF-II stimulates cell proliferation via the type I IGF receptor. The type I IGF receptor mediates IGF-II induced autocrine neuroblastoma cell growth. **(10*)**

Ambrose observed that the interaction of insulin-like growth factors with the IGF-I receptor is an important step in the control of cell proliferation and development. In particular, IGF-I and IGF-II are key regulators of central nervous system development and may modulate the growth of glial tumors. **(11*)** Nielsen noted that the transcription of IGF-II genes leads to the production of significant amounts of IGF-II which stimulate the proliferation of MSRCT (cancerous growths) by interaction with IGF-I receptors on the cells. **(12*)**

FDA, based upon Monsanto's research, continues to proclaim that IGF in milk has no effect on human metabolism. IGF-I is a mitogenic growth factor. Prager found rat cells responding to in vitro IGF-I treatment by increased proliferation and DNA synthesis. Tumor cell assays confirmed continued expression of IGF-I receptors. Raile observed similar effects. **(13*)** Insulin-like growth factor I and II were implicated in the growth promotion of in vivo tumors and tumor cells in vitro. Tumor cells responded to an addition of exogenous insulin growth factor with an increase of DNA synthesis. **(14*)**

Langford found that IGF-I has multiple metabolic actions and effects on a the differentiation and proliferation of a wide variety of cell types. **(15*)**

IGF IN MILK SURVIVES DIGESTION

FDA continues to accept the premise made by Monsanto that IGF-I is degraded by digestive enzymes and is not active in the upper gastrointestinal tract. FDA's conclusion is echoed by most respected observers.

Yet, according to Olanrewaju, recently published in the *American Journal of Physiology*, infusion of IGF in rats (in levels similar to those in bovine milk) increases the cellularity of the intestinal mucosa. **(16*)** Data indirectly supports the hypothesis that dietary IGF-I may be absorbed. This was supported by Baumrucker at the Department of Dairy and Animal Science at Pennsylvania State University who wrote that dietary IGF-I may be absorbed and causes transient systemic effects in the newborn calf. **(17*)**

Taylor reports that insulin-like growth factors have a potent mitogenic effect on the bowel. **(18*)**

Playford reports that milk proteins prevent digestion of luminal growth factors, allowing them to stimulate intestinal growth. **(19*)** Casein acts as an enzyme inhibitor. Unlike IGF-I in serum, IGF-I secreted into the gastrointestinal lumen is not bound to insulin-like growth factor I binding proteins. Since the growth factor is not protein bound, its concentration in the gut lumen may be high enough to exert biological activity. IGF is actually absorbed in a similar manner to EGF and passes through the digestive system undigested.

Rat milk soluble fraction (RMSF) protects milk borne peptides in the gastro-intestinal lumen by inhibiting in vitro the luminal peptidolysis, according to Rao. **(20*)**

Oster presented evidence that bovine xanthine oxidase is entrapped in liposomal form by the milk homogenization process. In this form milk resists gastric digestion and becomes biologically available. **(21*)** As a result of unnatural micronization (homogenization) the number of fat globules are increased and the size of those globules reduced. This enhances hormonal carrier potential and the permeability of intestinal mucosa increases as does hormonal absorption.

FDA is incorrect in assuming that IGFs are broken down in the gut, and therefore cannot affect animal or human metabolic functions. The evidence overwhelmingly contradicts this conclusion.

NATURALLY OCCURRING IGF IN THE HUMAN BODY

Human blood and saliva does contain IGF-I. That IGF-I is bound to proteins and receptors, and are building components of cellular material. An analogy must be made to the levels of IGF-I present in the human body. If one were able to analyze the average home, one could make the statement that the home contained a 55-gallon drum of glue. One could not walk through the house and find that glue; it would be present in the carpet, sheetrock, tiles, furniture, etc. If an individual walked into that house with a bucket of free flowing unbound glue, splashing that bucket as he walked through the house, he would be creating great damage.

Free IGF works the same way. The actual levels of free IGF-I are relatively quite small. They have been measured; most recently by Frystyk who found that IGF-I levels in humans were inversely proportional to age ranging from 950 ng/L (20-30 years of age) to 410 ng/L (60+ years of age). Levels of IGF-II were independent of age, being 1480 ng/L. **(22*)**

SYNERGISM OF IGF WITH OTHER HORMONES

The mediating effects of IGFs appear to be greatly enhanced and are synergistic when combined with other factors. Kachra found that when glucagon and GH (growth hormone) are combined with rBGH (50 ng/ml), they augmented increased levels of IGF-I up to 12-fold. **(23*)**

Frodin demonstrated that the combined effect of IGFs and bFGF (bovine follicle growth factor) is synergistic. **(24*)** The degree of synergism was two-to-four-fold in neonatal chromaffin cells and ten-to-twenty-fold in adult chromaffin cells compared with the effect of each growth factor alone. IGF-I and IGF-II acted in synergy with bFGF to stimulate proliferation and survival of chromaffin cells. Romagnolo found that the induction of IGF-I cells with dexamethasone (DEX0 triggered a 29.5-fold increase in the secretion of IGF-I. **(25*)**

IGF AND CANCER

IGF-I and II have been identified as autocrine and endocrine growth regulators which accelerate various types of carcinomas. IGF-I is considered to play an important role in the proliferation of pancreatic cancer cells, according to Gillespie **(26*)**.

Glick noted that IGFs play an important role in the regulation of glucose metabolism in central nervous system (CNS) tumors. **(27*)** It was reported by Atiq that IGF is associated with human primary colorectal tumors and colin carcinoma cell lines. **(28*)**

Yashiro found that IGF-bp (IGF binding protein) activity was significantly higher in cancer extracts, suggesting that higher IGF-bp activity in cancer tissue is involved in regulating growth of thyroid papillary carcinoma cells. **(29*)**

Robbins (Genentech, Inc.) found that IGF-I increased lymphocyte numbers in all of the peripheral lymphoid organs examined. This increase had functional significance, and Robbins concluded that IGF-I produced locally by thymic and bone marrow cells may be a natural component of B- and T-cell lymphopoiesis. **(30*)**

Yun demonstrated that IGF transcripts were 32-64-fold more abundant in Wilms tumors than in the adjacent uninvolved kidneys. IGF-II is suggested as playing a role in transforming growth factor in Wilms tumorigenesis. **(31*)**

Minniti concluded that insulin-like growth factor II (IGF-II) acts as an autocrine growth and motility factor in human rhabdomyosarcoma cell lines. Analyses of tumor biopsy specimens demonstrate high levels of IGF-II mRNA expression. All tumor specimens examined expressed the gene for IGF-II, and this expression was localized to the tumor cells and not to surrounding stroma. These data suggest that the IGF-II autocrine loop may be operating not only in vitro but also in vivo. **(32*)**

Developing osteogenic sarcoma were researched by Kappel who wrote that this type of cancer is the most common bone tumor of childhood and typically occurs during adolescent growth spurts when growth hormone and insulin-like growth factor-I (IGF-I0 may be at their highest lifetime levels. He noted that human osteogenic sarcoma cell lines are dependent on signaling through IGF-I receptors for in vitro survival and proliferation. Furthermore, they suggest modulation of the growth hormone IGF-I axis may affect the growth of these tumors in vivo. **(33*)** Lippman, as early as 1991, had implicated IGF-I as being critically involved in the aberrant growth of human breast cancer cells. **(34*)** Lee observed the processing of insulin-like growth factor by human breast tissue and commented:

> This indicates that oestrogen regulation of IGF-I peptide
> in breast cancer cells would support the hypothesis that
> IGF-II has an autocrine regulatory function in breast cancer. **(35*)**

Chen noted that IGFs are potent mitogens for malignant cell proliferation in the human breast carcinoma cell line. **(36*)** Figueroa confirmed that insulin-like growth factors (IGFs) are potent mitogens for breast cancer cells and their activity I modulated by high affinity binding proteins. **(37*)** Li treated breast cancer cells (MCF-7) with IGF-I and observed a 10-fold increase in mRNA levels of cancer cells and concluded that IGF-I modulation of gene expression appears to be an important step in cellular proliferation. **(38*)**

Krasnick furnishes another clue to this puzzle by revealing that IGF-I may have a role in the regulation of human ovarian cancer. His data support a role for IGF-I in proliferation of ovarian cancer and suggests that IGF-I and estradiol interact in a synergistic manner and regulate this malignancy. **(39*)** Musgrove states that growth factors play a major role in the control of human breast cancer cell proliferation. **(40*)**

THE MISSING LINK

On November 8, 1994, the *New York Times* published a story (written by Gina Kolata) which revealed:

1) There is good reason to believe that many very early cancers never become clinically significant.
2) Although 1 percent of women between the ages of 40 and 50 are diagnosed with breast cancer, autopsy studies reveal that 39 percent of women in that age group have breast cancer.
3) 46 percent of men between the ages of 60 and 70 have prostate cancer although only 1 percent are clinically diagnosed.
4) Virtually all people over 50 have thyroid tumors.
5) Cancerous tumors are the ones that have somehow thrown off the usually tight genetic controls on unwanted growth. **(41*)**

COMMENTS AND CONCLUSIONS

Milk? What have we done to it? We've taken a substance that was intended for the infant of a species, already loaded with fat, cholesterol and hormones. We've changed its constitution by genetically engineering it. We've simmered away its goodness through pasteurization. We've re-created its components through homogenization, a treatment in which fat droplets are shattered into droplets one tenth their original size and suspended in solution.

FDA now has information indicating that data was manipulated and withheld from peer review. In addition, new information has surfaced indicating that the product which was approved for use after so many years of testing is not the same product that is now being used. Most critically important are the facts presented in the previous 2 years of research which indicate that IGF in milk is absorbed intact and exerts proliferative growth effects.

Armed with the knowledge that virtually all humans have tumors waiting to proliferate, and milk hormones (IGFs) cause proliferation of cancer, and that treatment of cows with recombinant bovine growth hormone causes an increase in IGF levels in milk, it is now time for science, industry and FDA to re-investigate and re-evaluate this controversy.

It is also appropriate that FDA immediately place a moratorium on the use of rBST until appropriate testing can be completed.

FDA Did Not Review Key Research

Before the April 21, 1995 meeting, I requested that I be allowed to bring a tape recorder or arrange for a court stenographer to take a transcript of the discussion. Teske responded to my request by leaving a long message on my telephone answering machine. The summary of his response was that his people would tend to be more open if an "off the record" conversation were to occur. I would be allowed to bring a tape recorder if I wish, but his instincts told him that it would be better not to present the "pressure" of a tape recorder. I saw his point and agreed. I now regret that decision.

Dr. Teske is part of a "good ole' boy" network which exists to insulate and rationalize decisions, personnel and FDA policy. If a mistake is made by FDA, Teske would be the first to explain that night was really day, and the last to admit to any error.

At one point during our meeting, I offered Teske an opportunity to save face when I said, "I understand how you could have missed certain things in Monsanto's data. After all, they presented 53,000 pages of documents to you in their application." Teske angrily responded, "We not only checked every work, but we checked them twice." I remember smiling and commenting, "Wasn't once good enough?" I then turned to Condon and asked, "Did you check the specific data of the organ weights of those rats treated with BST?"

Teske did not allow Condon to respond. He answered, "Dr. Condon was responsible for checking the data and for detailed statistical analyses. He checked the numbers and found no irregularities." I looked directly at Condon and said to him, "I asked Dr. Condon, and I'd like to hear his answer." I studied Condon's face, looking for a twitch or a some subtle sign which would indicate to me whether or not his reply would be a truthful one. A poker player would call this a tell. I again asked, "Did you, Dr. Condon, personally review the data?" Condon's eyes looked directly into mine. "No, I did not." The table was quiet, and nobody spoke for a few seconds. Condon and I held our gaze. Marnane broke the silence. Although we were not operating under Robert's Rules of Order, Marnane made a motion. "For the record, I propose that Dr. Condon review the subject data."

He looked around for somebody to second his proposal. Teske turned to Condon. "Bob, is that okay with you?" Condon nodded his agreement. Teske turned to me and continued. "Dr. Condon is quite busy with new drug applications. This might take some time."

I foolishly said, "Take as much time as you need," basking in a minor victory. More than two months passed before Dr. Condon would call me at my home to discuss exactly the data that I wished to see analyzed. He promised that the work would be performed in early July. I was satisfied that Condon would focus on the "science" and ignore the "politics."

Is the Milk Different?

"Do you still consider rBST-treated milk and non-rBST treated milk to be indistinguishable?" I asked. "It doesn't matter," answered Teske. "Let me phrase the question differently. Do levels of IGF increase in milk after rBST treatment?" The group of scientist agreed that it did. "Is there evidence that IGF survives digestion?" One of the scientists responded to my question by answering, "Some IGF does survive digestion. However, I believe that the levels of IGF that bypass digestive processes are insignificant when compared to the total levels of naturally occurring IGF in the human bloodstream." I told him that I was aware that there were 500,000 ng of IGF present in the typical adult and only about 2000 ng in one glass of milk. I then told him that IGF was already bound to other proteins, just like the glue in a rug is bound to carpet fibers and thereby de-activated. I then informed him that recent research by Frystyk (reference #22 in the paper which I had just presented) indicated that the average adult has approximately 2000 ng of unbound IGF in his bloodstream. "Check my references," I offered. "I will," Teske promised.

It's Milk, Stupid!

At this point Teske looked at me with a smile. "Mr. Cohen," he asked. "Would you be willing to testify before a Senate committee that an individual might do more harm by drinking two glasses of normal untreated milk, then say, one glass of rBST-treated milk?" I didn't hesitate with my answer. "Absolutely!" Teske looked surprised by my admission. "Don't get me wrong," I explained. "I am not against genetic engineering. One day we will figure out the genetic code and not make these kinds of mistakes. If Monsanto designed rBST and the resultant product decreased the levels of IGF, I would be the first to pin a medal on the folks at Monsanto!" Teske and the others look stunned.

"IGF is the bad guy here," I said.

Teske responded. "It is our belief that levels of IGF are within normal statistical ranges and that most of the IGF is deactivated by strong digestive enzymes in the stomach. The small quantities of IGF getting through have no biological effects."

Shhh! Don't Let Nursing Mothers Know!

"Do you then not believe that a nursing mother does any biological good for her infant?" A scientist spoke. "I believe that a nursing mother offers nurturing, bonding and psychological comfort to her infant. Nothing more. The hormones do not work. They are not orally active." "You mean nursing doesn't work?" I asked. The meeting ended with the answer to that final question, unresolved. The implications of human breast feeding not working made every scientist in that room uncomfortable. Teske walked me to the door. We had pleasant words. I sent him a certified letter two weeks later requesting that he confirm my version of the summary of our meeting.

The paper which I requested from Monsanto and FDA, researched by G.D. Searle, a subsidiary of Monsanto, authored by D. Richard, G. Odaglia and P. Deslex, would answer a lot of questions if it would only be released for analyses. Reference # 44 of the *Science* article listed 32 organs and tissues in which the laboratory animals were exhibiting symptoms of developing leukemias. When the entire list of organs is finally released it will confirm that laboratory animals get cancer when treated with rBST.

The paper which Condon was going to review contained data indicating that laboratory animals had biological reactions from oral ingestion of rBST. Six years earlier, FDA had accepted Monsanto's conclusion that rBST could not have oral effects on laboratory animals. The data were never reviewed because scientists at FDA believed scientists at Monsanto. It was my belief, after observing biological effects for each of the four organs listed in the Juskevich and Guyer paper, that the twenty-eight other organs and tissue samples cited as reference #45 would clarify this debate and uphold my conclusion.

Two Monsanto scientists, Hammond and Collier, had previously presented their conclusion that no toxicology studies were necessary because rBST and IGF could not possiblly be orally active. It was long overdue, but the data would finally be reviewed. This review would indicate that laboratory animals were developing cancers.

Seven months before my meeting and less than two weeks after I filed my original petition, Sundlof, director of CVM, and Fred Shank, Ph.D,. and director of the Center For Food Safety and Applied Nutrition, issued a joint statement before a congressional subcommittee on human resources. The subject was food safety. One of the issues covered by this communiqué was the National Drug Residue Milk Monitoring Program (NDRMMP). In the statement, FDA's role in setting animal drug tolerances and withdrawal times was discussed. According to the authors, the FDA requires animal drug manufacturers to show that each new drug is safe. Toxicology, residue and basic metabolism studies must be performed and the manufacturer must submit a reliable test for measuring traces of the drug in animal tissues. That test is referred to as an assay.

Monsanto, however, never developed an assay for rBST. This was a violation of FDA rules. In spite of the fact that levels of IGF increase after milk is treated with rBST, there is no assay for measuring levels of IGF either. With no detection assay available, they trumpeted the "no difference" lie. The reason no such test was developed was that FDA explained in their landmark *Science* paper that nearly all BST was destroyed when milk is pasteurized. On page 878 of the Juskevich and Guyer paper, the authors cite reference #47, written by Jerome Moore, and published in the *Journal of Endocrinology.*

> [T]he need to pursue more definitive studies has already been
> stated as unnecessary because (BST) is biologically inactive in
> humans and orally inactive. Additionally, it has also been
> determined that at least 90 percent of (BST) activity is destroyed upon
> pasteurization of milk. Therefore, (BST) residues do not
> present a human food safety concern.

Moore never researched pasteurization. His area of expertise is in the field of the human growth hormone (GH). His research was performed on monkeys. The authors also missed a golden opportunity to correct an incorrect conclusion which FDA has reached about human growth hormone. Dwarves were treated with GH in the 1950s. FDA has repeatedly pointed to those treatments as proof of human safety of such treatment. However, Moore reveals in the opening paragraph of his paper that hGH was suspected in the occurrence of Jacob-Creutzfeldt (JC) disease in the dwarves so "successfully" treated. JC disease is similar to Alzheimer's disease with one exception. The onset of JC takes a couple of days as opposed to Alzheimer's gradual long-term onset. The reference was incorrectly cited. Another important fact was missed.

Groenewegen is the scientist who they should have cited. He was listed in the reference section as #49. Groenewegen measured levels of BST in regular milk and rBST-treated milk. The usual milk pasteurization protocol includes three methods, according to Groenewegen. One method is heating the milk for one second at a temperature of 192°F. Another is heating the milk for 15 seconds at a temperature of 161°. The third method calls for heating milk for 30 **minutes** at 145°F. Instead of heating milk for exactly 30 minutes, Groenewegen heated the milk for between 25 and 30 minutes (how un-scientific) at 160°F. 160 degrees! One degree less than the recommended temperature for the 15-second method. Groenewegen may have hoped that the BST would disappear after 30 minutes. His conclusion was:

> [H]eat treatment effectively reduced the immunoreactive
> quantities of BST in milk.

Groenewegen's fraud was reviewed in chapter 3 (*Science* article). He fooled almost everyone. Here are his results, from page 517 of his paper:

1) BST in milk from control cows averaged 3300 ng/L.
2) BST in milk from BST-treated cows averaged 4200 ng/L.
3) BST in pasteurized milk from control cows = 2700 ng/L.
4) BST in pasteurized milk from BST-treated cows = 3400 ng/L.

Levels of BST did not decrease by 90 percent. They decreased by exactly 18.10 percent (control milk) and 19.05 percent (BST-treated milk). Unfortunately, human safety was sacrificed because FDA concluded that BST disappeared when milk was pasteurized. There was no longer a need for additional studies.

Scientists close to this research and FDA had to know these incriminating data were more than just coincidence. The readers of the prestigious journal *Science* demonstrated their faith placed in Monsanto, St. Louis, Missouri. Missouri's state motto should be emblazoned on the wall of this pharmaceutical giant:

> "*Salus populi suprema lex esto*" (The welfare of the people
> shall be the supreme law).

The FDA feels morally justified in stating that the two milks are indistinguishable. But there's no test for rBST. They know there's a difference. Since Monsanto never developed a test (although they were required to by FDA), they know that you cannot distinguish the difference! Sundlof of the CVM testified before the Subcommittee of Human Resources and Intergovernmental Relations Committee on Government Operations. Even though FDA did not require Monsanto to develop a test to discriminate genetically engineered milk from untreated milk, Sundlof had the audacity to say:

Toxicology, residue and metabolism studies are also required.
If the product will cause residues in tissues, manufacturers
must also submit a reliable assay method for detecting drug
residues in edible tissues of slaughtered animals and milk. (16)

No assay was required because of the "pasteurization fraud." FDA
"insiders" had to know that these hormones were not destroyed by pasteurization.
By declaring that these hormones were destroyed they also declared that the two
milks were indistinguishable. This lie opened up the "door" to a new technology,
genetic engineering. Taylor received a promotion to under-secretary of USDA
after the GAO investigation. He testified before the same committee as Sundlof
and Shank. Taylor had previously resigned as Monsanto's attorney to become a
senior FDA employee and was investigated by Congress for a conflict of interests.
Less than two weeks after I filed my citizen petition, Taylor issued his own
statement. He wrote:

In determining whether a compound is likely to result in a residue, we
are able to rule out compounds that meet the following criteria:
There is a zero-day withdrawal period established by FDA or EPA. (17)

The translation for this is that BST does not work because pasteurization
destroys it. Collier and Hammond of Monsanto convinced FDA that there was no
need for toxicology studies or assays because there were no biological effects from
oral ingestion of rBST. Furthermore, they reasoned, rBST is destroyed when milk
is pasteurized. FDA did not review the Monsanto data because of Monsanto's
representations. The data published in *Science* indicated that there were biological
effects from oral ingestion of rBST. Additional data from twenty-eight organs and
tissues would indicate the scope of the biological effects. The last referenced
organ in the science paper is "and other lesions." "Other lesions" is a scientist's
manner of revealing **cancer**.

If Monsanto does release this paper, they may surrender their $600 million
biotechnology investment. If the American people get to read this paper, they
might realize just how government and big business work together in the same
boardroom, and go to sleep in the same bedroom. On November 24, 1994, I
received a letter from Linda Grasse of the Communications and Education Branch
of the CVM. Through Grasse I have come to understand that most of the FDA
employees are totally dedicated individuals with unwavering moral principles. By
her own admission, Grasse does not have an extensive scientific background. She
has the greatest amount of trust and faith in her colleagues. I had sent an earlier
version of my paper to Grasse. In her November 24, 1995 letter, she wrote to me:

I am writing to let you know that I received your paper

yesterday and read it last night. I appreciate the time you took
to research and write the paper. I expect you are waiting to learn
(a) whether I understood all the points you made, and (b) if I now
agree with your assessment on bovine somatotropin. The answer to
both questions is no. I am still confused by your scientific arguments.
In addition, I am convinced that the scientists in FDA would not
have approved the product if it were unsafe to humans. I believe that
our scientists are both knowledgeable and dedicated to protecting the
public health. (18)

Grasse edits two FDA publications, the *FDA Backgrounder* and the *FDA
Veterinarian*. In the May/June 1994 issue of the *FDA Veterinarian*, page 7,
column 3, there are a number of questions and answers. Here's my favorite.

QUESTION: ***What about the possibility that insulin-like growth factor-I
in milk from treated cows will lead to increased rates of
breast cancer and other human health problems?***

ANSWER: FDA and other scientific and regulatory bodies have
thoroughly examined the safety of milk produced by rbST-
treated cows and have concluded that it is safe. There is
absolutely no possibility that the consumption of milk
from rBST-treated cows could increase the risk of breast
cancer.

When I first came across this paper I called Grasse and asked her who was
responsible for this line. This is when I learned that she was the editor. I then
asked, "Who told you to write this?" Her response was, "Dr. Margaret Miller."
Miller. The same scientist who told Juskevich what to write in her landmark
Science article. The same Miller who at one time worked for Monsanto
Agricultural Company. The same Miller who was investigated by Congress and
the GAO for conflicts of interest in the approval process for rBST! And, finally,
the same Miller, who was cited as one of the authors of reference #74 in the
Science article, writing with Monsanto's Collier, who pointed out that :

The concentration of IGF-I in milk from the rbGH-treated (BST) cows
was significantly increased across the ten injection cycles.

How did this same scientist perform research at Monsanto, discovering that
levels of the powerful growth hormone, IGF, increase after rBST-treatment, and
then get a job at the FDA determining policy of labeling of milk containing rBST?
I recently posed this question to Gerald Guest, Ph.D., who was the director of
CVM during the term of the Monsanto rBST application. "Why did you hire

Margaret Miller?" I asked. "She was qualified, although I didn't make the decision to hire her," he answered. "That was done by Tom Mulligan, who at the time was the FDA director of toxicology."

Mulligan responded to my voice mail message with one of his own. "Margaret Miller started at FDA before I did, so I had absolutely nothing to do with hiring her. " Although I left many messages on Miller's voice mail regarding this subject, she no longer returns phone calls to me. Everybody denies hiring Miller. I suspect that Monsanto did the hiring and made the job placement. Miller's conclusion is that the rBST-treated milk is indistinguishable from normal milk. Her words on the top of page 883 of that *Science* paper refute this conclusion. Her research reveals that levels of IGF-I in milk always increase after cows are treated with rbST. Miller's research was biased. Instead of measuring the effects of rBST immediately after the birth of a calf, she began administering rBST treatment 60 days post-partum. It is well accepted that the most dramatic measurements of IGF are obtained in the days following the birth of a calf.

This would make sense to nursing mothers who have been told by pediatricians that the first milk, the colostrum, is very rich in hormones. Dairy farmers are prohibited by law from selling this "colostrum" to the public because of the extremely high levels of hormones which this milk contains. It is not logical to prohibit the sale of this hormone-rich milk. FDA believes that milk hormones do not work. However, if hormones do work, then the ban on selling colostrum is justified. Miller and the rest of the Monsanto scientists sought to eliminate any measurable difference in IGF levels by beginning the experiment one month after the calves were born, when levels of IGF would be relatively low. When levels of IGF were measured, FDA compared high levels of IGF in rBST-treated milk by saying, "It is well within the normal range." They eliminated the "normal range" and then included it when it suited their predetermined conclusions. The average level of IGF in milk of control animals was 3500 ng/L (about 1 quart). The milk from cows receiving subcutaneous injections of rBST measured 6100 ng/L. A 74 percent increase! Normal range? No. Ten cycles were averaged!

How in good conscience can FDA continue to say that there was no increase in levels of IGF? Indistinguishable? The are only two things that are indistinguishable. One is the question of where Miller's true loyalties lie -- with her former employer, Monsanto, or with an unbiased analyses of IGF issues and safety as it affects the American people. There is a thin timeline drawn between Miller's tenure at Monsanto and her employment at FDA. The second indistinguishable matter is separating fantasy from truth at FDA conclusions. The milk is obviously different. Levels of IGF have increased. I know that Monsanto openly donates money to members of Congress who vote on rBST issues. I wonder, what happens behind closed doors when Monsanto meets FDA? Could events similar to the well publicized Canadian bribe scandal which aired on the *Fifth Estate* television broadcast be standard operating procedure in our country?

(Canadian Ministers reported multimillion dollar bribes to the Royal Canadian Mounted Police. Monsanto had offered $2 million dollars if rBST were approved in Canada).

As we approached noon, signaling the end of our meeting, I requested that we summarize the major points of agreement or disagreement. Having taken careful notes, I reviewed the previous three hours. Few Americans were familiar with the controversy of the new genetically engineered bovine protein and they continued drinking their milk and eating dairy products from cows treated with these new biotech hormones. Some of those who became aware of the issues called food producers such as Kraft, Burger King and Pizza Hut on special 800-hotline numbers, voicing their concerns and asking questions. Most of these companies relied upon FDA's approval and the American Medical Association's clean bill of health for this new food additive. As far as these companies knew, such confirmation was overwhelming.

Customer Satisfaction / 2100 Powers Ferry Road, Suite 200 / Atlanta, Georgia 30339-5014 / 1-800-948-8488

November 14, 1994

Mr. Robert Cohen

Dear Mr. Cohen:

Thank you for your letter regarding the use of the Bovine Growth Hormone *bovine somatatrophin,* commonly known as BST. We appreciate your taking the time to contact us.

Pizza Hut, Inc. is standing by the FDA's approval of BST. The FDA's extensive scientific research, as well as other independent studies, have proven BST to be completely safe for human consumption in milk, milk products and for livestock. Among the health industry organizations endorsing the use of BST are the American Medical Association, The American Dietetic Association, the National Institute of the American Academy of Pediatrics. The BST hormone is also used in 30 other nations.

Additionally, since there is no scientific test to differentiate between the natural hormone and the synthetic hormone, we cannot test to guarantee whether or not we are receiving dairy products from BST-supplemented cows. All tests for the presence of BST will be positive since the hormone occurs naturally in milk, therefore, we feel that it would be very misleading to our consumers to label our products, BST Free.

Thank you again for contacting us.

Sincerely,

Robert A. Doughty

"The public will believe anything, so long as it is not founded on truth."

Edith Sitwell

"Every great mistake has a halfway moment, a split second when it can be recalled and perhaps remedied."

Pearl Buck

"People lie because they don't remember clear what they saw. People lie because they can't help making a good story better than it was the way it happened."

Carl Sandburg

Chapter 7

The Fourth Estate: What America Was Told About the "New" Milk

---

The BST controversy was explained to America's citizens through newspaper and magazine articles and television news programs. Daily newspapers find it unnecessary to research or check references to a story published in distinguished periodicals such as the *Journal of the American Medical Association* (*JAMA*) or *Science*. Writers simply quote the source in their article and the newspaper's editors write the headlines. The stories are accepted as fact by readers and the information in those stories becomes part of our collective culture. If FDA says that something is safe, then it must be safe. If *JAMA* endorses the safety of a new drug, then it must be safe. If every major magazine in America repeats FDA's safety assessment, citing the American Medical Association publication, then that drug must be safe. If every newspaper and magazine and evening news commentator says that genetically engineered milk is indistinguishable from normal wholesome milk, then it must be true. In the case of rbST, there was overwhelming and absolute agreement between every scientific organization and every arm of the media that the new milk was safe to drink because it was exactly the same as the old milk. This is what every American learned.

A small group of scientists and activists began to criticize the conclusions reached by FDA. These critics exposed the conflicts of interest between FDA and the drug manufacturer. In doing so, these contrary voices also exposed a weakness in the way America works. Americans are proud of their freedoms. We have freedom of the press, and rely upon organizations such as FDA which are supposed to protect our interests. We also trust that the media will act as a watchdog should the "system" fail. In this case, every sentinel was asleep. Monsanto, aware of problems with their new genetically engineered product, stacked the deck at FDA with their ex-employees. They paid money to members of Congress who were debating milk labeling bills. They filed suit against dairies and processors who attempted to merchandize the fact that they would not accept milk from cows treated with genetically engineered hormones. The consciousness of America rationalized that rbST was safe. We were told this over and over again from many different sources until we accepted it as truth. Suddenly, newsletters such as *Consumers Reports* and *Health and Healing* began to reveal contrary research, including information concerning illness to cows treated with this drug, increased levels of hormones, antibiotics and bacteria in milk, and possible links to cancer.

The FDA represents that there are no differences between the milk of cows treated with rBST and normal "wholesome" milk that has not been treated. That lie was repeated in newspapers and magazines all across America in 1994. Residents of Seattle, Washington, saw these written words during the summer of 1994 when they appeared in their own *Seattle Times* newspaper:

> Milk from BST-treated cows contains no more of the hormones than
> milk from other cows...no difference has been shown, according to the
> FDA. (1)

A few weeks later a similar article appeared for the people of Sacramento, California to read:

> According to the Federal Food and Drug Administration, synthetic BST
> is completely safe, and there is no difference between milk from treated
> and untreated cows. (2)

Residents of Rochester, New York, and Vermont and Wisconsin were exposed to similar articles in their local papers informing them about the safety of milk in spite of the numerous BST-related controversies. So did all of America learn from their local newspapers that milk was safe. Labeling laws. Drug approval. Conflicts of interest. Mastitis and genetic deformities in cows. People all over the country, each time they read an article, assimilated bits and pieces of the BST story. Each time an article appeared, however, the FDA and Monsanto position was repeated.

The Collective Consciousness of America

Redbook told its readers that the new milk was just as safe and wholesome as the milk Americans had been drinking all their lives. (3) "BST-treated milk and normal wholesome milk are exactly the same," we were informed over and over again. "The two milks are indistinguishable." If you repeat a lie often enough it becomes a truth. If the FDA says it's safe, then we have nothing to worry about, concluded the collective understanding of a nation.

More words have been written about the BST controversy than any other new drug application in FDA's history. The U.S. Department of Health and Human Services has published a bibliography containing the background material encompassing the research conducted on BST between 1985 and 1990. (4) The materials covered in this bibliography include more than 1100 journal articles, monographs, dissertations, audiovisual aids, editorials, letters to the editor and abstracts from gatherings of scientists. This chapter sets aside those detailed scientific arguments, concerning itself more with nontechnical articles like the ones you might have read in the *New York Times* or *Newsweek* or *Good Housekeeping*. These are the stories which presented ideas that became a part of the public psyche. Which version of reality did the "Fourth Estate" present to America?

All the News that Fits...We Print

On May 18, 1994, Marian Burros, a food writer for the *New York Times*, wrote an article clarifying the labeling issue debate on milk containing BST. (5) Burros introduced the major critics of Monsanto's new drug. They included the GAO (the investigative branch of Congress), Hansen of Consumer's Union - publisher of Consumer's Reports, Rifkin - organizer of the Pure Foods campaign in Washington and a critic of the concept of genetic engineering, and Samuel Epstein, a well-published cancer spokesman and professor of environmental medicine at the University of Chicago.

The article was written three months before I began to closely examine the different issues of this controversy. One fascinating tidbit of information contained in the Burros story was the revelation that the International Dairy Foods Association and the Grocery Manufacturers of America both had close formal ties to Monsanto. Burros was hailed by activists for writing this article. She alerted her readers that such controversy existed. She gave equal time to Epstein, Rifkin and Hansen. At the time, many felt that consumers had a right to know whether their milk was genetically engineered, in spite of FDA assurances that there was absolutely no difference between BST-treated milk and normal wholesome milk.

In September 1994, I spoke to Epstein, who hinted that a reporter would be writing a major expose of the BST controversy. I informed Epstein that I had discussed the issues with Burros and that she had determined that BST was no longer a problem. She told me that it was safe and she would not write about it again. Epstein became upset and ended our conversation. A few minutes later he called me back. "I've known her for 15 years," he said. "She said she never spoke to you. You're a damned liar." Burros never wrote Epstein's long-awaited exposé.

I was phoning and faxing Burros constantly with new information, to the point of being a nuisance. Every Wednesday her column would be printed. Instead of a "BST Causes Cancer" headline, she would print (skillfully written) cooking recipes like "Rosemary Infused Pork." Occasionally, Burros would write about a serious health issue. She found a new hero to write about. Long after Taylor had performed his service to Monsanto, and shortly after the GAO investigation, Taylor was rewarded with a promotion to under-secretary at the Department of Agriculture.

Burros would occasionally cite Michael Taylor in one of her columns. Taylor became the new American hero. He really cared about the health and safety of our food supply, Burros would tell us. Burros was helping to build this "villain" of the BST issues into a hero. I sent a letter with my comments, "Look who **your** reporter is writing about," to Sam Epstein. Epstein's secretary wrote back. "Your letters are no longer appreciated, and will not be accepted by this office." During the GAO investigation of conflicts of interest by Taylor, ex-Monsanto attorney who was writing new laws partial to Monsanto, Marian Burros' son, an attorney, became the official spokesman for the GAO investigation of conflicts of interest regarding BST issues.

What drama! What coincidence! What a small world! And they say that Monsanto does not have a long reach. When Monsanto cannot buy congressmen and reward writers by magically pulling strings behind the scenes creating random series of events that are statistically improbable, they use their power to threaten and intimidate individuals and businesses. Monsanto has sued small dairies who dare to market their milk as being free of BST. The *Vermont Free Press* reported Monsanto's suits against two dairies:

> Monsanto Spokesman Tom McDermott said the company sued Swiss
> Valley Farms in Davenport, Iowa, and Pure Milk and Ice Cream
> Company in Waco, Texas, because their advertising used "false and
> misleading" information to tell customers that neither sold milk from
> cows treated with the company's product. (6)

Monsanto lobbies for state assemblies to pass agriculture disparagement acts which punish individuals for speaking or writing negative **ideas** about agriculture products. The *Springfield Illinois Register* reported:

The Monsanto Company which makes the bovine growth hormone is worried about persistent complaints affecting sales. Dairy farmers fear bad publicity could undermine confidence in the nation's milk supply.

Only in America?

In Illinois, an agricultural disparagement act was introduced into the state legislature. The bill's sponsor, Sen. Todd Sieben, possibly influenced by his new friends, the Monsanto lobbyists, stated:

There are groups out there that I believe are distorting the facts about agriculture. (7)

Sieben introduced a bill which:

[P]rovides for a criminal penalty and civil liability for defamatory statements concerning agricultural products. (8)

In other words, I could go to jail for telling the truth about milk hormones. I could go to jail for writing chapters one through seven of this book. If they read chapters eight through fourteen I'll be tarred and feathered, boiled in oil, shot, hung, electrocuted, crucified, and then they'll kill me! Illinois defeated this bill which never made it out of committee. Similar bills have been enacted into law in seventeen states. At the same time that Monsanto hired lobbyists to knock on the doors of every one of 435 Congressional offices, their strategists and lobbyists were also busy working hard at the State House and Senate level. Bills were introduced all over the country called "Agriculture Disparagement Acts." You can now be personally liable, for example, if you criticize a genetically engineered agricultural product. This sure was an effective way to intimidate the press from reporting possible negative effects of milk hormones or flavor saver tomatoes or genetically engineered soybeans which were resistant to herbicides like Monsanto's own Roundup pesticide. Monsanto determined that a message had to be sent to anybody audacious enough to not use their product and brag about it. Monsanto went after the "little guy." BST was not needed by America, which had a milk surplus. It was not desired by many farmers who produced milk naturally. When dairymen attempted to inform consumers that their product was BST-free, they were brought into expensive and intimidating litigation by Monsanto.

A Congressman Who Took on Monsanto and the FDA

Vermont Congressman Bernard Sanders was infuriated in February 1994 after Monsanto filed suits against Swiss Valley Farms Company in Davenport,

Iowa, and Pure Milk and Ice Cream Company in Waco, Texas. Monsanto sued these two manufacturers for giving out "false and misleading information" when they dared to advertise and market their milk as different (and better than BST-treated milk). Monsanto had FDA on their side. FDA continued to inform the world that the two milks were indistinguishable. The public had a right to know which milk they were buying. Milk purchasers were willing to spend more for a "healthier" product. Monsanto strategists simultaneously lobbied state assemblies to pass agricultural disparagement acts to silence criticism and stifle public debate which would, according to Monsanto, hurt sales of BST.

Monsanto Spokeswoman, Lisa Watson

Lisa Watson, Monsanto spokeswoman, reported on a Canadian television program, *The Fifth Estate*, that FDA and Monsanto received relatively few reports of cows experiencing mastitis from BST treatment. The health magazine, *Vegetarian Times*, reported that FDA was aware of only fourteen cases of mastitis after the first 6 months of BST approval. (9) FDA had admitted to only fourteen cases. However, an agricultural journal reported that contrary information had been received in a FOIA request:

> FDA says it received 500 reports representing health problems
> in more than 9,500 cows injected with genetically engineered
> bovine growth hormone. (10)

Rifkin of Pure Foods did not believe Monsanto or FDA. He filed the above FOIA request, and after many months his suspicions were confirmed. In February 1995, Rifkin learned that there were actually many more adverse reactions than FDA or Monsanto would admit to. There were nearly 10,000 sick cows, not fourteen! FDA attempted to explain away that number as being "acceptable," since 2,700,000 dairy cows were actually dosed. If the same percentage of Americans became very ill from a new drug, we would have nearly 880,000 sick men, women and children to consider.

America's female population was given the "seal of approval" for BST-milk consumption primarily as a result of a column in which Bob Arnott, M.D., answered questions from readers of *Good Housekeeping*. In the June 1994 issue of the magazine, the question was:

"Is genetic milk different from regular milk?"

Arnott evidently did not research the answer to this question by reading the abstract of the Juskevich and Guyer *Science* paper. Nor did he appear to review any of the research which indicated that levels of IGF increase in milk after BST treatment. He relied upon our trustworthy friends at FDA.

> According to FDA Commissioner, David Kessler,
> M.D., no current techniques can distinguish between
> the two. There is no more growth hormone in genetic
> milk than in regular milk, and no difference in nutritional
> value between the two.(11)

There are other sources standing by to echo the FDA conclusion. A 1994 *New York Times* article told us:

> The Food and Drug Administration, which approved
> the drug in November, says that it is safe and that
> milk produced by hormone-treated cows cannot be
> distinguished from untreated cows. (12)

Newsweek

December 6, 1993: "Small wonder. The new milk will be virtually indistinguishable from the old." (13)

Time

May 17,1993 (quoting Lisa Watson, Monsanto spokesperson): "Milk from treated and untreated cows is functionally and biologically the same." (14)

Time After Time

February 14, 1994 (quoting FDA's Kessler): "There's virtually no difference between treated and untreated cows." (15) Kessler says "virtually." By February 1994, Kessler had admitted to himself that there is a difference. Is this the doctor Kessler or the lawyer Kessler carefully wording his statement to reveal "virtually no difference?"

The Wall Street Journal

You would expect editorials from financial magazines and newspapers to favor biotechnological pharmaceutical companies. The *Wall Street Journal* was not kind to pure food activists:

The scare got started with Jeremy Rifkin, who goblinizes nearly every outgrowth of agricultural science since Johnny Appleseed... Let's encourage the truth...With the help of some truth-telling by scientists, this should permit technology to triumph and, in the process, hasten the end of anticompetitiveness in the dairy case. (16)

Indeed! The journal assumes that scientists tell the truth. We've already seen that this is not always the case."

Forbes Magazine & Science

Forbes magazine encompasses the entire milk controversy by blaming it all on the anti-BST activists:

(They) have launched passionate campaigns denouncing (BST) as a vile poison. Their strident and scientifically baseless objections have found willing ears. (17)

On December 14, 1990, nearly four months after publishing the Juskevich and Guyer article which details that IGF levels increase after BST treatment, *Science* editorialized:

The evidence **clearly** (emphasis added by this author) indicates that the overall composition and nutritional quality of milk and meat from rBST-treated cows is equal to that from untreated cows. (18)

Science explained that unpublished data cannot be released by law until the FDA makes a final decision in the BST approval process.

The Scientists and Activists

Betty Martini and Barbara Mullarkey

There are two women who are on my very short list of people with whom I could be marooned on a desert island and never spend a bored moment. By their actions, these two fascinating, well-educated, witty women seem to care more about your health and the safety of your children than the FDA. They are Betty Martini, from Atlanta, Georgia, and Barbara Mullarkey from Oak Park, Illinois. Mullarkey was most certainly the model for the screenwriters who created the movie, *I Love Trouble*. She was one of the few columnists in America who voiced opposition to the new genetically engineered milk hormone. As previously mentioned, the role of Barbara was played by Julia Roberts who co-starred with Nick Nolte in the fantasy story of a drug company marketing a genetically engineered cow hormone which the pharmaceutical giant knew created cancer in laboratory animals.

These two women have educated and inspired me to dedicate a large part of my life into researching the new genetically engineered Monsanto growth hormone, BST. I receive phone calls every day from new "activists" in small towns in Utah, Tennessee and all over the United States, and have spoken to scientists around the world regarding BST issues. However, these two women spend a great part of their day, seven days a week, communicating with other activists, members of Congress, doctors and journalists in attempting to learn truths and dispel scientific fraud. For them, this mission is a full-time endeavor. Each of these two women could teach Amway a thing or two about network marketing. If I give information to Mullarkey in Illinois, I often get a reporter from Minnesota or Texas calling me for confirmation. Martini discovered the joys of the Internet, and feels free to post my unlisted phone number to the scientists and activists on the World Wide Web.

The monthly health newsletter, *Health and Healing*, published by Julian Whitaker, M.D., supplied me with my first source of information on bovine somatotropin in July of 1994. I was quite impressed with the column written by Jane Heimlich. The newsletter manager, sensing my interest, gave me Betty Martini's number. Martini introduced me to Mullarkey who opened up a new world containing alternative health thoughts with individuals seeking options to replace many of our modern day medical practices and concepts.

I was initially "buried" under a pile of literature from Martini and Mullarkey that took me months to digest. Each issue became as important as the previous controversy. Aspartame, Alar, insecticides, pesticides. It seemed as if our food supply was tainted and contaminated by technology. I have always considered myself to be a man of science and I am excited by genetic engineering. Yet, through Martini and Mullarkey, I learned that we, as a society, were permitting enormous mistakes to occur. The stakes were high. So were the potential earnings for pharmaceutical companies. Through Martini and Mullarkey, I began to see a pattern. Pharmaceutical companies seemed to be continuously generating suspect research. In every new drug or technique I found evidence of data manipulation. Testimony before Congress, accounts in the *Congressional Record*, confidential letters from retired FDA employees. There was a disturbing "mountain" of accumulating evidence criticizing the "establishment's" inability to protect its citizens.

Each and every "activist" shares one common enlightenment. Each is familiar with the phrase, "out of pocket." It's an expensive nonbusiness. There is no income. There certainly are expenses. Every month the phone bill must be accompanied by sedatives. At times I imagine that the postal service would suffer a significant loss of cash flow if I and hundreds of others like me didn't mail dozens of envelopes and letters each week. Photocopies, office supplies, we are an industry with no income and enormous expenses.

William von Myer, president of Fairview Industries in Wisconsin, claims to have spent over $100,000 in attorney's fees related to FDA hearings. Von Myer organized large demonstrations and generated publicity when he invalidated the FDA approval process of BST before the New York City Council in 1993.

David Kronfeld, Ph.D., one of the early BST researchers and developers, has since become one of the "movement's" vocal voices of opposition. Kronfeld has felt Monsanto's sting. Monsanto has tried to exert pressure on the dean of the college where Kronfeld teaches. Kronfeld's superiors have been warned by Monsanto to "muzzle" him or they would not consider any future grant support. Kronfeld is one of the most respected men in his field at the Department of Animal Sciences at Virginia Tech. Yet, there is just so much pressure an academic institution can take. Freedom of speech sometimes takes a second seat to millions of dollars of potential research grants.

Kronfeld, with his vast knowledge of animal agriculture techniques, alerted FDA that Monsanto's biased research treated herds of dairy cows with nine antibiotics that were not approved by FDA for use on lactating cows. Kronfeld pointed out that overdosed cows in "perfectly" managed experimental herds were not fair measures of projected real world effects. His prediction that there would be widespread reports of increased incidences of mastitis came true shortly after BST received official approval from FDA.

Pete Hardin

Pete Hardin is the editor of *The Milkweed*, the farmer's milk marketing report. Hardin is a "truthmonger" (as opposed to a rumormongerer), a reporter of truth. When BST was a new controversy in January of 1990, Hardin's newsletter printed stolen FDA files proving that cows experienced health problems from BST. While the files were secret, the FDA acted irresponsibly. The data which regulatory agencies were continuously receiving from Monsanto should have been kept a secret. This experimental research was "trade protected." FDA simply could have, and should have said, "no comment" when asked how the cows were reacting from BST. Instead FDA lied by assuring the American people that there were no problems.

Hardin writes for the dairy farmer. His first love is his family; his second is the dairy industry. Hardin was one of the first to note that farmers did not want BST. Farmers feared BST. Many dairy farmers sensed that the Dairy Council did not represent their interests on this matter. These dairymen felt alienated. *The Milkweed* became a strong voice of protest and was cited by scientists and politicians when testimony was presented to Congress.

Sam Epstein

Sam Epstein often stood alone and took barrage after barrage, direct hits fired from Monsanto/FDA allies which often made Epstein look like an idiot. I've got to give the man credit, although we have argued and my communications are not welcome in his office. In 1993, an English veterinarian, Ben Mepham, sent a series of letters to the British journal, *The Lancet*. Those letters suggested that increased levels of IGF in BST-treated milk might be responsible for cancer of the gut. "Impossible," cried Epstein, before FDA or Monsanto had opportunity to answer. "It causes cancer of the breast, not gut!"

Epstein never publicly conceded that BST might cause an increased possibility of a vast array of cancers, including leukemia. BST and IGF had potential to exert system effects, and were not targeted to one specific organ or tissue. In December 1994 he submitted a paper for publication titled, *Insulin-like growth factor 1 in biosynthetic milk is a potential risk factor for breast and gastrointestinal cancers.* Epstein is a brilliant scientist but he never really got the point about hormones in milk. If IGF from biosynthetic milk was dangerous, so was IGF in normal wholesome milk. None of the scientists observed this fact or had the guts to make this statement. It was folly to challenge Monsanto and FDA for allowing more hormones to be placed in the milk supply. Was it insanity to go up against the entire dairy industry because of the naturally occurring levels of these hormones? Epstein wrote an article for the *Los Angeles Times* in which he listed his well-founded suspicions concerning IGF. Epstein commented:

> IGF is not destroyed by digestion and is readily absorbed
> across the intestinal wall. IGF induces rapid division and
> multiplication of normal human breast cells. IGF promotes
> transformation of normal breast epithelium to breast cancer.
> IGF maintains malignancy of human breast cancer cells and
> accelerates the spread of cancer to distant organs. (19)

Epstein demanded in his article that Congress insist that FDA ban the use of BST. Epstein concluded that Congress had this duty. Epstein worked with Congress and offered his testimony before many committees. At the very least, Epstein felt that consumers should have opportunity to choose for themselves. He lobbied for Congress to pass laws requiring BST-treated milk to be labeled. Monsanto did not allow Epstein's newspaper attack to go unanswered. Yet, they wanted to avoid a direct attack. They enlisted two hitmen for the task. One was Dennis Bier, M.D., who was a member of the National Institutes of Health (NIH) panel who did not review Monsanto data. Bier wrote a well-publicized letter to FDA's Commissioner Kessler. That letter was simultaneously released to the press, written on stationery from the Baylor College of Medicine.

The Dairy Coalition in Washington also issued a statement, which not only criticized Epstein, but cited Bier's letter to Kessler. So as to provide overkill, the popular and well-respected ex-Surgeon General Koop was the second public figure who Monsanto recruited to attack Epstein. Bier agreed with Epstein on the following: Pasteurization does not destroy IGF, some IGF does bypass digestive processes, IGF molecules in humans and bovines are identical, IGF causes cell division, all malignant cancer cells produce IGF. Some of Bier's disagreements were in error. Bier said:

> Most studies demonstrate that IGF concentrations in milk
> are not altered after rbST-treatment. IGF is eventually
> inactivated by proteolytic digestive enzymes. BST does not
> affect human breast cells because there are no receptors in
> human tissue for BST. (20)

There are no BST receptors in mammary glands of cows either! The Dairy Coalition said:

> Epstein is just another misinformed consumer activist that
> is contributing to a well orchestrated food activist campaign
> based in fear, not science...this deplorable form of consumer
> activism was also attacked recently by former U.S. Surgeon
> General Dr. C. Everett Koop, who said, ...it is necessary to
> condemn these attacks on the safety of milk for what they are:
> baseless, manipulative and completely irresponsible. (21)

The Dairy Coalition cited hundreds of Monsanto-funded studies reviewed by the American Medical Association, the American Association of Pediatrics and the American Dietetic Association. Funny, the Dairy Coalition neglected to mention Monsanto's role in funding these "prestigious" and well-respected organizations. Epstein exaggerated and misinterpreted numbers and statements. For example, Epstein wrote that:

> Eli Lilly admitted that rbGH milk may contain more than
> a 10-fold increase in IGF-1 concentrations. (22)

Eli Lilly Pharmaceutical Company did not say this. Lilly said that their BST milk "would not contain more than 50,000 nanograms per liter." In the defense of accuracy, Lilly had to note one study in which the baseline level of IGF in control milk was 28,400 ng/L. After BST-treatment that IGF level increased to 35,500 ng. That study, performed on only eight cows, indicated a 25 percent increase in IGF in milk. It was not more than 10-fold, and Eli Lilly did not admit to this, as Epstein indicated.

Epstein also wrote that IGF was one of the "smaller molecular weight polypeptides." At a molecular weight of 7800 daltons, IGF is not "small," particularly when peptides like thryrotropin-releasing factor (TRF) and gonadotropin-releasing hormone (GnRH) weigh under 1200 daltons. A dalton is a unit of mass equal to one-sixteenth of the mass of an atom of oxygen - named after John Dalton, the discoverer of color blindness. Epstein himself was partially blind to the scientific facts when he made that last point. Epstein wrote that FDA did not present data on IGF-I salivary and blood levels in human infants which is not true. FDA did present these data. In addition, Epstein comments on the absence of any published studies on the oral activity of IGF. However, Medline, a computer database containing abstracts of thousands upon thousands of scientific studies contains a number of available studies for review. Epstein exaggerates IGF-I levels in milk by claiming to observe 20-fold increases in levels of IGF.

Epstein came to this conclusion after observing a normal range of between 1000 and 5000 ng of IGF per liter of milk by day #200 in a cow's cycle, and the BST-treated range of 6,000 to 20,000 ng. Epstein performed data analyses in much the same biased way in which FDA twisted the numbers. He was fighting fire with fire. I do not approve of the way FDA does things and I do not approve of this "two wrongs make a right" mentality. I question his mathematical skills, which make his work and all of the legitimate protest questionable and open to criticism. Epstein kept this controversy on the front pages of our newspapers. He made many errors and suffered by playing the role of sacrificial lamb and receiving the brunt of scientific ridicule and criticism. Most of that criticism was unwarranted. Epstein is an American hero. He did not make money from this BST protest. He lost standing in the scientific community. He alienated friends and colleagues. But he did care about the American people. He suspected that something was very wrong about this new genetically engineered hormone. He was right. In my opinion Sam Epstein is a royal pain in the ass. But I respect him. And I admire him because Epstein is a man who kept his dignity.

Consumer's Union

Consumer's Union, located in Yonkers, New York, is the publisher of the monthly magazine, *Consumer Reports*. If you have a burning desire to know which is the best fire extinguisher to use or out in the cold on which air conditioner will most efficiently cool your 10-by-12-foot bedroom, you can simply call their 800 phone number and pay $24 for a subscription for twelve issues filled with evaluations on consumer products and issues.

Consumer's Union thrives on publicity and controversy. They, however, have subscriptions to sell and if they are not at the very center of that controversy their interest proportionately wanes. For example, I asked a number of executives in the chain of command at Consumer's Union to allow Michael Hansen, scientist and reviewer, to accompany me on my meeting with five FDA scientists at my April 21, 1995, visit. The request was denied, in spite of the fact that Hansen told me that he would have appreciated this opportunity to interact with the CVM by this unique learning and teaching experience where a free flow of ideas would be exchanged without the pressure of reporters and TV cameras.

Hansen, like Epstein, is also an American hero. He is, however, paid to be a hero by Consumer's Union. He is not obsessed with the day to day issues of BST. There are hundreds or thousands of issues which have become controversial to Consumer's Union, which finds Hansen, as a research scientist, constantly at the center of activity. Once an issue is published and debated, Hansen has little time to linger. There is always another issue to protest. On to the next one. He probably goes home after work and "has a life," unlike myself and a few other individuals I have met through this "campaign." I applaud the work which Hansen began. His bovine somatotropin protests were "milked" by Consumer's Union over a 4-year period in which Hansen paved paths for others to follow. Although his protests fizzled out, he kept the game alive long enough for others to join the ranks. I became involved as Hansen was moving on. Hansen left when the mastitis issue was solved by perfect dairy management. The cows were supposedly safe enough to come home to graze. Freedom of Information Act data supplied to Pure Food's Jeremy Rifkin exposed another FDA and Monsanto lie.

A report issued by the Federal Office of Technology Assessment recognized that the government must pay careful attention to consumer's concerns to the threat to food products from biotechnology. Consumers are skeptical, resisting conclusions from regulatory agencies. A few years earlier reports of the pesticide, Alar, used in apples, and cyanide grape poisoning stories had soured the public confidence in regulatory agencies' ability to protect or advise us.

Consumers Reports began covering these issues. In the middle of the BST controversy GAO urged the FDA to stop sales of milk from cows treated with BST. Consumer's Union educated consumers and added fuel to the fire of the controversy surrounding Monsanto and FDA. (23) On March 20, 1992, the *Los Angeles Times* reported on a landmark ruling by a group of state appellate judges. As a result of a suit filed by Consumers Union in 1985, the judiciary panel ruled that judges can now order warnings to be placed on consumer products. This ruling set precedent for possible BST lawsuits. (24)

On March 31, 1993, Hansen gave testimony to the Veterinary Advisory Committee on potential animal and human health effects of BST. His affidavit revealed that there would be a 76 percent increase in mastitis rates for primaparous cows (cows that have birthed one calf) and a 50 percent increase for mulitparous (more than one birth) animals. Hansen pointed out the absurdity of BST approval by his statement:

The drug admittedly increases disease rates. So what are its benefits? Is it a cure for cow AIDS(BIV)? No. Is it a cure for any known cow disease? No. What is its benefit? It increases output of an agriculture product that is already in surplus and has been for a least a decade. We see absolutely no justification for tolerating an increase in disease rates for a drug that increases milk production, and that the FDA cannot possibly determine to be safe. We draw the Committee's attention to the regulations spelled out in 21CFR514.1 which clearly state that a drug must be safe and effective for its labeled use. (25)

Hansen also offered data revealing that experimental cows treated with BST were contracting mastitis at a rate seven times that of control animals. He cited Monsanto studies conducted in Vermont and Europe which indicated increased levels of mastitis would occur in BST-treated animals.

Hansen also brought attention to the Congressional Committees the fact that the GAO report revealed up to 52 drugs that are known to be used as antibiotics to treat mastitis. According to Consumer's Union, only 30 of those antibiotics had been approved by FDA. I questioned FDA's Grassie and she told me that a number of those "illegal" 52 drugs were not illegal at all. Most were generic versions of the 30 approved substances. Occasionally, a small dairy farmer, out of panic, would grab something from his medicine cabinet intended for his pet dog. This type of "illegal residue" would occasionally show up in FDA-tested samples and was not indicative of widespread use. What concerned me was the increased levels of antibiotics approved by FDA's Miller.

Miller knew that BST caused an increase in mastitis. She also knew that if ten animals in a 1000-cow herd had visible signs of mastitis, then 150-400 additional animals (for each case of mastitis that farmers could see, there were between 15 to 40 that they could not) were squirting increased somatic cell counts of pus into milk. These farmers had no choice but to dose all of their animals with increased levels of drugs. By changing the numbers on a piece of paper, the milk became healthy again. Americans are lucky that FDA is there to protect the interests of its citizens. If it weren't for scientists like Hansen and institutes like Consumer's Union, you probably would not have received any alerts on milk safety.

On May 6, 1993, Hansen offered additional testimony before a joint meeting of the Veterinary Medicine Advisory Committee and the Food Advisory Committee on the issue of whether or not BST-treated milk should carry a warning label to consumers. Hansen reiterated his concerns expressed in his previous testimony. In addition, he presented documentation that the nutritional value of milk could be substantially altered. All of Hansen's comments were factually correct, but the FDA contradicted every argument by commenting that Hansen's observations were "well within the normal range."

In the late fall of 1993, the *Los Angeles Times* reported that California had approved a 14 percent hike in milk prices. (26) The timing couldn't have been more perfect. After all, BST use had just been approved by the FDA. Consumer's Union argued that milk is the most profitable item to the grocery store owner. Every government report issued between 1990 and 1992 had assured the American public that the price of milk would not increase. Dairy farmers had argued that an increase in farm prices doesn't necessarily mean retail prices will rise. Would that same logic apply if the price of a barrel of oil increases? Won't we see an increase in the cost of gas at the pumps?

There was no milk shortage. Supply and demand forces were not driving the price of milk prices upward. Lobbyists accomplished this deed with lots of government help. The same government which was subsidizing that industry by buying up the large surplus, and the even larger surplus to come from BST, financed by your tax dollars. Over a 4-year period, Consumers Union alerted their subscribers - 5 million strong - to the dangers in BST-treated milk. Milk consumption in 1995 increased by 4 percent over 1994 levels.

Eric Millstone

Eric Millstone, Ph.D., is a professor and researcher at the University of Sussex in England. Millstone performed analyses on the increased incidence of mastitis in cows treated with BST. Monsanto, aware that Millstone's research would be damaging, prohibited him from publishing the incriminating data. The courts sided with Monsanto, agreeing that they had a proprietary interest in that data. Millstone published the story of his inability to disclose the very significant data. His story finally appeared in *Nature* magazine. (27) The actual data are still unpublished.

Millstone argues in his article, entitled "Plagiarism or Protecting Public Health," that the controversy about BST remains unsolved. Rapid publication of all available data is essential if progress is to be made. Millstone noted that Monsanto's published data did not coincide with the data which it gave Millstone and his group to review. Data from ten cows that began a critical experiment were not included in the experiment's eventual analyses. Monsanto requested of Millstone that the data be kept confidential. Monsanto has litigated the proprietary nature of the exclusivity of this research, which is still unpublished. Millstone is troubled by the results and frustrated at the legal restraints Monsanto has placed on him regarding the publication of such data.

"My illness is due to my doctor's insistence that I drink milk, a whitish fluid they force down helpless babies."

W.C. Fields

"Every great advance in natural knowledge has involved the absolute rejection of authority."

Thomas Huxley

"These dairymen are organized; they're adamant, they're militant...And they, they're massing an enormous amount of money that they're going to put into political activities, very frankly."

Secretary of the Treasury John Connally, to President Richard Nixon, From "The Watergate Tapes," March 23, 1971

Chapter 8

(Not So) Wholesome Milk

Dairy farms are not at all like the tranquil scenes depicted on the sides of milk containers. Cows are milk machines and dairy management is big business. Yields per animal are carefully monitored and animals that do not perform are culled from the herd, and sold to the meat processor where they eventually end up as fast food. The dairy farmer's sole purpose is to get as much milk from his animals for as many years as possible. That applies to a small farmer who pools milk to a milk co-operative along with dozens or hundreds of small farmers in the county or state. That also applies to the "factory" farms in which dairy cows go many months at a time chained to a stall while standing on a concrete floor inside of a barn. The dairy industry begins with a cow and a dairy farmer. Along the way are the drivers of trucks hauling 50,000 pounds of milk at one time to a processor. Farmers pay 15 cents for every hundred pounds of milk produced for an association. This association collects the money and uses the funds to achieve policies which are in the best interests of the dairy farmer. Milk from one cow's production would generate less than $100 in a year. Milk from 10 million cows generates hundreds of millions of dollars for the marketing arm of the Dairy Industry. Many of these dollars pay agencies to design brilliant advertising campaigns. Billboards across America with famous athletes sporting "milkstaches" attest to the success of this strategy. These dollars have also trickled up to people in power. The money goes to members of Congress, and to senators and even to presidents of the United States. Milk prices are regulated by the government. Many people within the industry view payments to these regulators as the cost of doing business.

Those seeking insight from the Bible might well be interested in the wisdom of the scriptures. Quite often milk is referred to in a figurative or illustrative way. The land promised to the Israelites is a land "flowing with milk and honey." Certainly, milk and honey did not literally flow. This was a land of great abundance and that phrase denoted peace and prosperity.

A Land Filled with Milk and Honey

A long time ago a shepherd came upon a burning bush that called upon him to remove his sandals, as he was standing upon holy ground. I try to imagine what I would have done after a hot day of driving my sheep through the wilderness. I probably would have stood there feeling sheepish, but I suppose that's what shepherds do. I might have scrambled down the mountain. Thank goodness Moses had the composure to stand his ground and recognize that he was in the presence of the one true God, and not under the influence of magic mushrooms or desert heat. A Voice, forceful and commanding, directed the shepherd to lead the nation of Jewish slaves out of their bondage in Egypt and into a land good and spacious, to a land flowing with milk and honey. The shepherd, Moses, would lead the Jews to that new land. Would they find honey and milk? Assuredly, the Voice in that bush, almighty enough to cause a bush to burn without consuming fuel, would possess the omnipotence to analyze whether cow's milk was a product suitable for human consumption. Did God make a blunder? Is the basic premise of this book at odds with that age old promise made to Moses?

Sometime after performing numerous assorted miracles that included plagues, frogs, locusts and parting the waters of the Red Sea, Moses found himself before God to receive the Ten Commandments. While Moses was communing with God, Aaron, Moses's brother, encouraged the newly freed slaves to transgress the first commandment and build a statue to a pagan god. Perhaps some form of poetic irony inspired Aaron to lead the Jews into melting their gold and silver and constructing a false God in the image of a calf. Calves are born into a world flowing with milk, receiving that gift from their mothers. It is appropriate for them to do so in order to experience enormous weight gains in a short amount of time. God's promise of a land flowing with milk was mocked by His chosen Jews who erected a symbol of milk as their new God while Moses was on Mount Sinai taking the first step of entry into that promised land of milk and honey.

The New Testament: Who Should Drink Milk?

The New Testament refers to the promise that God made to Moses. In Hebrews, chapter 5:12, human beings are ridiculed for consuming milk. The Bible suggests that it is time for re-education. The scriptures state:

> You again need someone to teach you from the
> beginning the elementary things of the sacred
> pronouncements of God, and you have become such
> as need milk, not solid food. For everyone that partakes
> of milk is unacquainted with the word of righteousness,
> for he is a babe. But solid food belongs to mature
> people, to those who through use have their perceptive
> powers trained to distinguish both right and wrong.

The Bible makes a proclamation regarding just for whom milk was intended and offers a lesson about milk consumption that has long lapsed from our collective consciousness. Milk is appropriate for infants. Infants must experience dramatic weight gains. Adults should not. Milk was never intended to be consumed by adults. A "true" believer, finding comfort and inspiration in the truths contained in the Bible, would have to reject dairy products. According to the Bible, every individual who partakes of milk is "unacquainted with the word of righteousness" and is consuming a product that was intended for babies.

God's promise to Moses? A land flowing with milk and honey! A land of sweetness where the milk would flow. The milk for infants from the breasts of their mothers. A land free of persecution where slaves would no longer be tormented with the infanticide of their first born males. A land where a people would be unfettered by the shackles of bondage and have opportunity to give birth to incalculable numbers of children. The milk would surely flow in this land and the Israelites were destined to enjoy the sweet taste of the freedoms promised by their God.

Dietary Laws: They Make Sense!

Moses was given a list of instructions to follow upon entering that land of milk and honey. The dietary and health laws preceded modern technologies, and yet anticipated many of the problems caused by improper handling of foods. Although swarms of bacteria could not be seen, many parasites and bacterium were eliminated from the diets of those who placed their faith and trust in such laws. In Leviticus 11:41-43, God tells Moses that "every swarming creature that swarms upon the earth is a loathsome thing," and Moses is instructed, "Do not make your souls loathsome with any swarming creature that swarms, and you must not make yourselves unclean by them and actually get unclean by them." Thousands of years later, Monsanto Agricultural Company of St. Louis, Missouri, devised a way to isolate the swarming bacteria surviving within human feces in gastrointestinal tracts. Taking those swarming germs, Monsanto added natural cow hormones and created a "flock" of bacteria (*E. coli*) able to recombine the natural hormone into a new product which was a little bit different, and a little bit more powerful than the naturally occurring bovine growth hormone. When injected into cows this hormone would change milk. The consumption of this new genetically tampered milk would increase the risk of human cancer.

The Presumptuous: Let Them Eat Bacteria

King David, who was given much of the credit for writing the Psalms, sang of the Monsanto Agricultural Company. In Psalm 119, which blesses those who follow the laws of God, we are warned (verse 85), "The presumptuous have excavated pitfalls to get me, those who are not in accord with your law." Can you imagine those "presumptuous" Monsanto scientists carefully scraping (while holding their noses, of course) hordes of bacteria from human feces? Can you imagine them joking about creating new products for our food supply from this stuff? I propose that we change the names of the new Monsanto hormones created by this process - BST (bovine somatotropin) and IGF (insulin-growth factor) , to somatotropic-hormones-insulin-type, or simply S-H-I-T. That would be appropriate. Then we could leave the health and safety debate for our religious leaders. Is eating SHIT kosher? Imagine a stoned hippie drinking a tall glass of genetically engineered milk. "Man, this is good SHIT!"

Americans eat hormones, fat and cholesterol with their morning cereal and squirt a few drops into their first cup of coffee. Perhaps some cream cheese on your bagel? Healthy breakfast? How about some yogurt? Your body is drug free, but don't forget to bathe your cells with powerful growth hormones before leaving for the office. Lunch? A slice of pizza. A milkshake with your cheeseburger. Some ice cream for dessert. Milk. America's number one food industry.

There has been no voice speaking to me from a burning bush, nor have I consumed any of those hallucinogenic mushrooms. The mission of this book is to lead you away from the plagues of milk, society's angel of death. Milk and dairy products are responsible for a great number of the common ailments found in both children and adults. Many myths about the wholesomeness of milk have been carefully constructed as golden calves, monuments to the marketing geniuses responsible for selling milk and dairy products.

There is as much fat in a glass of lowfat milk as there is in three slices of bacon. Osteoporosis? Milk is actually the culprit. Real cows don't eat grass, but there is plenty of calcium in their normal diet just as there is enough calcium in the typical American diet. Excess calcium is actually the real cause of osteoporosis. Drink milk and break bones. Cholesterol? Remember, each day the average American consumes the equivalent amount of cholesterol contained in fifty-three slices of bacon from milk and dairy products.

Milk was designed for a purpose. That purpose is to enable an infant to receive nourishment, including hormones, that will direct and regulate growth. Enormous growth. A human infant will double its weight in three months. A cow will gain 500 pounds in just six months. Milk is a hormonal delivery system. It is an appropriate food for infants who must gain weight rather quickly. Such hormones are not appropriate for adults. Milk drinkers bathe their systems with the white liquid containing fat, cholesterol and hormones. Their cellular processes become regulated by powerful growth hormones. However, in adults those hormones are unable to stimulate the same cellular growth that infants experience. Instead, in adults those hormones can create a holy terror.

And On His Farm He Had a Cow, E-I-E-I-O

I recently visited my town library. I reviewed the listings on the library computer. There was only one children's milk book to review. Not even a choice of conflicting presentations for 8-year-olds. The computer noted that the book was presently on the library shelves.

On the front cover of the little book a pretty female child holds a glass of milk. Her smile is mirrored in the face of a cow looking human-like in its facial features. What a friendly book! The cow contentedly chews a mouthful of grass. Both the child and the cow stand in a green field amidst gently sloping hills. On the back cover is a young boy holding onto the back of another cow. This second animal also is eating grass and keeps company with sheep and insects, bees and a butterfly in the foreground alighting on a flower. The book is *Green Grass and White Milk*, written and illustrated by Brandenberg. What words of knowledge will the children glean?

> Cows graze in valleys and eat in good green pastures.
> When she finishes eating she lies quietly. She lives in a
> warm dark barn that smells from hay. (1)

The book is beautifully illustrated with drawings of cows smiling their people-like smiles surrounded by either children or baby farm animals. A garden of Eden.

Meanwhile, Back At the Farm...

This past summer I took my family to visit a real working dairy farm. As we approached our objective, we searched the fields for cows which to "moo" to from out of our windows. There were no cows to be seen. We saw the dairy barns. When we reached our destination and finally made our way into a dairy barn, we witnessed nothing like the tranquil setting described in the children's book. The "barn" seemed more like a factory warehouse than a barn, having a concrete slab floor with enormous quantities of bovine excrement and flies. This stuff didn't smell like hay. It was more like, hey, what the heck is that stench? The stalls did not appear to be very comfortable. Cows weren't eating grass. Thick galvanized steel bars formed the stalls which separated each animal. They were chained in a manner that made sitting, grazing, walking and turning impossible. This wasn't a happy place like the farm in *Green Grass and White Milk.*

A cow produces milk for one reason only, to feed her calf. A human mother produces milk for her human baby, a squirrel for her children and a whale for her calves. In nature, the milk continues to flow for as long as the infant continues to nurse. This tactile suckling sensation produces a hormonal messenger that sends instructions to the mother's brain. The message...keep producing milk! A short time after the sucking ceases, the milk delivery system shuts down until the process begins anew with the birth of another child.

At around 6 months of age, a human baby begins to eat solid food. As teeth develop, the child begins to teethe and chew a nipple, a process which can be quite painful to the mother. As different foods are introduced, human babies demonstrate a preference for solid foods. A calf will generally reject milk and replace it with solid food as it matures. During the nursing period, the mother's breasts or udders are continuously engorged with milk, ready for a demanding user. The cow with calf will feed her offspring continuously, sometimes two dozen feedings daily. When an infant has been "weaned" from his or her mother's breast (or from that bottle of formula), mom usually replaces the "good old stuff" with cow's milk. Imagine Elsie the cow doing the same for her infant if it were possible. Her calf in its natural and innate wisdom prefers to obtain nutrients and nourishment from solid food. Imagine that cow ambling down to a supermarket and buying her 6-month-old calf a dose of human breast milk. She would lug home a 5 gallon container with the rendering of a missing calf on the side. "Have you seen my child?" It is absurd to drink the milk containing hormones from another species of animal. It isn't logical that a cow drink our milk or that we drink hers. It just goes to demonstrate how great marketing and brainwashing can manipulate our behavior.

Daddy, Tell Me a Story

The evening after visiting Ronneybrook farm, my daughter called to me, "Daddy, tell me a story." I filled her imagination with a world where people didn't drank milk. Only six, she thought it funny to imagine drinking milk from a dog. After seeing an udder up close she found the concept of drinking milk from cows to be equally as absurd.

The Twilight Zone

You unlock this chapter with "the key of imagination. Beyond it is another dimension, a dimension of sound, a dimension of sight, a dimension of mind. You're moving into a land of both shadow and substance, of things and ideas. You've just crossed over into the twilight zone." (2) Presented for your review, a world just like our own in a parallel universe. Everything in that world is identical to ours except for one factor. That world has no dairy industry. There has never been a cow and there are no such food items as butter, cheese or yogurt. No lost children on milk containers. No pogs from the tops of milk bottles.

Now imagine a copyright patent clerk sitting inside a building in the capitol city of a great nation on this parallel world. She hears a knock on her door and rises to greet a man holding a Saint Bernard dog. "Yes?," she inquires, seeking to help the man and at the same time mask her curiosity.

"You're not going to believe this," he answers, turning the canine upside down revealing a healthy and pregnant bitch to be, teats engorged with nourishment intended for her pups, to be born shortly. "I don't think that you can patent that," the unamused clerk replies.

"Wait a second," he answers, and in one swift motion grabs the animal with one arm while his hand firmly takes hold of a nipple and tweaks a white liquid into a small bowl which he's placed on the table. He then places the dog on the floor while the astonished clerk, at a loss for words, looks on. "Here, try this." He offers the bowl to the clerk, who having seen enough screams, "Get the hell outta here." The surprised man grabs the dog and makes a hasty retreat from the office.

One week later we see the clerk sitting at her desk. A knock at the door. She looks up. He is holding a long leash. Attached to the end of the leash is a reindeer. He hardly has time to protest her swift action. She firmly grabs his elbow and leads him out of her office. She closes her door and turns the lock. "If you come back again with any more animals, I'm having you arrested," she screams, yelling at the door which she has closed.

One week later same office, same knock, same man. This time she opens the door and is greeted by the man and his ox. He has a paper in his hand. A court order. He is accompanied by his attorney and a woman with a stool and wooden bucket. The attorney advises, "We have a court order here." His client holds the paper. The clerk stares wide-eyed as the woman sits on the stool, places the bucket under the ox, grabs the udder and begins to pump out liquid which fills the bucket. "I'm calling it milk," the man informs the clerk. He hands her a set of application forms. "I've had it analyzed. It's loaded with fat and cholesterol and hormones. I'll sell it to underweight people and weight lifters. They'll never need to take steroids again." The clerk visibly relaxes and smiles. "Hmm. Sounds interesting."

"Want to try some?" He offers her a cup. She grimaces. "No, no! It's kind of a disgusting thought, drinking that stuff." "Do you think the public will buy it?" He asks. She shakes her head. "It takes all kinds," she says, referring to the man in front of her. "It sure does," replies the man, mentally spending the fortune which this patent will produce.

It is a disgusting thought, sucking from the udder of a bovine. Imagine the first human to think of such an idea? One wonders, did he have a bucket? Did he have a cup? Did he simply attach his mouth to the udder of his cow and mimic the behavior of her calf? Why do we find the lactating milk of a cow so delicious, and yet not the dog? Why do we consider the taking of milk from other animals to be a repulsive concept?

In many nations, the thought of drinking milk from a cow is abhorrent. Masai tribesmen in Africa routinely bleed their cattle for nourishment. They make small incisions in the necks of their animals and drink their blood for breakfast. The thought of Americans drinking milk is enough to make these people physically ill. The entire concept of drinking cow's milk is absurd. Ever smell the underside of a cow? You wouldn't want to touch anything coming out of spouts that looked that ugly. I enjoy watching baby pigs suckling or lambs bleating for the milk which they demand. The thought of people suckling that substance is disgusting to me.

Milk is filled with dead cells, sloughed off in the milk as protein matter in the name of cuisine. Milk is loaded with pus from cows that have mastitis which is treated with antibiotics. Milk is chock-full of pesticides. Milk contains bacteria, which in spite of numerous wonder drugs with which cows are treated, is not entirely destroyed. Fat and cholesterol? No other food contains such a "one-two punch." Milk contains the same exact hormone, genetically structured, as the human equivalent hormone, IGF-I, the powerful growth factor. Show me one man or woman who would knowingly take a pill containing equal doses of this "drug" contained in one glass of milk. Why should adults drink these hormones? How did we so successfully block out from our minds any conceptualization of the origin of the product contained in those gallon jugs in supermarkets? Picture the likeness of happy cows grazing in beautiful fields so artfully portrayed on their containers of milk.

Next time you drink a glass of milk pretend that it comes from a Saint Bernard dog or a pig or a deer. That thought is enough to gag on. Only a random quirk of human sociological development enabled the cow industry to develop as large as it has. It could have easily been the dog industry instead, and we'd all be milking our own pet dogs, and be just as naive and unbothered by dog milk as we are by cow milk. Come to think of it, dog milk might be healthier, as the IGF is a different type and wouldn't affect us. Who has taught us to drink milk from cows, continuously reinforcing that message? The wealthiest and most powerful food industry lobby in America, that's who.

The Dairy Industry

One of the greatest efforts in American investigative journalism resulted in the book, *Milking the Public*, written by Michael McMenamin and Walter McNamara in 1980. (3) This reference work was published by Nelson-Hall in Chicago and thanks is given to the publisher, particularly Steven Long, for permission authorizing use of the following passages. This book is still in stock and may be ordered directly from the publisher at 312-930-5903.

You have previously read how twelve members of the Dairy Sub-committee of the House Agriculture Committee received $711,000 in bribes, called PAC money, directly from various agriculture interest groups. Those dollars were mere droplets in the milk bucket when compared to the enormity of the grand total paid out to influential individuals by the dairy coalition. If you read McMenamin's book you will reach the conclusion that Watergate was a third-degree burglary compared with the grandest heist in America's history. Who were the victims? The American public, who paid billions of dollars more for their milk as a result of "brilliant marketing." Who were the conspirators? One was Richard Nixon, who received more than $3 million dollars from this powerful lobby.

Watergate Tapes: President Nixon Was Bribed

The transcript from one of the Watergate tapes made on March 23, 1971, reveals a president (Nixon) carefully choosing his words for the men delivering an enormous bribe. If only the walls of the Oval Office could talk, what secrets they would reveal. Here, then, the transcript of President Richard M. Nixon's meeting with milk producer cooperatives:

Uh, I know...that, uh, you are a group that are politically
very conscious...And you're willing to do something
about it. And, I must say a lot of businessmen and others...
don't do anything about it. And you do, and I appreciate
that. And, I don't have to spell it out.

Here, caught on tape is a president receiving a bribe. Later on, after these milk producers have left, Nixon, alone with advisor John Connally, says:

They are tough political operatives. This is a cold political deal.

Who was getting the money, who was getting the price increases, who was paying the bribe and who was actually footing the bill? The authors of the milk industry book carefully lay out all of the details. The dairy industry learned, throughout the administrations of four presidents that they could buy presidential decisions with both legal and illegal cash contributions. They learned that they can buy the votes of members of congressional committees. They successfully bribed one secretary after another. They learned to avoid antitrust litigation and they learned how to regulate price controls for their milk.

Today farmers pay 15 cents to this coalition for every hundred pounds of milk that they produce. That may sound like just pennies, but it all adds up. The USDA reports that 400 million pounds of milk are produced every single day. When the numbers are tabulated, they run into the hundreds of millions of dollars. In chapter four of *Milking the Public*, the authors demonstrate how easily a president could rely upon his dairy coalition friends. In 1967, Lyndon Johnson was still running for re-election, a decision which changed after $90,711 was invested in a "Salute to the President" book that was to be sold to help finance that campaign. When Johnson announced his intention not to run, that ended all value to the book which had been printed. Who would pay for that book? As it turned out, favors were called in by Johnson, who knew where and how to get the bills paid.

On March 29th, 1967, the Johnson administration increased milk prices by 7 percent. The cost of living for the previous 12 months was 2.8 percent. Three invoices totaling $90,711 were paid by the Central Arkansas Milk Producers Association ($30,250), the North Texas Producer's Association ($28,500) and the remaining $31,000.96 was paid by the Milk Producer's Inc. (MPI). Hubert Humphrey was another matter. Thousands of dollars in illegal donations were paid to Humphrey from Dairy Coalition sources. The New York-based ad agency, Lennen and Newell, billed the Humphrey campaign for services and then sent the invoices to the Associated Milk Producers Inc., c/o Bob Lilly, New Ulm, Minnesota.

Crooks, Crooks and More Crooks

Hundreds of donations, attempts at influence, hundred dollar bills stuffed into attache cases, then transferred to wall safes, then co-mingled with other money from dairy groups. The names and dates and players all carefully researched and spelled out by McMenamin. Haldeman, Erlichman, John Mitchell, Republicans and Democrats, presidents and congressmen. There are more dollars available today. Has the dairy coalition learned to use more discretion? Does anybody believe that the same practices no longer occur? When the Executive Branch of the federal government wrote that dairy prices would decrease after milk was genetically engineered because there would be a greater supply of milk, did anybody really believe this?

The Just Plain Yogurt Industry

The Dannon Company spelled out their philosophy in regards to BST-treated milk, a position similar to other major milk industry producers and manufacturers.

Dear Mr. Cohen,   *September 27, 1994*

Thank you for your recent inquiry regarding our position on bovine somatotropin, commonly known as BST. As you may know, after decades of extensive research, the Food and Drug Administration (FDA) approved the use of BST in November, 1993. The sale of BST is permitted beginning February 4, 1994. By way of background, BST is a natural protein hormone produced by a cow and trace amounts are contained in all milk--whether from supplemented or unsupplemented cows. BST is what stimulates the conversion of feed into milk production. When supplemental BST is given to a cow, it can enhance the energy conversion process and, hence, can increase a cow's productive capacity. Some estimates put this increase in the range of 8% to 15%.

The FDA, the agency responsible for ensuring the safety of the nation's food supply, has tested and studied the effect of BST on human and animal health for many years. FDA declared milk from cows who receive supplemental BST safe for human consumption in 1985, over seven years ago. Many other credible scientific and medical groups throughout the world have also reviewed the data and made the same finding--milk and meat from BST supplemental cows is safe.

The milk from cows given supplemental BST is the same as--actually indistinguishable from--the milk from unsupplemental cows. There is no increase in the level of BST in the milk and the nutrient composition of the milk is unchanged.

Some of the BST controversy deals with BST's alleged impact on milk prices and the small dairy farmer. It is important to note that those concerns do not extend to human health or food safety. At the same time, much controversy is generated by those who are opposed to the use of biotechnology in all forms, including animal and plant agriculture.

*With this background in mind, Dannon, along with the **National Yogurt Association**, has taken the following position:*

*1) Dannon, along with the **National Yogurt Association**, support the adoption of new production technologies that contribute to the efficiency and productivity of our food production system so long as these technologies have been approved as safe after rigorous scientific evaluation and analyses by government agencies responsible for ensuring the safety of the American food supply.*

*2) Dannon, along with the **National Yogurt Association**, neither advocates nor opposes the use or approval of BST. The choice to use BST will be made at the dairy farm level by individual producers, just as dairy farmers choose other technologies that increase efficiency and make their work easier. Dannon, does not participate in this decision making process.*

3) Because of the industry practice of pooling milk from many farmers, it would be virtually impossible for any dairy processors or distributors to state accurately and consistently that their product comes from herds that have not received supplemental BST. In addition no test exists to distinguish between milk from supplemental and nonsupplemental herds. We do not believe that claims on our part or on the part of our milk suppliers that our milk does not come from cows given additional BST could be substantiated with any credible evidence and we will not misrepresent the facts.

*4) For this same reason, Dannon, along with the **National Yogurt Association**, will not label its dairy products as "not from BST-treated herds." The milk is indistinguishable and to label it would be misleading. Legal experts who have evaluated the issue have concluded that processors or retailers "will be running a substantial risk of violating federal law if they choose to state in labels or on store posters that their products do not contain milk from cows given BST.*

I hope this clarifies our position on BST. As the agency responsible for the approval of BST, questions or concerns regarding its potential use can be addressed directly to the FDA. The FDA contact is:

Mary-Alice Miller, Chief Education and Communications Branch, Center For Veterinary Medicine, 456 Metro Park North II, 7500 Standish Place, Rockville, MD, 20855 Telephone: (301) 594-1740.

You may also call the Dairy Industry BST Infoline at (202) 682-1678 with any question on BST.

I hope that this information is helpful to you.

Sincerely
M. Sturgis
Consumer Response Representative (800) 321-2174

The National Yogurt Foundation

Dannon mentions the National Yogurt Association four times, but they do not offer their phone number or address. McLean, Virginia, home of the National Yogurt Association, was less than two miles from downtown Washington, D.C., home of Congress. Companies like Dannon Yogurt have learned that it is profitable to create associations and locate them "close to the real action."

The Dairy Coalition, which includes the National Milk Producers Federation, the International Dairy Foods Association, and the International Dairy Federation (IDF), is committed to educating consumers about the safety of the nation's milk supply. The Coalition's official policy is to neither endorse nor oppose BST. However, they incorrectly issued a press statement in March of 1995 that Consumer's Union had "backed off claims that milk from BST-supplemented cows poses a health threat to humans." Consumer's Union promptly issued a statement saying that their position on BST had not changed and that labeling of BST products should be mandatory. However, let's examine the impartiality of the IDF.

Dale Bauman, Cornell University Scientist

In December 1993, the IDF issued a bulletin on somatotropin, a technical report. The senior author of that report was Dale Bauman, a Cornell University researcher who had worked closely with Miller, the Monsanto scientist who became subject of a GAO conflict of interest investigation. Among other lies, this technical report states:

Furthermore, pasteurization eliminates 85-90 percent of immunoreactive BST in milk . (4)

Unlike Juskevich and Guyer, Bauman correctly cited Groenewegen. However, Juskevich and Guyer stated that 90 percent of the BST was destroyed by pasteurization. Bauman takes liberty by writing 85-90 percent. Do scientists like Bauman make up numbers out of thin air? Perhaps. Groenewegen's actual numbers were 18.10 percent for normal milk and 19.05 percent for BST-treated milk. And, Groenewegen tried very hard to deactivate all of the BST by using the 30-minute pasteurization method with the high heat used in the 15 second pasteurization treatment. One of Bauman's specialties is the study of mastitis. Actual publication of additional incriminating data, were nearly published by Erik Millstone at the Science Policy Research Unit, Sussex University, Brighton, England. That publication was blocked by Monsanto. Bauman wrote about mastitis:

These summaries indicated that treatment with BST had
no effects of biological importance on mastitis-related
variables. (5)

Try to figure that one out! That means they had effects, just none of
biological importance, whatever the heck that means. If I had udders filled with
milk and covered with ulcers, that would be biologically significant to me. Moo!
Bauman said that they "had no effect on mastitis related variables," whatever those
"variables" are. BST increased mastitis. BST made cows sick. BST increased
the levels of hormones in milk. Thankfully, our variables were safe.

Mastitis: Ulcers On Cow's Udders

If a farmer wakes up Monday morning and sees the tell-tale signs of
mastitis, ulcerations of the udders, of ten of his cows in a herd of 1000 animals,
then 150 to 400 of those cows also have mastitis which is internal, and their milk
contains increased levels of pus. The farmer must treat his entire herd with
increased levels of antibiotics which are permitted into your milk by a stroke of the
pen from a Monsanto scientist. This must be what dairy scientist Dale Bauman
means when he writes "no biological importance." This is why the Dairy Coalition
feels justified in repeating that milk is safe. Because the FDA says so. Nowhere in
his report does Bauman say that BST-treated milk is indistinguishable from normal
untreated milk.

America Purchases Surplus Milk

In a 1991 story, Consumers Union (CU) reported that the United States
purchased the equivalent of 9 billion pounds of surplus milk from dairy producers
in 1990. (6) Why was it so important to produce more milk? Why did the dairy
industry lobby for BST and higher milk prices? Who would be hurt by this
insanity? At the same time that America was developing a hormone to make more
milk, and purchasing the surplus milk which was flooding the market, we were
also paying more that $1.3 billion dollars to dairymen to slaughter more than 1
million cows which were producing this surplus.

Dairymen were taught a valuable lesson by the Washington bureaucracy.
By buying more cows to produce more milk they would receive more subsidies. If
we could genetically engineer a hormone that would yield even more milk, there
would be greater subsidies. An article in *National Review* beautifully expressed
the system which we have created. This article reviewed a book written by James
Payne called *The Culture of Spending: Why Congress Lives Beyond Our Means.*
The author points out the enormity of the Dairy Coalition lobbying effort. There is

no antidairy coalition, no such counter-lobby, so members of Congress only get one side of the story, a biased presentation. Payne writes:

> Sheer conviviality and direct personal contact are important
> factors in the spending culture. The congressman has lunch
> with pro-spending lobbyists every day. He almost never has
> lunch with opponents of spending (who, politically, can hardly
> be said to exist). The whole situation is terribly one-sided. (7)

Major scandals have thrust the dairy industry into the national spotlight. The last occurred during the Nixon White House years. Millions of dollars were donated to Nixon's election committee which resulted in price controls for milk which benefited the dairy industry. More than 25 years ago, dairy groups were recorded on the "Watergate tapes" in making payments and donations which purchased influence at the highest levels of our government.

A Doctor Who Makes "Free" Housecalls

Welcome to the world of the Internet. And welcome to the home page of Alan Greene, M.D., a pediatrician who takes questions and in answering them offers detailed advice dispensed with caring bedside manner. You can visit Dr. Greene at:

http://www.drgreene.com

I asked Dr. Greene a question which he posted to his website:

> Recently I met with top scientists at the FDA in Rockville,
> Maryland, discussing among other things, breastfeeding. It
> was their collective opinion that breastfeeding offered psych-
> ological nurturing benefits, but nothing more. No immunological
> factors, etc. Their logic was that all proteins are broken down
> by strong digestive enzymes. What do you think?

Dr. Greene agreed that milk buffered gastric pH and created an environment in which proteins survive digestion. Then, with just a bit of sarcasm and a lot of wit, and plenty of references based upon research published in accredited journals, Dr. Greene wrote an answer to my question. That answer, with his blessing, appears here.

Dr. Greene Wrote:

I applaud the critical thinking and intellectual curiosity of these scientists. When immunoglobulins were first discovered in breast milk, the appealing and simple conclusion was drawn that these immunoglobulins would directly improve the immune status of the baby. Indeed specific antibodies against respiratory and intestinal bacteria and viruses are found in human breast milk. These have been thought to increase a child's resistance to infection. Apparently, the aforementioned scientists have pointed out that this reasoning is overly simplistic. In fact, the strong digestive enzymes in the infant and the acid bath awaiting the antibodies in the stomach would tend to denature and digest these antibodies, rendering them useless.

While I admire their reasoning and believe that this line of thinking deserves further exploration, not all proteins are digested before they affect the babies health. Some proteins even make it intact through the stomach. Based on the available evidence, I vehemently disagree with the conclusion that breast milk is essentially no different than formula.

Many studies comparing the frequency of illness between breast and formula-fed infants have demonstrated fewer illnesses and less severe illnesses in breast-fed infants (Garza et al, Special Properties of Human Milk, Clinics of Perinatology, *14: 11-32, 1987). While it is very difficult to separate all of the many variables of parenting style and environment, mounting evidence shows a striking reduction in the incidence and seriousness of gastrointestinal infections, respiratory infections, and* <u>ear infections</u> *in breast-fed babies (Duncan et al, Exclusive Breast Feeding for at Least Four Months Protects Against Otiis Media,* Pediatrics, *91: 867-872, 1993). Other studies have shown a decrease in non-infectious diseases such as eczema and asthma. If the immunoglobulins are rendered useless by digestion, how could this be?*

Psychological Factors

You mentioned that these scientists suggest that the only difference between formula and breast milk is psychological. I strongly disagree that this is the only difference, but I agree that the psychological difference can have profound implications. Over the last decade-and-a-half the developing field of psychoneuroimmunology has demonstrated repeatedly that an individual's psychological state has a direct effect on his or her immune function. Perhaps the nursing experience by itself does directly improve the immune status of the infants.

Immunoglobulins

All types of immunoglobulins are found in human milk. The highest concentration is found in colostrum, the pre-milk which is only available from the breast the first three to five days of the baby's life. Secretory IGA, a type of immunoglobulin that protects the ears, nose, throat and the GI tract, is found in high amounts in breast milk throughout the first year. Secretory IGA does its work before it would be digested in the stomach. Secretory IGA attaches to the lining of the nose, mouth and throat and fights the attachment of specific infecting agents. Breastmilk levels of IGA against specific viruses and bacteria increase in response to a maternal exposure to these organisms. Thus, human milk has been called environmentally specific milk, which the mother provides for her infant to protect specifically against the organisms that her infant is most likely to be exposed to.

Lactoferrin

Lactoferrin is an iron-binding protein that is found in human milk, but not available in formulas. It limits the availability of iron to bacteria in the intestines, and alters which healthy bacteria will thrive in the gut. Again, it is found in the highest concentrations in colostrum, but persists throughout the entire first year. It has a direct antibiotic effect on bacteria such as staphlocci and E. coli.

Lysosomes

Human breast milk contains lysosomes (a potent digestive ingredient) at a level thirty times higher than in any formula. Interestingly, while other contents of breast milk vary widely between well-nourished and poorly nourished mothers, the amount of lysosome is conserved, suggesting that it is very important. It has a strong influence on the type of bacteria which inhabit the intestinal tract.

Growth Factors

Human breast milk specifically encourages the growth of Lactobacillaceae, helpful bacteria which can inhibit many of the disease-causing gram-negative bacteria and parasites. In fact, there is a striking difference between the bacteria found in the guts of breast and formula-fed infants. Breast-fed infants have a level of lactobacillus that is typically 10 times greater than of formula-fed infants. Both the presence of the lactobacilli and the action of the lactoferrins and lysosomes help protect the infant.

Allergic Factors

The cows' milk protein used in many formulas is a foreign protein. When babies are exposed to non-human milk, they actually develop antibodies to the foreign protein. Research has shown that without exception the important food allergens found in milk and soybean formulas are stable to digestion in the stomach for as long as 60 minutes (as compared to human milk protein which is digested in the stomach within 15 minutes). Thus, the foreign proteins pass through the stomach and reach the intestines intact, where they gain access and can produce sensitization. While research in this area is still relatively in the beginning stages, this early exposure to foreign proteins may be the pre-disposing factor in such illnesses as eczema and asthma. The effects of early exposure to foreign protein are explored in three abstracts in the Journal of Allergy and Clinical Immunology, *from January of 1996.*

Carnitine

While carnitine is present in both breast milk and formula, the carnitine in breast milk has higher bioavailability. Breast-fed babies have significantly higher carnitine levels than their counterparts. Carnitine is necessary to make use of fatty acids as an energy source. Other functions of carnitine have been hypothesized, but have not yet been proven.

Lipid Differences

The main long-chain fatty acids found in human milk are still not present in formulas in the United States. These lipids are important structural components, particularly in the substance of the brain and the retina. Significantly different amounts of these ingredients have been found in the brains and retinas of breast-fed versus formula-fed infants. <u>This difference may have other subtle effects on the cell membrane integrity in other parts of the body as well.</u>

Apart from the specific properties that I have mentioned above, it is important to emphasize that breast milk is a dynamic fluid that changes in composition throughout the day and throughout the course of lactation. It provides for the baby the specific nutrients that are needed at each age and in each situation. The early data about breast milk was obtained from the pooled breast milk of many mothers. At that time it was not understood how unique human breast milk is for each individual infant (Lawrence, P.B., Breast Milk, Pediatric Clinics of North America, *Oct. 1994). (Parenthetically, breast milk tastes different from feeding to feeding, another advantage over formula, as it prepares babies for the wide variety of foods to which they will be exposed in the future.*

The suggestion you heard from these prominent scientists serves as a good reminder that the mysteries of this dynamic fluid have not, by any means, been fully deciphered. Nevertheless, it becomes clearer year by year, that human milk is precisely designed for human babies. There may well be other important micro-nutrients or factors that we don't even have instruments to measure yet. Not many decades ago, immunoglobulins weren't even imagined. While formulas are an excellent alternative when breast feeding is not possible, human breast milk is the superior food for human babies for many, many reasons.

THANK YOU, DR. GREENE!

What are the implications? Clearly, proteins in milk survive digestion. Nursing mothers believe this. Their pediatricians certainly believe this. The only ones who do not believe this are the FDA scientists. If proteins in human milk survive digestion, then proteins in cow milk survive digestion. If IGF-I is the most powerful growth hormone in the human body, and if cow IGF-I is identical to human IGF-I, then every time we drink a glass of milk or eat a slice of cheese we take hormones into our body. Indeed, protein hormones do survive digestive processes. Milk is a hormonal delivery system.

Mark Goldman, CEO of Farmland Dairies, the largest dairy distributor in Bergen County, New Jersey, has maintained a heroic position regarding the genetically engineered bovine protein. His company has been rewarded with increased sales of its products because Goldman refuses to accept milk from cows that have been treated with rbST. That policy, brilliantly marketed, reflects consumer's concerns about these hormones.

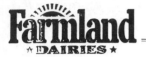

FARM FRESH SINCE 1914

FARMLAND DAIRIES
POLICY STATEMENT ON rBST/rBGH

Farmland Dairies strongly opposes use of the drug
rBST/rBGH (recombinant Bovine Somatotropin/recombinant
Bovine Growth Hormone) on dairy cows. Farmland Dairies
has requested and received written pledges from all dairy
farmers shipping to Farmland that they will not administer this
drug to their cows.

On Skim Plus, where Farmland adds additional non-fat milk
solids, those solids are obtained from farmers and/or
organizations who also do not use this drug.

520 Main Avenue, P.O. Box 3340, Wallington, NJ 07057
Tel 201 777 2500 • Fax 201 777 7648

"I feel strongly that the blanket statements which appeared in the press that there is a direct and causative relation between smoking of cigarettes, and the number of cigarettes smoked, to cancer of the lung is an absolutely unwarranted conclusion."

Dr. Max Cutler (NY TIMES, 4/14/54)

"There is still no positive proof of a casual relationship between the use of thalidomide during pregnancy and malformations in the newborn."

Frank Getman, President of Merril Co., manufacturer of Thalidomide, 2/21/62

"If your eyes are set wide apart you should be a vegetarian, because you inherit the digestive characteristics of bovine ancestry."

Dr. Linard Williams, London, 1932

Chapter 9

Milk Consumption: A Second Opinion from the Medical Establishment

Doctors have little time nor inclination to analyze their patient's dietary or nutritional needs. Rarely does a doctor ask a patient what foods he or she eats. Temperatures and blood pressures can be taken along with x-rays and blood analysis. Results of such clinical tests can be measured against charts containing statistical standards. A typical visit to a doctor's office often results in a long wait before seeing the doctor. More often than not, the patient is there seeking a diagnosis and cure for his particular ailment. The medical practitioner often writes a prescription for a medication and then makes arrangements for follow up visits and re-analyses of symptoms. Doctors try to cure disease by eliminating the symptoms. They rarely seek the cause of the disease. Patients complaining of migraines or epileptic episodes are given EEGs and referred to neurologists. They are rarely asked whether they drink diet soda or use aspartame, both of which have been associated with headaches and seizures. Patients reporting mucous, earaches and constant colds and congestive problems have blood work and chest x-rays. A doctor rarely explores the relationship between disease and possible reaction to casein in milk, one of nature's strongest glues. Food additives such as monosodium glutamate (MSG) have caused terrible reactions in thousands of individuals. Sleep patterns have been interrupted because of digestive problems while doctors rarely explore the specific foods being eaten.

Alternative medical practitioners and herbalists have long recognized the link between good diet and good health. Billions of people on planet Earth rely upon pharmacies that carry herbal remedies to cure illness, such as ginseng root and chamomile tea. Most Americans and their doctors look at such practice and custom with blighted hope and cynicism, unaware that many of America's pharmaceuticals are developed from herbs and rare plants found in the Amazon region or from the barks of rare trees. Recently, a few doctors have been exploring the connection between diet and human disease. Two of these doctors, Neal Barnard, M.D., and Robert Kradjian, M.D., have recognized that milk and dairy products might represent an enormous contributory influence towards illness in America.

In high school, young bright scholars become inspired to go to the best colleges where they pursue an undergraduate course of study concentrated in the sciences, biology, chemistry, physics and calculus. If all goes well and their grades are superior to their fellow students, the competition, they might elect to go on to medical school. An intense course of study follows. Anatomy, physiology, histology, one "ology" after another of intense memorization and study. Later on, these elite students intern in hospitals and one day become medical doctors. It takes dedication, motivation and commitment to become a doctor. Some doctors are naturally brilliant. Others, using tools of study properly learned in primary school, including discipline, achieve that same medical degree. For some, it's easy, for others, not so easy. For all, it's the same degree.

All doctors are not alike. Some have time to read one journal per week and some have time to read twenty. Some work every day of the year and some vacation every other weekend. Some, not many, make house calls. Many doctors are so busy, their waiting rooms filled by patients seeking consultation for varieties of illness, that there is little time for anything for them to do but attend to their patient's immediate needs. If you have ever sat for one hour in a standing-room-only waiting room, you understand when the doctor rushes through your exam, gives you 30 seconds of chit chat, writes a prescription, and rushes out the door towards another examination room. Doctors are not in business to practice preventative medicine. Their priority is to properly diagnose and then safely medicate. They are taught in medical school their proper role in our society. Nutrition often plays no role in their training.

"Doctor, should I drink milk?" you ask. What knowledge do they base their response upon? Did they study about milk in medical school? Do they even think about the hormones or antibiotics, fat or cholesterol, bovine proteins which trigger allergies? Most doctors suggest that everybody should drink milk. Robert M. Kradjian, M.D., in response to a patient's question, began to explore the milk and dairy influence on our culture. His investigation and review of the scientific literature resulted in a letter written to his patient.

Dr. Robert Kradjian's Letter to his Patients

"Milk." Just the word itself sounds comforting! "How about a nice cup of hot milk?" The last time you heard that question it was from someone who cared for you - and you appreciated their effort.

The entire matter of food and especially that of milk is surrounded with emotional and cultural importance. Milk was our very first food. If we were fortunate, it was our mother's milk. A loving link, given and taken. It was the only path to survival. If not mother's milk, it was cow's milk or soy milk "formula"--rarely it was goat, camel or water buffalo milk.

Now, we are a nation of milk drinkers. Nearly all of us. Infants, the young, adolescents, adults and even the aged. We drink dozens or even several hundred gallons a year and add to that many pounds of "dairy products" such as cheese, butter and yogurt.

Can there be anything wrong with this? We see reassuring images of healthy, beautiful people on our television screens and hear messages that assure us that, "Milk is good for your body." Our dietitians insist that: "You've got to have milk, or where will you get your calcium?" School lunches always include milk and nearly every hospital meal will have milk added. And if that isn't enough, our nutritionists told us for years that dairy products make up an "essential food group." Industry spokesmen made sure that colorful charts proclaiming the necessity of milk and other essential nutrients were made available at no cost for schools. Cow's milk became "normal."

Milk Makes Most People Sick!

You may be surprised to learn that most of the human beings that live on planet Earth today do not drink or use cow's milk. Further, most of them can't drink milk because it makes them ill.

There are students of human nutrition who are not supportive of milk use for adults. This is from the March 1991 Medical Reader:

If you really want to play it safe, you may decide to join the growing number of Americans who are eliminating dairy products from their diets altogether. Although this sounds radical to those of us weaned on milk and the five basic food groups, it is eminently viable. Indeed, of all mammals, only

humans--and then only a minority, principally Caucasians--
continue to drink milk beyond babyhood.

Are You Confused?

Who is right? Why the confusion? Where best to get our answers? Can we trust milk industry spokesmen? Can you trust any industry spokesmen? Are nutritionists up to date or are they simply repeating what their professors learned years ago? What about the new voices urging caution?

Where to Find Answers

I believe that there are three reliable sources of information. The first, and probably the best, is a study of nature. The second is to study the history of our own species. Finally we need to look at the world's scientific literature on the subject of milk.

Let's look at the scientific literature first. From 1988 to 1993 there were over 2,700 articles dealing with milk recorded in the "Medicine" archives. Fifteen hundred of these had milk as the main focus of the article. There is no lack of scientific information on this subject. I reviewed over 500 of the 1,500 articles, discarding articles that dealt exclusively with animals, esoteric research and inconclusive studies.

A Horror Story

How would I summarize the articles? They were only slightly less than horrifying. First of all, none of the authors spoke of cow's milk as an excellent food, free of side effects and the "perfect food" as we have been led to believe by the industry. The main focus of the published reports seems to be on intestinal colic, intestinal irritation, intestinal bleeding, anemia, allergic reactions in infants and children as well as infections such as salmonella. More ominous is the fear of viral infection with bovine leukemia virus or an AIDS-like virus as well as concern for childhood diabetes. Contamination of milk by blood and white (pus) cells as well as a variety of chemicals and insecticides was also discussed. Among children, the problems were allergy, ear and tonsillar infections, bedwetting, asthma, intestinal bleeding, colic and diabetes. In adults, the problems seemed centered more around heart disease and arthritis, allergy, sinusitis, and the more serious questions of leukemia, lymphoma and cancer.

I think that an answer can also be found in a consideration of what occurs in nature - what happens with free living mammals and what happens with human groups living in close to a natural state as "hunter-gatherers."

Our Paleolithic ancestors are another crucial and interesting group to study. Here we are limited to speculation and indirect evidences, but the bony remains available for our study are remarkable. There is no doubt whatever that these skeletal remains reflect great strength, muscularity (the size of muscular insertions show this), and total absence of advanced osteoporosis. And if you feel that these people are not important for us to study, consider that today our genes are programming our bodies in almost exactly the same way as our ancestors of 50,000 to 100,000 years ago.

What is Milk?

Milk is a maternal lactating secretion, a short term nutrient for new-borns. Nothing more, nothing less. Invariably, the mother of any mammal will provide her milk for a short period of time immediately after birth. When the time comes for "weaning," the young offspring is introduced to the proper food for that species of mammal. A familiar example is that of a puppy. The mother nurses the pup for just a few weeks and then rejects the young animal and teaches it to eat solid food. Nursing is provided by nature only for the very youngest of mammals. Of course, it is not possible for animals living in a natural state to continue with the drinking of milk after weaning.

Is All Milk the Same?

Then there is the matter of where we get our milk. We have settled on the cow because of its docile nature, its size, and its abundant milk supply. Somehow this choice seems "normal" and blessed by nature, our culture, and our customs. But is it natural? Is it wise to drink the milk of another species of mammal?

Consider for a moment, if it was possible, to drink the milk of a mammal other than a cow, let's say a rat. Or perhaps the milk of a dog would be more to your liking. Possibly some horse milk or cat milk. Do you get the idea? Well, I'm not serious about this, except to suggest that human milk is for human infants, dogs' milk is for pups, cow's milk is for calves, cats' milk is for kittens, and so forth. Clearly, this is the way nature intends it. Just use your good judgment on this one.

Milk is not just milk. The milk of every species of mammal is unique and specifically tailored to the requirements of that animal. For example, cow's milk is very much richer in protein than human milk. Three to four times as much. It has five to seven times the mineral content. However, it is markedly deficient in essential fatty acids when compared to human mothers' milk. Mothers' milk has six to ten times as much of the essential fatty acids, especially linoleic acid.

(Incidentally, skimmed cow's milk has no linoleic acid). It simply is not designed for humans.

Food is not just food, and milk is not just milk. It is not the proper amount of food but the proper qualitative composition that is critical for the very best in health and growth. Biochemists and physiologists - and rarely medical doctors - are gradually learning that foods contain the crucial elements that allow a particular species to develop its unique specializations.

Clearly, our specialization is for advanced neurological development and delicate neuromuscular control. We do not have much need of massive skeletal growth or huge muscle groups as does a calf. Think of the difference between the demands made on the human hand and the demands on a cow's hoof. Human newborns specifically need critical material for their brains, spinal cord and nerves.

Does Mothers' Milk Increase Her Baby's IQ?

Can mother's milk increase intelligence? It seems that it can. In a remarkable study published in the Lancet *during 1992 (Vol. 339, pp. 261-264), a group of British workers randomly placed premature infants into two groups. One group received a proper formula, the other group received human breast milk. Both fluids were given by stomach tube. These children were followed up for over 10 years. In intelligence testing, the human milk children averaged 10 IQ points higher! Well, why not? Why shouldn't the correct building blocks for the rapidly maturing and growing brain have a positive effect?*

In the American Journal of Clinical Nutrition *(1982) Ralph Holman described an infant who developed profound neurological disease while being nourished by intravenous fluids only. The fluids used contained only linoleic acid - just one of the essential fatty acids. When the other, alpha linoleic acid, was added to the intravenous fluids the neurological disorders cleared.*

In the same journal five years later, Bjerve, Mostad and Thoresen, working in Norway found exactly the same problem in adult patients on long term gastric tube feeding.

In 1930, Dr. G.O. Burr in Minnesota working with rats found that linoleic acid deficiencies created a deficiency syndrome. Why is this mentioned? In the early 1960s pediatricians found skin lesions in children fed formulas without the same linoleic acid. Remembering the research, the addition of acid to the formula cured the problem. Essential fatty acids are just that and cow's milk is markedly deficient in these when compared to human milk.

Well, at Least Cow's Milk is Pure

Or is it? Fifty years ago an average cow produced 2000 pounds of milk per year. Today the top producers give 50,000 pounds! How was this accomplished? Drugs, antibiotics, hormones, forced feeding plans and specialized breeding; that's how.

The latest high-tech onslaught on the poor cow is bovine growth hormone or BGH. (BST) This genetically engineered drug is supposed to stimulate milk production, but, according to Monsanto, the hormone's manufacturer, does not affect the milk or meat. There are three other manufacturers: Upjohn, Eli Lilly, and American Cyanamid Company. Obviously, there have been no long-term studies on the hormone's effect on the humans drinking the milk. Other countries have banned BGH because of safety concerns. One of the problems with adding molecules to a milk-cow's body is that the molecules usually come out in the milk. I don't know how you feel, but I don't want to experiment with the ingestion of a growth hormone. A related problem is that is causes a marked increase (50 to 79 percent) in mastitis. This, then, requires antibiotic therapy, and the residues of the antibiotics appear in the milk.

It seems that the public is uneasy about this product and in one survey 43 percent felt that growth hormone-treated milk represented a health risk. A vice-president for public policy at Monsanto was opposed to labeling for that reason, and because the labeling would create an "artificial distinction." The country is awash with milk as it is, we produce more milk than we can consume. Let's not create storage costs and further taxpayer burdens, because the law requires the USDA to buy any surplus of butter, cheese or non-fat dry milk at a support price set by Congress! In fiscal 1991, the USDA spent $757 million on surplus butter, and one billion dollars a year on yearly average for price supports during the 1980s (Consumer Reports, May 1992: 330-332).

Drink Milk and Drink Toxins

Any lactating mammal excretes toxins through her milk. This includes antibiotics, pesticides, chemicals and hormones. Also, all cow's milk contains blood! The inspectors are simply asked to keep it under certain limits. You may be horrified to learn that the USDA allows milk to contain from one to one and a half million white blood cells per milliliter. (That's only 1/30 of an ounce). If you don't already know this, I'm sorry to tell you that another way to describe white cells where they don't belong would be to call them pus cells. To get to the point, is milk pure or is it a chemical, biological, and bacterial cocktail? Finally, will the Food and Drug Administration (FDA) protect you? The United States General Accounting Office (GAO) tells us that the FDA and the individual states are failing to protect the public from drug residues in milk. Authorities test for only 4 of the 82 drugs in dairy cows.

As you imagine, the Milk Industry Foundation's spokesman claims it's perfectly safe. Jerome Kozak says, "I still think that milk is the safest product we have."

Other, perhaps less biased observers, have found the following: 38% of milk samples in ten cities were contaminated with sulfa drugs or other antibiotics. (This from the Center for Science in the Public Interest and The Wall Street Journal, *December 29, 1989). A similar study in Washington, D.C. found a 20 percent contamination rate (*Nutrition Action Healthletter, *April 1990).*

What's going on here? When the FDA tested milk, they found few problems. However, they used very lax standards. When they used the same criteria, the FDA data showed 51 percent of milk samples showed drug traces.

Let's focus in on this because it's so critical to our understanding of the apparent discrepancies. The FDA uses a disk-assay method that can detect only 2 of the 30 or so drugs found in milk. Also, the test detects only at the relatively high level. A more powerful test called the "Charm II test" can detect 40 drugs down to 5 parts per billion.

Bon Apetit! There's Pus in Your Milk!

One nasty subject must be discussed. It seems that cows are forever getting infections around the udder that require ointments and antibiotics. An article from France tells us that when a cow receives penicillin, that penicillin appears in the milk for from 4 to 7 milkings. Another study from the University of Nevada, 'Reno tells of cells in "mastic milk," milk from cows with infected udders. An elaborate analyses of the cell fragments, employing cell cultures, flow sytometric analysis, and a great deal of high tech stuff. Do you know what the conclusion was? If the cow has mastitis, there is pus in the milk. Sorry, it's in the study, all concealed with language such as, "..macrophages containing many vacuoles and phagocytosed particles."

It Gets Worse

Well, at least human mother's milk is pure! Sorry. A huge study showed that human breast milk in over 14,000 women had contamination by pesticides! Further, it seems that the sources of the pesticides are meat and - you guessed it - dairy products. Well, why not? These pesticides are concentrated in fat and that's what's in these products. (Of interest, a subgroup of lactating vegetarian mothers had only half the levels of contamination).

A recent report showed an increased concentration of pesticides in the breast tissue of women with breast cancer when compared to the tissue of women with fibrocystic disease. Other articles in the standard medical literature describe problems. Just scan these titles:

1. *"Cow's Milk as a Cause of Infantile Colic Breast-Fed Infants"* Lancet *2 (1978): 437*
2. *"Dietary Protein-Induced Colitis in Breast-Fed Infants"* J. Pediatr. *101 (1982): 906*
3. *"The Question of the Elimination of Foreign Protein in Women's Milk"* J. Immunology *19 (1930): 15*

There are many others. There are dozens of studies describing the prompt appearance of cow's milk allergy in children being exclusively breast-fed! The cow's milk allergens simply appear in mother's milk and are transmitted to the infant.

American Academy of Pediatrics: Opinion

*A committee on nutrition of the American Academy of Pediatrics reported on the use of whole cow's milk in infancy (*Pediatrics, *1983: 72-253). They were unable to provide any cogent reason why bovine milk should be used before the first birthday, yet, continued to recommend its use! Doctor Frank Oski from the Upstate Medical Center Department of Pediatrics, commenting on the recommendation, cited the problems of occult gastrointestinal blood loss in infants, the lack of iron, recurrent abdominal pain, milk-borne infections and contaminants, and said:*

> *Why give it at all - then or ever? In the face of uncertainty about many of the potential dangers of whole bovine milk, it would seem prudent to recommend that whole milk not be started until the answers are available. Isn't it time for these un-controlled experiments on human nutrition to come to an end?*

In the same issue of Pediatrics *he further commented:*

> *It is my thesis that whole milk should not be fed to the infant in the first year of life because of its association with iron deficiency anemia (milk is so deficient in iron that an infant would have to drink an impossible 31 quarts a day to get the RDA of 15 mg), occult gastrointestinal bleeding, and various manifestations of food allergy. I suggest that unmodified*

whole bovine milk should not be consumed after infancy
because of the problems of lactose intolerance, its contribution
to the genesis of atherosclerosis, and its possible link to
other diseases.

What Would (the Late) Doctor Spock Say?

In late 1992, Dr. Benjamin Spock, possibly the best known pediatrician in
American history, shocked the country when he articulated the same thoughts and
specified avoidance for the first two years of life. Here is his quotation:

I want to pass on the word to parents that cow's milk from
the carton has definite faults for some babies. Human milk
is the right one for babies. A study comparing the incidence
of allergy and colic in the breast-fed infants of omnivorous
and vegan mothers would be important. I haven't found
such a study; it would be both important and inexpensive.
And it will probably never be done. There is simply no
academic or economic profit involved.

Other Problems

Let's just mention the problems of bacterial contamination. Salmonella, E.
coli, *and* staphylococcal *infections can be traced to milk. In the old days*
tuberculosis was a major problem and some folks want to go back to those times
by insisting on raw milk on the basis that it's "natural." This is insanity! A study
from UCLA showed that over a third of all cases of salmonella infection in
California, 1980-1983 were traced to raw milk. That'll be a way to receive good
old brucellosis again and I would fear leukemia, too. (More about that later). In
England, and Wales where raw milk is still consumed, there have been outbreaks
of milk-borne diseases. The Journal of the American Medical Association *(251:*
483, 1984) reported a multi-state series of infections caused by Yersinia
enterocolitica in pasteurized whole milk. This is despite safety precautions.

Juvenile Diabetes

All parents dread juvenile diabetes for their children. A Canadian study
reported in the American Journal of Clinical Nutrition, *Mar. 1990, describes a*
"...significant positive correlation between consumption of unfermented milk
protein and incidence of insulin dependent diabetes mellitus in data from various

countries. Conversely, a possible negative relationship is observed between breast feeding at age 3 months and diabetes risk."

*Another study, from Finland, found that diabetic children had higher levels of serum antibodies to cow's milk (*Diabetes Research *7(3): 137-140 March 1988). Here is a quotation from this study:*

> *We infer that either the pattern of cow's milk consumption is altered in children who will have insulin dependent diabetes mellitus or, their immunological reactivity to proteins in cow's milk is enhanced, or the permeability of their intestines to cow's milk protein is higher than normal.*

Scientists Missed the Point!

The April 18, 1992 British Medical Journal *has a fascinating study contrasting the difference in incidence of juvenile insulin dependent diabetes in Pakistani children who have migrated to England. The incidence is roughly 10 times greater in the English group compared to children remaining in Pakistan! What caused this highly significant increase? The authors said that "the diet was unchanged in Great Britain. Do you believe that? Do you think that the availability of milk, sugar and fat is the same in Pakistan as it is in England? That a grocery store in England has the same products as food sources in Pakistan? I don't believe that for a minute. Remember, we're not talking here about adult onset, type II diabetes which all workers agree is strongly linked to diet as well as to genetic predisposition. This study is a major blow to the "it's all in your genes" crowd. Type I diabetes was always considered to be genetic or possibly viral, but now this? So resistant are we to consider diet as causation that the authors of the last article concluded that the cooler climate in England altered viruses and caused the very real increase in diabetes! The first two authors had the same reluctance too admit the obvious. The milk just may have had something to do with the disease.*

Do Children Get Diabetes from Milk?

The latest in this remarkable list of reports, a New England Journal of Medicine *article (July 30, 1992), also reported in the* Los Angeles Times. *This study comes from the Hospital for Sick Children in Toronto and from Finnish researchers. In Finland there is:*

> *[T]he world's highest rate of dairy product consumption and the world's highest rate of insulin dependent diabetes. The disease*

*strikes about 40 children out of every 1,000 there contrasted with
six to eight per 1,000 in the United States. Antibodies produced
against the milk protein during the first year of life, the
researcher's speculate, also attack and destroy the pancreas
in a so-called auto-immune reaction, producing diabetes in
people whose genetic makeup leaves them vulnerable...142
Finnish children with newly diagnosed diabetes. They found
that every one had at least eight times as many antibodies
against the milk protein as did healthy children, clear evidence
that the children had a raging auto immune disorder.*

*The team has now expanded the study to 400 children and is starting a trial
where 3000 children will receive no dairy products during the first nine months of
life. "The study may take 10 years, but we'll get a definitive answer one way or
the other," according to one of the researchers. I would caution them to be
certain that the breast feeding mothers use of cow's milk in their diets be withheld
or the results will be confounded by the transmission of the cow's milk protein in
the mother's breast milk.*

The World Must Be Crazy!

*Now, what was the reaction from the diabetes association? This is very
interesting! Dr. F. Xavier Pi-Sunyer, the president of the association says:*

*It does not mean that children should stop drinking milk or that
parents of diabetics should withdraw dairy products. These are
rich sources of good protein.*

*My God, it's the "good protein" that causes the problem! Do you suspect
that the dairy industry may have helped the ADA in the past?*

Leukemia? Lymphoma? This May Be The Worst: Brace Yourself!

*I hate to tell you this, but the bovine leukemia virus is found in more than
three of five dairy cows in the United States! This involves about 80 percent of
dairy herds. Unfortunately, when the milk is pooled, a very large percentage of
all milk produced is contaminated (90 to 95 percent). Of course, the virus is
killed in pasteurization - if the pasteurization was done correctly. What if the milk
is raw? In a study of randomly collected raw milk samples the bovine leukemia
virus was recovered from two-thirds. I sincerely hope that raw milk dairy herds*

are carefully monitored when compared to the regular herds. (Science 1981; 213:1014).

There is a world-wide problem. *One lengthy study from Germany deplored the problem and admitted the impossibility of keeping the virus from infected cow's milk from the rest of the milk. Several European countries, including Germany and Switzerland, have attempted to "cull" the infected cows from the herds. Certainly the United States must be the leader in the fight against leukemic dairy cows, right? Wrong! We are the worst in the world with the former exception of Venezuela according to Virgil Hulse, M.D., a milk specialist who also has a B.S. in Dairy Manufacturing as well as a Master's degree in Public Health.*

Chicago: 1985, 4 Die, 150,000 Sickened from Milk

As mentioned, the leukemia virus is rendered inactive by pasteurization. Of course. However, there can be Chernobyl-like accidents. One of these occurred in the Chicago area in April, 1985. At a modern, large milk processing plant an accidental "cross connection" between raw and pasteurized milk occurred. A violent salmonella outbreak followed, killing 4 and making an estimated 150,000 ill. Now the question I would pose to the dairy industry people is this: "How can you assure the people who drink this milk that they were not exposed to the ingestion of raw, unkilled, fully active bovine leukemia viruses?" Further, it would be fascinating to know if a "cluster" of leukemia cases blossoms in that area in 1 to 3 decades. There are reports of "leukemia clusters" elsewhere, one of them mentioned in the June 10, 1990 San Francisco Chronicle *involving Northern California.*

What happens to other species of mammals when they are exposed to bovine leukemia virus? It's a fair question and the answer is not reassuring. Virtually all animals exposed to the virus develop leukemia. This includes sheep, goats and even primates such as rhesus monkeys and chimpanzees. The route of transmission includes ingestion (both intravenous and intramuscular) and cells present in milk. There are obviously no instances of transfer attempts to human beings, but we know that the virus can infect human cells in vitro. There is evidence of human antibody formation to the bovine leukemia virus; this is disturbing. How did the bovine leukemia virus particles gain access to humans and become antigens? Was it as small denatured particles?

1 + 1 = 2

If the bovine leukemia virus causes human leukemia, we could expect the dairy states with known leukemic herds to have a higher incidence of human leukemia. Is this so? Unfortunately it seems to be the case! Iowa, Nebraska, South Dakota, Minnesota and Wisconsin have statistically higher incidence of leukemia than the national average. In Russia and in Sweden, areas with uncontrolled bovine leukemia virus have been linked with increases in human leukemia. I am also told that veterinarians have higher rates of leukemia than the general public. Dairy farmers have significantly elevated leukemia rates. Recent research shows lymphocytes from milk fed to neonatal mammals gains access to bodily tissues by passing directly through the intestinal wall.

The Good News and the Bad News

An optimistic note from the University of Illinois, Urbana, from the Department of Animal Sciences shows the importance of one's perspective. Since they are concerned with the economics of milk and not primarily the health aspects, they noted that the production of milk was greater in the cows with the bovine leukemia virus. However, when the leukemia produced a persistent and significant lymphocytosis (increased white blood cell count), the production fell off. They suggested, "...a need to re-evaluate the economic impact of bovine leukemia virus infection on the dairy industry." Does this mean that leukemia is good for profits only is we can keep it under control? You can get the details on this business concern from Proc. Nat. Acad. Sciences, U.S., Feb. 1989. *I added emphasis and am outraged that a university department feels that this is an economic and not a human health issue. Do not expect help from the Department of Agriculture or the universities. The money stakes and the political pressures are too great. You're on your own.*

What does this all mean? We know that virus is capable of producing leukemia in other animals. It is proven that it can contribute to human leukemia (or lymphoma, a related cancer. Several articles tackle this one:

1. *"Epidemiologic Relationships of the Bovine Population and Human Leukemia in Iowa."* Am. Journal of Epidemiology, *112 (1980): 80*
2. *"Milk of Dairy Cows Frequently Contains a Leukemogenic Virus."* Science, *213 (1981): 1014*
3. *"Beware of the Cow." (Editorial)* Lancet, *2 (1974) : 30*
4. *"Is Bovine Milk a Health Hazard?"* Pediatrics; *Suppl. Feeding the Normal Infant. 75:182-186; 1985*

Something's Rotten...in Norway

In Norway, 1422 individuals were followed for 11 and one-half years. Those drinking two or more glasses of milk per day had 3.5 times the incidence of cancer of the lympathatic organs. British Med. Journal, *61: 456-9, March 1990.*

One of the more thoughtful articles on this subject is from Allan S. Cunningham of Cooperstown, New York. Writing in the Lancet, November 27, 1976 (page 1184), his article is entitled, "Lymphomas and Animal-Protein Consumption." Many people think of milk as "liquid meat" and Dr. Cunningham agrees with this. He tracked the beef and dairy consumption in terms of grams per day for a one year period, 1955-1956, in 15 countries. New Zealand, United States, and Canada were highest in that order. The lowest was Japan followed by Yugoslavia and France. The difference between the highest and lowest was quite pronounced: 43.8 grams/day for New Zealanders versus 1.5 for Japan. Nearly a 30-fold difference! (Parenthetically, the last 36 years have seen a startling increase in the amount of beef and milk used in Japan and their disease patterns are reflecting this, confirming the lack of "genetic protection" seen in migration studies. Formerly the increase in frequency of lymphomas in Japanese people was only in those who moved to the USA)!

An interesting bit of trivia is to note the memorial built at the Gyokusenji Temple in Shimoda, Japan. This marked the spot where the first cow was killed in Japan for human consumption! The chains around this memorial were a gift from the U.S. Navy. Where do you suppose the Japanese got the idea to eat beef? The year? 1930.

Cunningham found a highly significant positive correlation between deaths from lymphomas and beef and dairy ingestion in the 15 countries analyzed. A few quotations from the article follow:

> The average intake of protein in many countries is far in excess of the recommended requirements. Excessive consumption of animal protein may be one co-factor in the causation of lymphomas by acting in the following manner. Ingestion of certain proteins results in the absorption of antigenic fragments through the gastrointestinal mucous membrane.

> This results in chronic stimulation of lymphoid tissue to which these fragments gain access...Chronic immunological stimulation causes lymphomas in laboratory animals and is believed to cause lymphoid cancers in men...The gastrointestinal mucous membrane is only a partial barrier to the absorption of food antigens, and circulating antibodies to food protein is common-place, especially potent lymphoid stimulants. Ingestion of cow's milk can produce generalized lymphadenopathy, hematosplenomegaly, and profound adenoid hypertrophy. It

has been conservatively estimated that more than 100 distinct
antigens are released by the normal digestion of cow's milk
which evoke production of all antibody classes. This may
explain why pasteurized, killed viruses are still antigenic
and still cause disease.

Cancer's the Answer: Got Milk?

Here's more. A large prospective study from Norway was reported in the British Journal of Cancer *61 (3):456-459, March 1990. (Almost 16,000 individuals were followed for 11 and one-half years). For most cancers there was no association between the tumor and milk ingestion. However, in lymphoma, there was a strong positive association. If one drank two glasses or more daily (or the equivalent in dairy products), the odds were 3.4 times greater than in persons drinking less than one glass of developing a lymphoma.*

Mad Cow Disease

There are two other cow-related diseases that you should be aware of. At this time they are not known to be spread by use of dairy products and are not known to involve man. The first is bovine spongiform encephalopathy (BSE), and the second is the bovine immunodeficiency virus (BIV). The first of these diseases, we hope, is confined to England and causes cavities in the animal's brain. Sheep have been known to suffer from a disease called scrapie. It seems to have been started by the feeding of contaminated sheep parts, especially brains, to the British cows. Now, use your good sense. Do cows seem like carnivores? Should they eat meat? This profit-motivated practice backfired and bovine spongiform encephalopathy, or Mad Cow Disease, swept Britain.

The disease literally causes dementia in the unfortunate animal and is 100 percent incurable. To date, over 100,000 cows have been incinerated in England in keeping with British law. Four hundred to 500 cows are reported as infected each month. The British public is concerned and has dropped its beef consumption by 25 percent, while some 2,000 schools have stopped serving beef to children. Several farmers have developed a fatal disease syndrome that resembles both BSE and CJD (Creutzfeldt-Jacob-Disease). But the British Veterinary Association says that transmission of BSE to humans is "remote." The USDA agrees that the British epidemic was due to the feeding of cattle with bone meal or animal protein produced at rendering plants from the carcasses of scrapie-infected sheep. They have prohibited the importation of live cattle and zoo ruminants from Great Britain and claim that the disease does not exist in the United States.

A Rose By Another Name is Still a Rose, or, Mad Cow Disease = Downer Cow Syndrome

However, there may be a problem. "Downer cows" are animals who arrive at auction yards or slaughter houses dead, trampled, lacerated or too ill from viral or bacterial diseases to walk. Thus, they are "down." If they cannot respond to electrical shocks by walking, they are dragged by chains to dumpsters and transported to rendering plants where, if they are not already dead, they are killed. Even a "humane" death is usually denied them. They are then turned into protein food for animals as well as other preparations. Minks that have been fed this protein have developed a fatal encephalopathy that has some resemblance to BSE. Entire colonies of minks have been lost in this manner, particularly in Wisconsin. It is feared that the infectious agent is a prion or slow virus possibly obtained from the ill "downer cows."

Don't Eat the Cat Food!

The British Medical Journal *in an editorial whimsically entitled, "How Now, Mad Cow?" (BMJ vol. 304, 11 Apr. 1992: 929-930) describes cases of BSE in species not previously known to be affected, such as cats. They admit that produce contaminated with bovine spongiform encephalopathy entered the human food chain in England between 1986 and 1989. They say, "The result of this experiment is awaited." As the incubation period can be up to three decades, wait we must.*

AIDS Too, Brute?

The immunodeficiency virus is seen in cattle in the United States and is more worrisome. Its structure is closely related to that of the human AIDS virus. At this time we do not know if exposure to the raw BIV proteins can cause the sera of humans to become positive for HIV. The extent of the virus among American herds is said to be "widespread." (The USDA refuses to inspect the meat and milk to see if antibodies to this retrovirus is present. It also has no plans to quarantine the infected animals). As in the case of humans with AIDS, there is no cure for BIV in cows. Each day we consume beef and dairy products from cows infected with these viruses and no scientific assurance exists that the products are safe. Eating raw beef (as in steak Tartare) strikes me as being very risky, especially after the Seattle E. coli deaths of 1993.

A report in the Canadian Journal of Veterinary Research, *October 1992, Vol. 56, pp. 353-359 and another from the Russian literature tell of a horrifying development. They report the first detection in human serum of the antibody to a* *bovine immunodeficiency virus protein. In addition to this disturbing report, is another from Russia telling us of the presence of virus proteins related to the bovine leukemia virus in 5 of 89 women with breast disease (*Acta Virologica *Feb. 1990 34(1): 19-26). The implications of these developments are unknown at present. However, it is safe to assume that these animal viruses are unlikely to "stay" in the "animal" kingdom.*

Other Cancers - Does it Get Worse?

Unfortunately, it does. Ovarian cancer - a particularly nasty tumor- was associated with milk consumption by workers at Roswell Park Memorial Institute in Buffalo, New York. Drinking more than one glass of whole milk or equivalent daily gave a woman a 3.1 times risk over non-milk users. They felt that the reduced fat milk products helped reduce the risk. This association has been made repeatedly by numerous investigators.

Harvard Medical School Study

Another important study, this from the Harvard Medical School, analyzed data from 27 countries mainly from the 1970s. Again, a significant positive correlation is revealed between ovarian cancer and per capita milk consumption. These investigators feel that the lactose component of milk is the responsible fraction, and the digestion of this is facilitated by the persistence of the ability to digest the lactose (lactose persistence) - a little different emphasis, but the same conclusion. This study was reported in the American Journal of Epidemiology *130 (5): 904-910, Nov. 1989. These articles come from two of the country's leading institutions, not the* Rodale Press *or* Prevention Magazine.

Lung Cancer

Even lung cancer has been associated with milk ingestion. The beverage habits of 569 lung cancer patients and 569 controls again at Roswell Park were studied in the International Journal of Cancer, *April 15, 1989. Persons drinking whole milk 3 or more times daily had a 2-fold increase in lung cancer risk when compared to those never drinking whole milk.*

For many years we have been watching the lung cancer rates for Japanese men who smoke far more than American or European men but who develop fewer lung cancers. Workers in this research area feel that the total fat intake is the difference.

Prostate Cancer

There are not many reports studying an association between milk ingestion and prostate cancer. One such report though, was of great interest. This is from the Roswell Park Memorial Institute and is found in Cancer *64 (3): 605-612, 1989.* They analyzed the diets of 371 prostate cancer patients and comparable control subjects:

> Men who reported drinking three or more glasses of whole milk
> daily had a relative risk of 2.49 compared with men who reported
> never drinking whole milk...the weight of the evidence appears to
> favor the hypothesis that animal fat is related to increased risk
> of prostate cancer. Prostate cancer is now the most common
> cancer diagnosed in U.S. men and is the second leading cause of
> cancer mortality.

Is there any health reason at all for an adult human to drink cow's milk? It's hard for me to come up with even one good reason other than simple preference. But if you try hard, in my opinion, these would be the best two: milk is a source of calcium and it's a source of amino acids (proteins).

Calcium

Let's look at the calcium first. Why are we concerned at all about calcium? Obviously, we intend to build strong bones and protect us against osteoporosis. And no doubt about it, milk is loaded with calcium. But is it a good calcium source for humans? I think not. These are the reasons. Excessive amounts of dairy products actually interfere with calcium absorption. Secondly, the excess of protein that the milk provides is a major cause of the osteoporosis problem. Dr. Hegsted in England has been writing for years about the geographical distribution of osteoporosis. It seems that the countries with the highest intake of dairy products are invariably the countries with the most osteoporosis. He feels that milk is the cause of osteoporosis. Reasons to be given below.

Numerous studies have shown that the level of calcium ingestion and especially calcium supplementation has no effect whatever on the development of osteoporosis. The most important such article appeared recently in the British Journal of Medicine where the long arm of our dairy industry can't reach. Another study in the United States actually showed a worsening in calcium balance in post-menopausal women given three 8-ounce glasses of cow's milk per day (Am. Journal of Clin. Nutrition, *1985).* The effects of hormone, gender, *weight bearing on the axial bones, and in particular, protein intake, are critically important. Another observation that may be helpful to our analysis is to note the absence of any recorded dietary deficiencies of calcium among people living on a natural diet without milk.*

The Key to Osteoporosis

For the key to the osteoporosis riddle, don't look at calcium, look at protein. Consider these two contrasting groups. Eskimos have an exceptionally high protein intake estimated at twenty-five percent of total calories. They also have a high calcium intake at 2500 mg/day. Their osteoporosis is among the worst in the world. The other instructive group are the Bantus of South Africa. They have a twelve percent protein diet, mostly plant protein, and only 200 to 350 mg/day of calcium, about half our women's intake. The women have virtually no osteoporosis despite bearing six or more children and nursing them for prolonged periods! When African women immigrate to the United States, do they develop osteoporosis? The answer is yes, but not quite as much as Caucasian or Asian women. Thus, there is a genetic difference that is modified by diet.

If Not Milk, Where Do You Get Your Calcium?

To answer the obvious question, "Well, where do you get your calcium?" The answer is: "From exactly the same place the cow gets the calcium, from green things that grow in the ground," mainly from leafy vegetables. After all, elephants and rhinos develop their huge bones (after being weaned) by eating green leafy plants; so do horses. Carnivorous animals also do quite nicely even without leafy plants. It seems that all of earth's mammals do well if they live in harmony with their genetic programming and natural food. Only humans living an affluent lifestyle have rampant osteoporosis.

If animal references do not convince you, think of the several billion humans on this earth who have never seen cow's milk. Wouldn't you think osteoporosis would be prevalent in this huge group? The dairy people would suggest this but the truth is exactly the opposite. They have far less than that seen in the countries where dairy products are commonly consumed. It is the subject of another paper, but the truly significant determinants of osteoporosis are grossly excessive protein intakes and lack of weight bearing on long bones, both taking place over decades. Hormones play a secondary, but not trivial role in women. Milk is a deterrent to good bone health.

The Protein Myth

Remember when you were a kid and the adults all told you to "make sure you got plenty of good protein?" Protein was the nutritional "good guy" when I was young. And of course, milk fits right in.

As regards protein, milk is indeed a rich source of protein - "liquid meat," remember? However, that isn't necessarily what we need. In actual fact, it is a source of difficulty. Nearly all Americans eat too much protein.

For this information we rely on the most authoritative source that I am aware of. This is the latest edition (10th, 1989; 4th printing, Jan. 1992) of the "Recommended Dietary Allowances" *produced by the National Research Council. Of interest, the current editor of this important work is Dr. Richard Havel of the University of California in San Francisco. First to be noted is that the recommended protein has been steadily revised downward in successive editions. The current recommendation is 0.75 g/kilo/day for adults 19 through 51 years. This, of course, is only 45 grams per day for the mythical 60 kilogram adult. You should also know that the World Health Organization estimated the need for protein in adults to be 0.6g/kilo per day. (All RDA's are calculated with large safety allowances in case you're the type who wants to add some more to "be sure.") You can "get by" on 28 to 30 grams per day if necessary!*

Now, 45 grams a day is a tiny amount of protein. That's an ounce and a half! Consider too, that the protein does not have to be animal protein. Vegetable protein is identical for all practical purposes and has no cholesterol and vastly less saturated fat. (Do not be misled by the antiquated belief that the plant proteins must be carefully balanced to avoid deficiencies. This is not a realistic concern.) Therefore, virtually all Americans, Canadians, British and European people are in a protein overloaded state. This has serious consequences when maintained over decades. The problems are the already mentioned osteoporosis, atherosclerosis and kidney damage. There is good evidence that certain malignancies, chiefly colon and rectal, are related to excessive meat intake. Barry Brenner, an eminent renal physiologist was the first to fully point out the dangers of excess protein for the kidney tubule. The dangers of the fat and cholesterol are known to all. Finally, you should know that the protein content of human milk is about the lowest (0.9%) in mammals.

Is That All of the Trouble?

Sorry, there's more. Remember lactose? This is the principal carbohydrate of milk. It seems that nature provides newborns with the enzymatic equipment to metabolize lactose, but this ability often extinguishes by age four or five years.

What is the problem with lactose or milk sugar? It seems that it is a disaccharide which is too large to be absorbed into the blood stream without first being broken down into monosaccharides, namely galactose and glucose. This requires the presence of an enzyme, lactase, plus additional enzymes to break down galactose into glucose.

Let's think about this for a moment. Nature gives us the ability to metabolize lactose for a few years and then shuts off the mechanism. Is Mother Nature trying to tell us something? Clearly, all infants must drink milk. The fact that so many adults cannot seems to be related to the tendency for nature to abandon mechanisms that are not needed. At least half of the adult humans on this earth are lactose intolerant. It was not until the relatively recent introduction of dairy herding and the ability to "borrow" milk from another group of mammals that the survival advantage of preserving lactase (the enzyme that allows us to digest lactose) became evident. But why would it be advantageous to drink cow's milk? After all, most of the human beings in the history of the world did. And further, why was it just the white or light skinned humans who retained this knack while the pigmented people tended to lose it?

Some students of evolution feel that white skin is a fairly recent innovation, perhaps not more than 20,000 or 30,000 years old. It clearly has to do with the Northward migration of early man to cold and relatively sunless areas when skins and clothing became available. Fair skin allows the production of vitamin D from sunlight more readily than does dark skin. However, when only the face was exposed to sunlight, that area of fair skin was insufficient to provide the vitamin D from sunlight. If dietary and sunlight sources were poorly available, the ability to use the abundant calcium in cow's milk would give a survival advantage to humans who could digest that milk. This seems to be the only logical explanation for fair skinned humans having a high degree of lactose tolerance when compared to dark skinned people.

*How does this break down? Certain racial groups, namely blacks, are up to 90 percent lactose intolerant as adults. Caucasians are 20 to 40 percent lactose intolerant. Orientals are midway between the two groups. Diarrhea, gas and abdominal cramps are the results of substantial milk intake in such persons. Most American Indians cannot tolerate milk. The milk industry admits that lactose intolerance plays intestinal havoc with as many as 50 million Americans. A lactose-intolerance industry has sprung up and had sales of $117 million in 1992 (*Time, May 17, 1993*).*

*What if you are lactose intolerant and lust after dairy products? Is all lost? Not at all. It seems that lactose is largely digested by bacteria and you will be able to enjoy your cheese despite lactose intolerance. Yogurt is similar in this respect. Finally, and I could never have dreamed this up, geneticists want to splice genes to alter the composition of milk (*Am. J. Clin. Nutr. *Suppl. 302s*).*

One could quibble and say that milk is totally devoid of fiber content and that its habitual use will predispose one to constipation and bowel disorders.

The association with anemia and acute intestinal bleeding in infants is known to all physicians. This is chiefly from the lack of iron and milk's irritating qualities for the intestinal mucosa. The pediatric literature abounds with articles describing irritated intestinal lining, bleeding, increased permeability as well as colic, diarrhea and vomiting in cow's milk-sensitive babies. The anemia gets a double push by loss of blood and iron as well as deficiency of iron in the cow's milk. Milk is also the leading cause of childhood allergy.

Low Fat Milk

One additional topic: the matter of "low fat" milk. A common and sincere question is: "Well, low fat milk is OK, isn't it?"

The answer to this question is that low fat milk isn't low fat. The term, "low fat," is a marketing term used to mislead the public. Low fat milk contains from 24 to 33 percent fat as calories. The 2 percent figure is also misleading. This figure refers to weight. They don't tell you that, by weight, the milk is 87 percent water!

No Fat Milk

"Well then, you kill-joy, surely you must approve of non-fat milk!" I hear this quite a bit. (Another constant concern is: "What do you put on your cereal?") True, there is little or no fat, but now you have a relative overburden of protein and lactose. If there is something that we do not need more of it is another simple sugar-lactose, composed of galactose and glucose. Millions of Americans are lactose intolerant to boot, as noted. As for protein, as stated earlier, we live in a society that routinely ingests far more protein than we need. It is a burden for our bodies, especially the kidneys, and a prominent cause of osteoporosis. Concerning the dry cereal issue, I would suggest soy milk, rice milk or almond milk as a healthy substitute. If you're still concerned about calcium, "Westsoy" is formulated to have the same calcium concentration as milk.

Summary

To my thinking, there is only one valid reason to drink or use milk products. That is just because we simply want to. Because we like it and because it has become part of our culture. Because we have become accustomed to its taste and texture. Because we like the way it slides down our throat. Because our parents did the very best they could for us and provided milk in our earliest training and conditioning. They taught us to like it. And then probably the very best reason is...ICE CREAM! I've heard it described, "...to die for."

I had one patient who did exactly that. He had no obvious vices. He didn't smoke or drink, he didn't eat meat, his diet and lifestyle was nearly a perfectly health promoting one; but he had a passion. You guessed it, he loved rich ice cream. A pint of the richest would be a lean day's ration for him. On many occasions he would eat an entire quart - and yes, there were some cookies and other pastries. Good ice cream deserves this after all. He seemed to be in good health despite some expected "middle age spread" when he had a devastating stroke which left him paralyzed, miserable and helpless, and he had additional strokes and died several years later never having left a hospital or rehabilitation unit. Was he old? I don't think so. He was in his 50s.

So don't drink milk for health. I am convinced on the weight of the scientific evidence that it does not "do a body good." Inclusion of milk will only reduce your diet's nutritional value and safety.

Most of the people on this planet live very healthfully without cow's milk. You can too. It will be difficult to change; we've been conditioned since childhood to think of milk as "nature's most perfect food." I guarantee you that it will be safe, improve your health and it won't cost anything. What can you lose?

Dr. Kradjian is a man of great wit, intelligence, perspective and passion. He is the author of, "Breast Cancer." Robert Kradjian, once chief of breast surgery at Seton Medical Center near San Francisco, has recently retired from his medical practice.

All of your life you've been hearing and reading the dairy industry's opinion about milk. A second opinion was beautifully presented in Kradjian's well- documented letter. A third opinion is offered by Dr. Neal Barnard.

A Third Opinion from Neal Barnard, M.D.

Neal Barnard, M.D., is president of Washington, DC-based "Physicians Committee for Responsible Medicine" (PCRM). Founded in 1985, PCRM is supported by over 6000 physicians and 60,000 laypersons. Its advisory board includes 26 medical doctors from a broad range of specialties.

Dr. Barnard is a popular speaker and the author of many best-selling books, including *Food for Life*. PCRM promotes preventive medicine through innovative programs. Among those programs are:

1) The Cancer Prevention and Survival Fund.
2) The Gold Plan, a healthy eating program for businesses, hospitals and schools.

3) The New Four Food Groups, a proposal for new federal nutrition policies.
4) Saving Lives Public Service Announcements, such as the series featuring Dr. Henry Heimlich's "maneuver."

Recently, Barnard and PCRM issued a nutrition bulletin, portions of which, with their permission, are published here. PCRM can be reached at 202-686-2210.

Milk: No Longer Recommended or Required

A substantial body of scientific evidence raises concerns about health risks from cow's milk products. These problems relate to the proteins, sugar, fat, and contaminants in dairy products, and the inadequacy of whole cow's milk for infant nutrition.

The American Academy of Pediatrics recommends that infants under a year of age not receive whole cow's milk. (1)

Cow's milk products are very low in iron. (2) To get the U.S. Recommended Daily Allowance of 15 mg of iron, an infant would have to drink more than 31 quarts of milk per day. Milk can also cause blood loss from the intestinal tract, which, over time, reduces the body's iron stores. Researchers speculate that blood loss may be a reaction to proteins present in milk. (3)

Milk Proteins and Diabetes

Studies of various countries show a strong correlation between the use of dairy products and the incidence of diabetes. (4) A recent report in the New England Journal of Medicine *(5) adds substantial support to the long standing theory that cow's milk proteins stimulate the production of antibodies (6) which, in turn, destroy the insulin-producing pancreatic cells (7).*

Milk Sugar and Health Problems

Many people, particularly those of Asian and African ancestry, are unable to digest the milk sugar, lactose. The result is diarrhea and gas. For those who can digest lactose, its breakdown products are two simple sugars: glucose and galactose. Galactose has been implicated in ovarian cancer (8) and cataracts (9, 10).

Contaminants

Milk contains frequent contaminants, from pesticides to drugs. About a third of milk products have been shown to be contaminated with antibiotic traces.

The vitamin D content in milk has been poorly regulated. Recent testing of 42 milk samples found only 12% within the expected range of vitamin D content. Testing of 10 samples of infant formula revealed seven with more than twice the vitamin D content reported on the label, one of which had more than four times the label amount. (11) Vitamin D is toxic in overdose. (12)

Osteoporosis

Dairy products offer a false sense of security to those concerned about osteoporosis. Studies have shown little effect of dairy products on osteoporosis. (13) In postmenopausal women, most studies show little effect of calcium intake on the bone density of the spine. There is also little or no effect on bone at the hip, where very serious breaks can occur. Some studies have found an effect of calcium intake on bone density in the forearm. (14) Studies of postmenopausal women have likewise shown that calcium intake has relatively little effect on bone density. (15, 16) Science *magazine of August 1, 1986, noted "the large body of evidence indicating no relationship between calcium intake and bone density." (17)*

A recent report in the American Journal of Clinical Nutrition *found that calcium absorbability was actually higher for kale than from milk, and concluded, "greens such as kale can be considered to be at least as good as milk in terms of their calcium absorbability." (18) Beans are also rich in calcium. Fortified orange juice supplies large amounts of calcium in palatable form. (19) Calcium is only one of many factors that affect the bone. Other factors include hormones, phosphorus, boron, exercise, smoking, alcohol and drugs. (14, 16, 20, 21) Protein is also important in calcium balance. Diets that are rich in protein, particularly animal proteins, encourage calcium loss. (22, 23, 24)*

Recommendations

In summary, there is no nutritional requirement for dairy products, and there are serious problems that can result from the proteins, sugar, fat and contaminants in milk products. Therefore, the following recommendations are offered:

1. *Breast feeding is the preferred method of infant feeding.*
2. *Parents should be alerted to the potential risk to their children from cow's milk use.*
3. *Cow's milk should not be required or recommended in government guidelines.*
4. *Government programs, such as school lunch programs should be consistent with these recommendations.*

"The casein content of cow's milk is 300 percent more than is contained in mother's milk. Casein is a milk by-product used as one of the most tenacious glues for gluing wood together."

Dr. N.W. Walker

"Discovery consists of seeing what everybody has seen and thinking what nobody has thought."

Albert Szent-Gyorgyi

Chapter 10

An Analysis: What is in Milk

A sip of milk contains hundreds of different substances, each one having the potential to exert a powerful biological effect when taken independently of the others. Together, this bouillon of proteins and hormones and fat and cholesterol, viruses and bacteria, pesticides with vitamin D added, combine to affect its users in ways that can never be fully understood.

Milk. It's pure and it's white, just like refined sugar and the ten gallon hat worn by a good-guy cowboy and the stallion he rode in on. Like the newly fallen blanket of January snow and like a sparkling ray of light before it enters into a prism. Like the viscous liquid in a newly opened can of latex paint. Ask a child what color results from mixing all other colors together and instinctively he'll answer, black. He'll be wrong. Mix blue and green and yellow and red and thousands of other colors together and you'll end up with white. Merge violet and indigo, blue and green, yellow, orange and red lights together and you'll end up with a pure beam of white light. And there's more! Don't forget infrared and ultraviolet light. You cannot see them but they're part of white light too. There are many things in milk you cannot see. Scientists believe that there are many things in milk that are yet to be discovered.

There are so many things contained in beautiful white milk whose appearance is illusory and misleading, deceptive in its appearance. Milk is wholesome. Milk is pure. There's no need to inventory a list of ingredients on the side of a milk carton. Ingredients? Why, pure wholesome milk of course! Right? Wrong! When we pasteurize milk we destroy the vitamins. We have to put back an artificial version of the vitamin D destroyed by heat, Vitamin D-3. Most containers will not divulge, "Vitamin D added." They'll ingenuously disclose,

"Milk, Vitamin D." What is in milk? What do we drink in that glass of white liquid? What do we consume in our yogurt, our cheese and our butter?

Milk, The Basics, According to the USDA

    The United States Department of Agriculture publishes data revealing the nutritional contents of foods. (1) Since 454 grams equal one pound, and the average American eats approximately 2.5 pounds per day (1135 gr) of milk and dairy products, one simply multiplies 11.35 times each item to come to the average daily intake of various components of items found in milk. According to the USDA publication, 100 gr of whole milk (3.7 percent fat) contains the following:

Item		Amount of "Item" in 100 Gr		Amount in Average Daily Diet
Water (percent)	=	87.2 percent	=	water
Calories	=	66.0 cal	=	749.10 cal
Protein	=	3.5 gr	=	39.73 gr
Fat	=	3.7 gr	=	42.00 gr
Carbohydrate	=	4.9 gr	=	55.62 gr
Calcium	=	117.0 mg	=	1,327.95 mg
Phosphorus	=	92.0 mg	=	1,044.20 mg
Iron	=	Trace	=	TRACE
Sodium	=	50.0 mg	=	567.50 mg
Potassium	=	140.0 mg	=	1,589.00 mg
Vitamin A	=	150.0 I.U.	=	1,702.50 I.U.
Thiamine	=	0.03 mg	=	0.34 mg
Riboflavin	=	0.17 mg	=	1.93 mg
Niacin	=	0.10 mg	=	1.14 mg
Ascorbic Acid	=	1.00 mg	=	11.35 mg

    Beside the many elements not listed, the chart reveals that the average American receives 749 calories each day from milk and dairy products and 42 gr of fat.

    The human body requires cholesterol and manufactures what it needs. Most doctors and dietitians would advise their clients to limit the consumption of foods containing cholesterol. According to the *Dictionary of Sodium, Fats and Cholesterol*, whole milk (3.5 percent fat) contains 34 mg of cholesterol per 8.6 ounce cup. (2) Taking into account the fact that the average American eats 2 1/2 pounds of dairy product per day (40 ounces), the average daily cholesterol eaten each day from milk and dairy products is equivalent to 158 mg of cholesterol. Let's translate that into an easily understood food equivalent. Bacon. Walk into a diner, order a side of bacon with your eggs, and the waitress could just as easily yell out, a side of cholesterol. With good reason. Each piece of broiled, fried, crisp drained bacon (based upon Oscar Mayer, 18-26 slices per pound) contains 3 mg of cholesterol. Now, compare the bacon with the milk. Calories are calories and fat is fat and cholesterol is cholesterol.

Welcome to the World of Heart Disease!

If your dairy intake is equal to the average American's, you are eating the same cholesterol contained in 53 slices of bacon every single day. If you are 54 years old, you've been doing this for 52 years. Through milk, you've eaten the equivalent cholesterol contained in 19,345 slices of bacon per year. After 52 years you've consumed the same amount of cholesterol contained in over 1 million slices of bacon! Doctors have no clue as to the cause of America's number one killer, heart disease. Ask your medical practitioner if he or she would recommend that you eat 1 million slices of bacon over a lifetime.

Protein

Milk has been called liquid meat. It contains the same amino acids and protein as meat. Weight lifters will stop at nothing to attain the perfect physique and have now discovered that bovine hormones are powerful growth factors. Two weight lifters actually injected themselves with Monsanto's bovine protein, according to an adverse reaction report obtained through the Freedom of Information Act. (3) Weight lifters soon learned that genetically engineered versions of naturally occurring human and bovine IGF-I were readily available from research laboratories. (4) Athletes learned that this hormone, when injected, promoted muscular growth and weight gain.

The best part about this hormonal treatment was that it was not detectable. Remember, IGF-I in cows and humans is identical, 70 amino acids, same gene sequence. FDA allowed Monsanto to genetically engineer versions of these protein hormones without the responsibility of developing an assay. Therefore, there was no way to test an athlete for the presence of a hormone that normally occurs. In the Summer Olympics held in Atlanta in 1996, there was one female athlete, a swimmer from a European nation, who was repeatedly tested by Olympic officials for the presence of growth hormones. Her husband, a weight lifter, must have been aware of this therapy. It was common knowledge among weight lifters that the growth properties were incredible. Page 29 of the *New*

Scientist quotes one weightlifting athlete (in *Muscle Media 2000*) who injected IGF-I:

> I got ripped. It was really noticeable. I stay pretty lean most of the time, but this took it to a different level. Veins in my abs. That sort of thing. (5)

This European athlete's swimming performances improved so dramatically from her previous year's times that officials and fellow athletes suspected that something was terribly wrong. If the swimmer had been using IGF-1 she would never have tested positive because there is no test to discriminate genetically engineered IGF-I from normal IGF-I. Officials tested her many times for the presence of other hormonal factors. There being no test for IGF-I, they could not detect its presence.

More Proteins

In 1877, a scientist identified and described a process to isolate three milk proteins, casein, lactalbumin and lactoglobulin. (6) Today at least eight different types of casein have been identified along with the group of whey proteins which include lactoglobulins, lactalbumins and immunoglobulins. (7) Endocrinologist Clark Grosvenor published a review of the known hormones and growth factors in milk for the Endocrine society in 1982. (8) Each sip of white liquid meat (milk) does include pituitary, hypothalamic, pancreatic, thyroid, parathyroid, adrenal, gonadal, and gut hormones. The list does not include other important milk factors such as prostaglandins and neuropeptides. The bioactive substances taken from Table One of Grosvenor's paper include:

PITUITARY HORMONES (PRL, GH, TSH, FSH, LH, ACTH Oxytocin)

STEROID HORMONES (Estradiol, Estriol, Progesterone, Testosterone, 17-Ketosteroids, Corticosterone, Vitamin D)

HYPOTHALAMIC HORMONES (TRH, LHRH, Somatostatin, PRL- inhibiting factor, PRL- releasing factor, GnRH, GRH)

GASTROINTESTINAL PEPTIDES (Vasoactive intestinal peptide, Bombesin, Cholecystokinin,Gastrin, Gastrin inhibitory peptide, Pancreatic peptide,Y peptide, Substance P, Neurotensin)

THYROID AND PARA-THYROID HORMONES	(T3, T4, rT3, Calcitonin, Parathormone, PTH peptide)
GROWTH FACTORS	(IGFs (I and II), IGF binding proteins, Nerve growth factor, Epidermal growth factor and TGF alpha, TGF beta, Growth Inhibitors M.D.GI and MAF, Platelet derived growth factor)
OTHERS	(PGE, PGF2 alpha, cAMP, cGMP, Delta sleep inducing peptide, Transferrin, Lactoferrin, Casomorphin, Erythropoietin)

All of this in your morning cereal! It still appears white and pure.

Hormones and Growth Factors

Cow's milk contains a variety of proteins and protein hormones besides IGF-I. The functions of many of these bioactive substances are largely unknown and remain to be interpreted. In 1956, evidence of corticosteroids was discovered in cow's milk. (9) Since that date hundreds of other protein and steroid hormones, estrogen, progesterone, calcitonin have been detected in bovine milk. The most critically important piece of the milk puzzle was supplied by Klagsburn (10), who in 1978 determined that growth hormones in cow and human milk stimulated cellular growth. It took mankind thousands of years to realize that milk contained powerful growth hormones. Nearly 20 years after Klagsburn's observation, we are still in denial that milk is an effective delivery system for powerful growth hormones.

Insulin-Like Growth Factor-I (IGF-I)

IGF-I has been called the key factor in the growth and proliferation of cancer in humans by more than one microbiologist and cancer researcher. (See the detailed comments in the paper submitted to FDA in Chapter 6). IGF-I, the most powerful growth hormone in the human body is identical to cow IGF-I. IGF-I makes cells grow. You will not grow an extra finger and your earlobe will remain the same shape. If you drink milk your belly might grow, but that's probably due to all of the fat and calories in dairy products. Most organs and appendages of your body are genetically coded with restrictions so that they do not alter their basic configurations. There are, for the most part, built-in genetically determined limits on growth not true of cancer. The last thing a human adult body needs is a powerful growth hormone instructing cells to grow. Got milk? Then you've got hormones. The hormones work.

The X-O Factor

Kurt Oster, M.D., and Donald Ross, Ph.D., called their book, first printed in 1983, *The X-O Factor* and included the following descriptive phrase on the book's cover: "a triumph over the most serious threat to life today." (11) Oster and Ross did not consider insulin-like growth factor when researching and writing about bovine hormones. This hormone was not well known at the time and Monsanto's BST research was in a top-secret mode. Profit comes before the sharing of knowledge. Without a profit potential, pharmaceutical companies could not justify spending hundreds of millions of dollars to develop new technologies. BST and IGF were exciting concepts which should have been shared with the scientific community.

Oster and Ross performed heart research. Ross resides in Connecticut. Oster died in 1992. Ross and Oster met at St. Vincent's Hospital in Bridgeport, Connecticut where Ross was the director of the chemistry laboratory. Oster, who practiced internal medicine and cardiology at the same hospital, received his medical training in Germany. It was there that Oster first learned about plasmologen, the phospho-lipid-cholesterol-like substance which surrounds each of the cells making up normal heart and arterial wall fibers. This membrane, according to Oster and Ross, is responsible for a number of different functions including the transport of oxygen, calcium and potassium ions, and other enzymes and nutrients to the interior of cells. Thirty percent of the phospholipid membrane in human heart muscle cells is composed of plasmologen.

Plasmologen

Plasmologen was discovered by a German biochemist, Robert Feulgen, in the 1930s. It was at the University of Cologne that Oster met and studied with Fuelgen and his team of researchers. The presence of plasmologen is essential to the structure of heart muscle tissue. The authors of *The X-O Factor* use the following analogy to demonstrate just how vital plasmologen is:

> The presence of plasmologen within the component of the cell
> membrane is essential to the integrity of the cell in much the same
> way that mortar is an ingredient of a brick wall. One could imagine
> what would happen to a brick wall if 30 percent of the mortar fell out.

While Oster and Ross were primarily concerned about the heart, they observed that plasmologen is also present in the myelin sheaths enveloping nerves, the outer covering of the "wires" which transmit electrical signals in the body. Plasmologen is also present in the kidneys and in the mucous membrane of the large intestine. Oster and Ross had no way of guessing that the plasmologen factor might affect the permeability of IGF across the intestinal wall. Their work has serious implications for the survivability of bovine hormones, and absorption rates over and across intestinal lumen. While observing laboratory tissues from heart attack victims, histological clues, Oster and Ross noted the absence of plasmologen. The laws of nature required the presence of this "mortar" and yet it was absent. They wrote:

> [E]arly disappearance of plasmologen suggests the possibility
> that the pain associated with myocardial infarction (heart attack)
> might be a manifestation of enzymatic action on the phospho-
> lipid-rich myelin sheath of sensory nerve endings in the heart.

Some enzyme was dissolving the plasmologen within heart tissue. Oster observed that heart tissue in heart attack victims was different than normal heart tissue. After much research and analyses, Oster focused upon an enzyme called xanthine oxidase (X-O). X-O is found in virtually every animal, and is produced by the liver. This substance can change or oxidize plasmologen to a different substance. There was very little research in the scientific literature about X-O.

This was when Oster met Ross. Together they examined histological samples of heart tissues and found the clue which provided an answer to Oster's puzzle. Tissue samples sectioned from diseased arteries not only contained X-O, but the X-O was still biologically active. Oster observed the enzymatic action of X-O breaking down tissues. The results of this research were published in the *Proceedings of the Society For Experimental Biology and Medicine* in 1973. Since normal human serum does not contain large amounts of X-O, Oster and Ross proposed a potential source, which became the theory pursued in future research:

> Another potential source of the enzyme X-O...bovine milk is
> presently under investigation by this laboratory since it has
> been shown that milk antibodies are significantly elevated in
> the blood of male patients with heart disease.

The Homogenization Factor

Oster and Ross focused upon homogenized milk because of work which they had performed for pharmaceutical companies. Oster had previously observed that the size of a chemical crystal had great effect on its biological availability. The difference between success of one drug versus success of another was micronization, reducing the size of the drug. Homogenization was a process of micronization, the fat molecules were reduced by a factor of at least 10 times. Oster then compared WHO death rates from atherosclerotic and degenerative heart disease with consumption of milk, butter and cheese. He surveyed thirteen countries and observed a correlation between nations which homogenize milk and death rates from degenerative heart disease.

Large fat globules are not easily passed through the intestinal wall. However, homogenization reduces the size of the fat globules by evenly dispersing them throughout the milk when they are forced through a fine filter at pressures equal to 4500 pounds per square inch. After homogenization the fat molecules, which are now one-tenth their original size, are more resistant to digestion Oster and Ross recognized that X-O would be easily carried across intestinal membranes. They did not consider that IGF would also "hitch the same free passage" through the gut and into the bloodstream. Ross and Oster were now faced with finding actual proof that milk was the culprit. X-O was, after all, produced naturally in the body. Their research team developed a reliable method of studying antibodies to detect the possible presence of proteins from cow's milk.

If the FDA and Monsanto were correct in concluding that milk proteins cannot possibly pass through the stomach and intestines and survive, then there would not be any possibility of antibodies produced as a defense against these "foreign invaders." However, if Oster and Ross detected antibodies to milk proteins, then this would be the evidence needed to demonstrate that milk proteins survived digestion. Oster and Ross did not suspect that the normal cow hormone would be genetically engineered and the levels of IGF would increase in milk. If milk proteins survived digestion and milk proteins exerted powerful growth effects, then mankind was in for great trouble if and when these proteins survived digestion.

Oster and Ross performed a double blind experiment on a group of heart attack survivors. They eliminated any suggestion of personal bias by designing research in which drinks were given to patients by a nurse having no clue as to which patient received milk containing milk hormones, and which group received no milk. They then tested the patients' blood for the presence of milk antibodies. Within a few weeks those patients who had received milk containing bovine milk xanthine oxidase (BMXO) produced human antibodies to the BMXO. This would have been impossible if bovine hormones were broken down by digestion. Oster and Ross concluded that:

> X-O from cow's milk (BMXO) may be absorbed and may enter the
> cardiovascular system. People with clinical signs of atherosclerosis
> have greater quantities of BMXO antibodies. BMXO antibodies

are found in greater quantities in those patients who consume the largest volumes of homogenized milk and milk products.

This observation was later confirmed independently by a team of researchers at the University of Delaware who hypothesized that small quantities of BMXO absorbed over an individual's lifetime might hold great biological significance. Oster and Ross described the role of homogenization in permitting the increased biological availability of bovine hormones. Little research has been performed by the dairy industry in this field. The mistake of homogenization, and not IGF itself, might be the greater part of this problem. By separating the cream, they have removed the potential goodness. Instead of the cream rising to the top, we have unleashed the demons of illness and death.

In this chapter, we investigated the components of milk. Let's now consider what a wholesome glass of milk does to your stomach. You've just finished a delicious well balanced dinner. The first course was a nutritious salad, mixed greens with tomatoes, shredded carrots, radishes and cabbage. The main course was filet mignon accompanied by a baked potato and sautéed mushroom caps. You ate the accompanying broccoli and one small dinner roll. For dessert there's a rich slice of chocolate cake. What goes down well with cake? Got milk?

Inside of your stomach is a hard to digest protein mash consisting of partially digested starch from the potato and bits and pieces of multi-colored carbohydrates. Your powerful stomach enzymes are beginning to degrade this pulpy mass of food. The gases produced in such an acid bath would qualify as a hazardous materials operation if it were spilled on a factory floor. Suddenly, the entire process of digestion and degradation is interrupted by twelve ounces of ice cold milk.

Milk! What a surprise to the contents of your stomach. Digestion is halted, a lot more acid is needed, the time to digest this mixture of starch, carbohydrate, protein and acid is now increased by many hours. The milk has counterbalanced the effects of the digestive acids. As the new acid is squirted into the stomach you feel the first ominous signs of discomfort. Got milk? Get Tums!

"There's a high rate of cancer among my friends. It doesn't mean anything."

Dr. Frances Clifford
Health Commissioner of Niagara County, New York, home of the Love Canal, a
toxic waste site for the Hooker Chemical Company

"There is absolutely no possibility that the consumption of milk from rbST-
treated cows could increase the risk of breast cancer."

Linda Grasse, FDA Veterinarian, May/June 1994

Chapter 11

Cancer: The Link Between Growth Hormones in Milk and Dairy Consumption

---

A diagnosis of cancer can be a death sentence. Occasionally, a victim receives a reprieve by being "cured" through radiation treatment or traditional chemotherapies. Technology offers hope for a cure by leading edge scientific techniques including the use of interferons or procedures still considered experimental research by FDA and not yet approved for use by the entire population. Often, alternative therapies are successful in halting the spread of a tumor. Sometimes cancers disappear entirely after one or a combination of the above treatments are applied. Once a cancer is diagnosed there is little emphasis placed upon how the individual got the cancer in the first place. The only significant issue becomes treatment and cure, not prevention.

When a cell dies the body has to make new cells to replace the old ones. Many substances or circumstances kill cells. Most of the body's cells are programmed to die and be replaced. The body is often invaded by chemicals or events that cause damage and increase cellular replication. What kills cells? Sunlight, x-rays, ultraviolet rays, microwaves, pollution, cigarette smoke, just to name a few. It is well accepted that cigarette smoking is one of the biggest contributors toward the development of lung cancer. Science has yet to describe the actual process of how cancers grow. A cancer is a mistake. Since it is the body's own mistake, the cancer is not attacked by the body's normal immune system. A cancer begins with one cell. A cancerous liver cell or lung cell has something wrong in its code. It grows but does not retain the characteristics of the cell it is replacing. Instead, it just keeps growing and growing. In 3 months that one cell doubles to become two cells. Every 3 months the number of cells doubles. Three months later the two become four. After 1 year the cancer has 16 cells.

After two years the cancer has 256 cells. In 5 years the cancer is 1 million cells strong. The actual cancer may not be detected for many years to come. The cancer may at some time stop growing. We have very tight and remarkable genetic controls that sometimes keep cancers from growing.

Every single cancer that has ever grown in every human so diagnosed has one thing in common. Every cancer relies upon the most powerful hormone in the human body for its growth. That hormone is IGF-I. Insulin-like growth factor does not cause cancer. It allows existing cancers to grow. Those existing cancers were caused by one event, and one event only: an error in cellular replication. Cigarette smoke does not contain IGF-I. Neither do dioxins or uranium-235. These toxins can cause cancer by killing cells and making new replication necessary, but in order for cancer to grow there must be IGF-I. Without IGF-I, the growth hormone, there is no cancer. We manufacture IGF-I in our bodies. We also consume IGF-I in dairy products. In milk, there are a number of elements which protect this hormone. Casein, milk's "glue," is one protective element. Another is the process of homogenization which creates more fat molecules and makes them smaller. These fat molecules carry IGF-I from milk through the stomach and gut into the bloodstream where they can circulate through the human body to exert powerful growth effects.

Cancer is a big business. One wonders what happens if we ever find a cure? Will we destroy an industry and put a lot of people out of work? Is it in the best interests of certain individuals to never find a cure for cancer? The American Cancer Society published a brochure entitled "Cancer Facts & Figures - 1994." In that document they state:

> Since there is no nationwide cancer registry, there is no
> way of knowing exactly how many new cases of cancer
> are diagnosed each year. (1)

How can there be no nationwide registry? Is this a part of the cancer industry's brilliantly devised plan? For a nation so developed with communications and computer technologies, it seems a crime that there are so little data available accompanied by cancer statistics. Cancer is a disease that many people, fearful of a confirming diagnosis, would rather not know that they have. Billions of dollars go into researching cures for cancer. Yet, society does not seem interested in who gets it and why and where and when.

There is no national cancer registry system. Statistics issued by governmental agencies are at least 3 years old. World health statistics are even worse. Data about cancers in nations all over the world are incomplete and questionable. It seems that some "power" has inefficiently designed a system intended not to reveal facts about cancer rates. IGF hormones increase in BST-treated milk and normal untreated milk contains high levels of IGF. Nobody has written or spoken about this obvious connection. One group of scientists understood the power of this growth hormone. A second group of scientists knew that this powerful growth hormone was present in milk. These scientists do not attend the same cocktail parties. There is no exchange of information. In milk, we drink IGF-I. If increased levels of IGF were poison to the human body, then naturally occurring levels of IGF were also a potential problem.

Why is There No Up-to-Date Cancer Registry?

The International Dairy and Breast Cancer Chart on pages 248 and 249 contains data which were taken from WHO mortality statistics per 100,000 of population by country. These data were obtained from a combination of different sources. Some of the data were published by WHO. Some data were gathered directly from embassies located in New York City. Other numbers and figures were available in the World Almanac. Some numbers were prepared by the Milk Industry Foundation and were published by the United States Department of Agriculture (USDA). With no other data source available, it should be accepted not as proof but rather as a clue. Population charts and breast cancer rates per 100,000 people are compared with national dairy consumption. One of the problems I had in building my charts was that some nations experienced high per capita cheese consumption rates and low milk consumption, while other nations were just the opposite. Accordingly, I developed a conversion factor, accepting the USDA published standard for relative equivalents. According to USDA, to make one pound of butter one requires 21.2 pounds of whole milk. To make one pound of whole milk cheese requires 10 pounds of whole milk.

I often ask people (when I control the conversation to include milk, genetic engineering and breast cancer), "What nation has the highest incidence of breast cancer rates in the world?" The most frequently heard response is the United States. We have been bombarded with warnings that one out of eight women alive today will be diagnosed with breast cancer during her lifetime. Two years ago that number was one out of nine. Three years ago one out of ten. I see a disturbing trend here. Holland, Austria, Norway, New Zealand, France, Great Britain and Ireland all have higher breast cancer rates than the United States. Those nations with higher breast cancer rates also consume more dairy than U.S. residents.

High Dairy Consumption Correlates to Breast Cancer Rates

Interestingly enough, Australia, Portugal, Spain, Romania, Korea have lower breast cancer rates than Holland, Austria New Zealand and France. Each of these nations in the first group consume less dairy than the nations in the second group. Nations with plenty of fat in their diet like East Germany suffered dairy shortages before the Berlin Wall came down. During the years previous to that political event, the reported incidence of breast cancer from East Germany was quite low. West Germans, on the other hand, had high rates of dairy consumption and cancer rates.

The International Dairy and Breast Cancer Chart

Country	Breast Cancer per 100m Women	Lbs Milk per Capita	Pints per Day Consumed
Hungary	28.50	241	0.7
England	24.23	389	1.1
Belgium	24.00	286	0.8
Netherlands	22.13	498	1.4
W. Germany	21.47	400	1.1
Austria	21.02	456	1.2
Italy	18.29	366	1.0
Sweden	18.12	513	1.4
Norway	17.88	588	1.6
New Zealand	17.85	583	1.6
France	17.79	511	1.4
Ireland	17.54	490	1.3
Canada	16.73	362	1.0
United States	**16.49**	**363**	**1.0**
Czechoslovakia	15.79	584	1.6
Finland	15.44	518	1.4
Australia	13.19	356	1.0

By no means was my study of data a scientific study. The data are often incomplete and the different methods of measuring, collecting and reporting data to the WHO is sometimes biased and different according to national differences. There is a need for better systems to collect these data, both worldwide and nationally. The data in this chart are breast cancer incidence, not death. By using this chart and checking mortality statistics there is a way of predicting death rates from breast cancer. The population statistics of a nation and the per capita consumption of milk, cheese and butter can describe how many women will die of breast cancer the following year in that nation.

Country	Breast Cancer per 100m Women	Lbs Milk per Capita	Pints per Day Consumed
Portugal	13.18	230	0.6
Greece	12.37	449	1.2
Spain	11.81	300	0.8
Poland	10.66	455	1.2
Romania	8.51	294	0.8
Chile	5.45	51	0.1
Japan	4.62	115	0.3
Brazil	3.12	124	0.3
Venezuela	2.93	74	0.2
Mexico	2.01	173	0.5
Peru	1.18	17	0.7
Argentina	1.12	217	0.6
Cuba	7.62		
Trinidad	7.00		
Singapore	6.35		
Guatemala	4.94		
Costa Rica	4.00		
Mauritius	3.09		
Guyana	2.62		
Bahrain	2.60		
Panama	2.50		
Kuwait	1.92		
Surinam	1.75		
Ecuador	1.72		
Paraguay	1.44		
Egypt	1.38		
Korea	1.26		
Dominican Rep.	1.09		
Zimbabwe	1.02		
El Salvador	0.21		

These nations all have extremely low per capita consumption of milk and dairy products. No milk data statistics were available because dairy consumption is considered to be extremely low.

Breast cancer rates are also on the low end when compared with nations consuming large amounts of milk, cheese and butter.

A standardized set of parameters needs to be applied when collecting data from different nations. The data contained here furnish another important clue as a partial answer to questions raised about milk. There exists a strong correlation between dairy consumption and breast cancer. In nations where per capita daily consumption of milk and dairy exceeds one-half pint, there is a high incidence of breast cancer. Conversely, where dairy consumption is less than one pint per day the breast cancer rates are considerably lower.

The Key Cancer-Causing Factor is Use of Dairy Products

It has been established that IGF-I is a powerful cellular growth hormone. IGF-I is identical in the number of amino acids and the amino acid sequence in humans and cows. Furthermore, IGF has been identified by many scientists performing microbiological research as the key factor in the growth and proliferation of cancer. (See Chapter Six, particularly pages 158-163.) IGF-I in milk survives digestion and enters into the bloodstream. IGF-I is a growth hormone. Drink milk and you are taking growth hormones into your body.

IGF-I is always present in every single type of human cancer. It is always there, initiating cellular growth and proliferation. Every single cancer researcher in the world is aware of the power of this hormone. IGF-I plays a role in every single cancer and every type of tumor known to medical science, and has done so forever and will continue to do so. That includes brain cancers and breast cancers and pancreatic cancers and lung cancers and prostate cancers. If you know somebody who has cancer they should be alerted to the dairy connection. Without the powerful growth effects exerted by IGF-I, there would not be cancer. With milk, we bathe our cells with IGF-I. Wouldn't it be prudent to eliminate the one dietary source of IGF-I from our bodies? Can sexy milk mustaches continue to cloud our vision and understanding of milk? Milk is a hormonal delivery system!

Cancer Treatment Center

The Cancer Treatment Centers of America (CTCA) manage cancer programs at hospitals and private medical facilities throughout the United States. CTCA's mission is to provide care, diagnosis and total body treatment for their patients. They recognize that diet and proper nutrition play a role in developing and defeating cancers. According to the people who run this organization, about one third of cancer deaths are related to the foods people eat. (2)

Breast Cancer and Dairy Products

Are there links between breast cancer and dairy products? Little has been written in popular magazines about the dairy-cancer connection. Popular magazines rely upon advertising revenue from the dairy industry. However, the scientific literature is filled with such references linking dairy consumption with cancer. Most doctors have observed no connection. For those who have, they link the high levels of fat and cholesterol in milk to cancer. Many doctors received their training before IGF-I was even identified as a cellular growth hormone. The scientists write about how cancers grow in the scientific journals. They sustain their grants from the government to continue their particular research. However, their observations are not "marketed."   There is no group that can benefit financially from such evidence.   Do you believe that dairy executives want you to know that hormones in milk make cancers grow?   They should come to terms with this sweeping deception, like the cigarette industry CEOs have recently done.

Breast Cancer Research

As you read about some of the recent breast cancer research, keep in mind the importance of IGF-I as a growth factor.   Recall that IGF-I is a protein hormone that we drink in milk.   Consider the fact that IGF-I from cows is identical to IGF-I normally produced in the human body.   The IGF-I in milk survives digestion and causes growth, just what it was designed to do.   Infants are supposed to experience rapid and dramatic growth.   Adults are not, and the breast tissue and breast cells of adults should not be "influenced" by hormones which initiate cellular growth and cellular proliferation.

Researcher Carlos Arteaga, M.D., has been developing a strategy to treat breast cancer. (3) He recognizes the importance of the entire IGF system and is attempting to learn the mechanisms of that system.   If he can develop a way to sensitize cells to the proliferative effects of IGF he believes that he can stop breast cancer cells from growing.   Unfortunately, Arteaga cannot get women to ignore the dairy industry message.   Women continue to eat dairy products, believing that the calcium in milk will help prevent bone disease.   That message is reinforced to women who continue to drink milk, believing that milk mustaches are beautiful.

Tamoxifen is a drug that is used to treat women who have breast cancer. Friedl noted that tamoxifen therapy works to inhibit the actions of IGF-I. (4) In his paper, published in the *European Journal of Cancer*, Friedl observes that IGF-I levels in breast cancer patients were suppressed after tamoxifen therapy.

IGF-I and Cancer

The paper presented to FDA on April 21, 1995 (Chapter Six), reviewed some of the research linking IGF-I and cancer.   IGF-I has been identified as a growth regulator which accelerates various types of cancers.   IGF-I is considered to play an important role in the proliferation of pancreatic cancer cells (5) and plays an important role in the regulation of glucose metabolism in CNS (central nervous system) tumors. (6)   Many scientists have recognized the IGF-I cancer link.   Atiq reported that IGF-I is associated with rectal tumors (7) while Yashiro found that IGF-bp (IGF binding protein) activity in cancer tissue is involved in regulating growth of thyroid tumors. (8)   Robbins found that IGF-I increased lymphocyte numbers in lymphoid organs examined.   This increase had functional significance, and Robbins concluded that IGF-I may be a natural component of bone cancer. (9)

Yun demonstrated that there was 32-64 times more IGF in cancerous kidney tumors than in the adjacent uninvolved kidneys. (10) Minniti concluded after analyses of tumor biopsy specimens that IGFs act as a growth factor in human cancers. Kappel wrote that osteogenic sarcoma is the most common bone tumor of childhood and typically occurs during adolescent growth spurts when growth hormone and insulin-like growth factor-I may be at their highest lifetime levels. (11) As early as 1991, Lippman had implicated IGF-I as being critically involved in the aberrant growth of human breast cancer cells (12), while Lee observed that IGF has a' regulatory function in breast cancer. (13) Chen noted, and Figueroa confirmed, that IGFs are potent mitogens for malignant cell proliferation in the human breast carcinoma cell line. (14, 15)

Li (16) treated breast cancer cells with IGF-I and observed a 10-fold increase in levels of cancer cells and concluded that IGF-I appears to be an important step in cellular proliferation. Krasnick furnished another clue to this puzzle by revealing that IGF-I may have a role in the regulation of human ovarian cancer. (17) His data supported a role for IGF-I in proliferation of ovarian cancer and suggested that IGF-I and estrogen interact in a synergistic manner and regulate this malignancy. Musgrove stated that growth factors play a major role in the control of human breast cancer cell proliferation. (18)

Do All Adults Have Cancer?

Cancer occurs more frequently than is commonly believed. Gina Kolata revealed, in her November 8, 1994, *New York Times* column (19), that virtually all adults have cancer, which normally stops growing as a result of tight genetic controls. That article also revealed, through autopsy studies of premature deaths not related to cancer, that although 1 percent of women between the ages of 40 and 50 are clinically diagnosed with breast cancer, 39 percent of those women who died premature deaths (from causes other than cancer) had undiagnosed cancers in their breasts. However, Gina Kolata did not explore the role of factors in breast cancer. To many scientists, IGF-I is the key factor in the growth and proliferation of human cancer.

The Leukemia Connection

What is the sound of a cotton ball dropping on the top of a helium-filled balloon and then crashing to the thick pile carpet below? What sound does a blade of grass make as it thrusts its way through the top layer of soil into the warmth of sunlight? What terrible and fearful sound, the flapping of an approaching butterfly wing to an aphid on the stalk of a dandelion?

What horrible discord is created by the birth of an abnormally formed white blood cell among healthy ones? A cacophony of offending sounds and warning alarms. Like the screeching of tires preceding a traffic accident or the honking voices of geese, alerting one another to the presence of a lurking predator, all occurring in a terrible microinstant of time.

The body produces an abnormally formed cell, an invader to its environment, offending other cells who run away and hide from the deformed stranger who sulks silently in a corner beginning to replicate, bubbling away creating more of its own demon offspring. The healthy cells, brave and yet fearful, mount a courageous attack but are repelled. The spleen in response to the first battle lost replicates champion warrior white cells to fight the invader who, with its new army, wins battle after battle, defeating the host. The spleen, now on full alert, is aware of its own mortality. Throwing caution to the cellular winds, it mobilizes. Responding to the enemy it grows enormously in size creating armies and hordes of sentries to fight a battle which has already been decided and lost.

The invader settles in the lymph nodes and then the bone marrow. Abnormal white cells overpower and rout the platoons of healthy blood cells sent to do battle. Leukemia. Overwhelming and usually fatal. Once upon a time rats were observed in a laboratory experiment. Their bowls of food were filled to the brim with milk containing recombinant genetically engineered bovine somatotropin. The experiment lasted 21 days and was too short in duration to have detected the birth of the first cells in an incipient disease. Twice upon a time rats were force-fed the same chemical for 90 days. No milk chaser in this trial. Another group, their brothers and sisters, were injected with the same drug. The scientists, gods of the laboratory in immaculate white coats, beheld glorious reactions to the group receiving injections under the flap of skin in their necks. The quietly suffering females had their spleens grow in size 39 percent more than the average control group female spleens. Ouch. These were creatures whose internal systems were in disarray. Silently screaming with pain, their spleens grew in size to fight the identical losing battle with the successful invader. Their brothers' spleens grew 46 percent. During the 3-month campaign, a silent war had waged inside of these tiny creatures, rats who nobody had reason nor compassion to care for, awaiting sacrifice and autopsy on their unlucky thirteen-week birthdays. And the scientists, they saw the spleens and measured the spleens and observed the exceptional growth.

Did they look for similar effects from the animals whose mouths were opened by a special tool called a gavage and force fed BST? Would it have been reasonable to assume that they too might have experienced a similar but delayed reaction to BST? Nobody looked, nobody talked. If they suspected a problem they did a good job of keeping their suspicions to themselves. The spleens were cut away, isolated from surrounding tissues and weighed, the numbers of 360 animals filling long columns in a laboratory notebook. When the data were finally printed, the scientists concluded that there were no biological effects from oral ingestion of this drug.

The numbers were published and the conclusions blindly accepted by the agencies and governing bodies of the world. Every potential critic pointed to the evidence and confirmed their innate belief that the drug would be deemed safe. There was no need to check the figures, the scientists had spoken the law of their God. Trust, faith in scientific data. Once published, "evidence" becomes gospel. And then one day, a doubter looked at the numbers. He stood on top of them and to the right, and then the left. He stood on his head and then noticed something wrong. A little voice from that heretic cried, "Forty-six percent." "What?" whispered the scientist in disbelief. "Forty-six percent," answered the skeptic. "Who is that?" demanded the government bureaucrat. "The animals," said the voice a bit louder and bolder. "The spleens. Look how the spleens grew. Aren't those biological effects?" "No," said the scientist and bureaucrat together, in two part harmony, their heads shaking and their fingers wagging in the face of the cynical questioner, their movements orchestrated to the string section of a symphony orchestra. The voice stopped, intimidated, and withdrew to recalculate his equations. "I'm right," the voice yelled. "You're wrong," he screamed, gaining strength and growing bolder. "I can't let you get away with this." And he didn't. And in his fairy tale, all of the people in the world, all of the animals in the labs and on the farms lived happily ever after.

Leukemia. Swollen lymph nodes. Increased spleen growth. Assorted gross lesions. The symptoms were developing in Monsanto's rbST animal study. The animals were sacrificed early enough to ignore the symptoms. But the data survived the animals and lived to tell their painful stories.

According to the Leukemia Society of America, leukemia causes more deaths among children ages 1 to 14 in the United States than any other disease. Leukemia and lymphomas are the fourth major cause of cancer deaths in men and women in the United States. Every twelve minutes, another child or adult dies from leukemia. (20) In leukemia, the body experiences a shortage of normal white blood cells and a profusion of abnormally developed white blood cells. Evidence suggests that increased levels of BST in laboratory animals were causing animals increased spleen growth in those animals. The body has chemical messengers called hormones. Many hormones are of the type that promote rapid growth. Insulin-like growth factor is one powerful growth hormone. When IGF was discovered, its growth properties were observed but its actual proliferative effects were not yet suspected. It acted like insulin, so it was called insulin-like.

Eat Growth Hormones and Get Leukemia

In February 1988, a letter from a Japanese researcher was published in *The Lancet* reporting the occurrence of leukemia in five Japanese children treated with growth hormone (GH) for GH deficiency. (21) GH programs in 17 European nations were then surveyed and a disturbing number of children were found to have contracted leukemia.

In May 1988, the Lawson Wilkins Pediatric Endocrine Society and the Human Growth Foundation met in Bethesda Maryland to discuss the increased incidence of hypo-pituitary children (those who were short because of low levels of growth hormones being secreted by the pituitary gland) getting leukemia as a result of being given treatments of human growth hormone. (22) *Science News* cited the Lawson Wilkins study and reported that:

> Short statured youngsters receiving human growth hormone
> treatments appear at increased risk of developing leukemia. (23)

However, there was no scientifically accepted controlled experiment because each child had a completely different set of circumstances. Some children, for example, were treated with natural growth hormone and others received a genetically engineered version. There was one scientific experiment in which laboratory animals ate growth hormones. These animals experienced enormous spleen increases. FDA noted no biological effects.

FDA and other agencies have told us that human GH treatments have been around since the 1950s. According to FDA and the scientific community, GH treatment is perfectly safe. Jerome Moore, one of the scientists cited by Juskevich and Guyer, was quoted in the *Science* paper as attesting to the safety of GH treatment on dwarves. However, when Moore's paper is examined, we learn that pituitary derived human growth hormone (hGH) was not safe. Treatment with hGH was suspected as causing the occurrence of Jacob-Creutzfeldt disease in some children treated with the hormone. (24)

Jacob-Cruetzfeldt is caused by a transmissible protein called a prion. This organic brain disease is debilitating, causing a loss of motor and mental skills. This neurological disease has been identified as one of the rare diseases which cows have transmitted to humans. A dairy farmer in England contracted the human equivalent of this bovine disease and his herd had to be destroyed. In the very first paragraph of his paper, Moore commented that dwarves caught the same disease from taking human growth hormone. Yet scientists and FDA point to the early 1950's treatment of dwarves as evidence that these growth hormones are safe and cause no harm. Growth hormones cause rapid and uncontrolled growth. When given at a time other than the human infancy, that growth is inappropriate. Keep drinking milk and you bathe your system with unwanted growth hormones.

Cows treated with rbST yield milk containing increased levels of powerful growth hormones. Monsanto's first biotech product, the genetically engineered bovine protein marketed as Posilac, is the largest selling dairy animal product in the United States, according to the *Dick Davis Digest*, one of Wall Street's most respected economic newsletters. The October 13, 1997 issue of this biweekly journal reported:

> About 25% of dairy cows are in herds that use Posilac to boost milk production. The product turned profitable at the end of 1996, as sales climbed 40% for the year. We see Posilac remaining in the black with further sales gains this year...With the company's strong growth prospects, the shares are a top choice for above average appreciation in the coming months. (25)

Every day the average American drinks milk and eats dairy products from cows treated with this genetically engineered bovine protein. Whole milk and skim milk, ice cream and yogurt, pizza, cheese and butter. Our milk has changed and the new milk contains increased levels of naturally occurring growth hormones.

"I would call milk perhaps the most unhealthful vehicle for calcium that one could possibly imagine, which is the only thing people really drink it for, but whenever you challenge existing dogma...people are resistant."

Neal Barnard, M.D.

"So don't drink milk for health. I am convinced on the weight of the scientific evidence that it does not 'do a body good.' Inclusion of milk will only reduce your diet's nutritional value and safety."

Robert M. Kradjian, M.D.

"Cow's milk in the past has always been oversold as the perfect food, but we are now seeing that it isn't the perfect food at all and the government really shouldn't be behind any efforts to promote it as such."

Benjamin Spock, M.D.

Chapter 12

The Truth About Calcium, Osteoporosis and Milk Allergies

Drug stores are stocked full of items to counteract the reactions brought about from consuming milk and dairy products. The casein in milk has been described as a primary cause of mucous and congestion. There are studies that have linked milk consumption with childhood earaches. Pills for headaches and sprays for nasal congestion line the shelves of America's drug stores and supermarkets. There are allergy capsules and antihistamines as well as laxatives to relieve irritable bowel syndrome. Three quarters of the human race cannot digest lactose in milk. All people produce antibodies to bovine proteins with anti-histamine production. The range of people's symptoms can be relieved by the products sold in pharmacies. There are stool softeners and medications to relieve intestinal gas, bloating and diarrhea. There are antacid tablets for indigestion that also contain dietary calcium in a form that is easily assimilated by the human body. There are so many manufacturers who benefit from diseases and symptoms caused by milk and these companies should be paying royalties on the sales of their remedies to the dairy industry. Without milk and dairy consumption, there might not be a need for many of these pharmaceuticals. Milk is responsible for an important part of the cash flow of drug stores. Without a strong milk industry, we might see many of these apothecaries fail.

Many diseases have been attributed to milk and dairy consumption. Not only have bovine proteins been linked with allergies but they've been implicated as the cause of serious diseases such as cancer, heart disease and osteoporosis. By consuming milk and dairy products we may be placing the final restraint on our ability to extend our longevity and live well over 100 years of age. By discontinuing the consumption of milk and dairy products, we might very well discover the "Fountain of Youth."

In his book, *The Allergy Discovery Diet*, John Postley, M.D., calls milk one of the common causes of food sensitivities. In addition to avoiding milk products, Postley recommends reading food labels for the "ubiquitous presence" of evidence of milk compounds such as whey solids or casein. (1) Harvey and Marilyn Diamond, in *Fit For Life*, the best selling book that changed the way people combine their foods, resulting in healthier eating, devoted a chapter to dairy products and concluded that there was nothing that would destroy a healthy diet regimen as successfully as milk and dairy products. The Diamonds give milk and dairy products credit for cholesterol problems as well as allergies and seriously challenge the enormous calcium myth perpetrated on the American public by the dairy industry. (2)

An indication of the lack of perception by the medical establishment linking human allergies to milk products can be illustrated by *Allergies: A-Z*. (3) The authors of this book tell the story of Hippocrates, the learned scholar whose name is attached to the oath that doctors recite but rarely adhere to. They note that Hippocrates was one of the first individuals to link milk consumption to allergic reactions such as hives and gastrointestinal disorders. Yet two sentences later, the authors report that the true incidence of cow's milk allergy is only one in 1000. Do these men who lack vision think that Hippocrates only knew 1000 people and was writing about that one individual? Maybe milk problems happened to more than one in a thousand. Maybe it was all Greek to them! Why do some scientists and doctors ignore the evidence, display no analytical common sense, and display a complete lack of logic in their analyses? And why, do many people believe everything that is written in black and white, particularly those things written by people with lots of letters attached to the end of their names?

Advice to Doctors from Doctors

Doctors, who had not placed strong emphasis on nutrition in medical school, were at last getting an accurate and unbiased message concerning milk. Many M.D.s who subscribe to the trade journal, the *Townsend Letter For Doctors*, drank their first sip of milk's great controversy. The *Townsend Letter* included a brief column on the dangers of cow's milk. This medical newsletter gave credit to good marketing by the dairy industry which informs us to drink milk because it is "wholesome and necessary." (4) The newsletter responds to this marketing message, "In reality, cow's milk, especially processed cow's milk, has been linked to a variety of health problems." Among those problems attributed to milk and dairy consumption by this medical newsletter written by doctors for doctors, include:

1) mucus production
2) hemoglobin loss
3) childhood diabetes
4) heart disease
5) atherosclerosis
6) arthritis
7) kidney stones
8) mood swings
9) depression
10) irritability
11) allergies

Nine months earlier, the seed to this story was planted in the August issue of *Natural Health*. In an article entitled "Don't Drink Your Milk!," author Nathaniel Mead describes "nature's perfect food" as being linked to a great number of serious health problems. Mead's article begins by including a quote from a Washington, D.C., pediatrician by the name of Russell Bunai, M.D. When asked his opinion on what single change in the American diet would produce the greatest health benefit, Bunai responded, "Eliminating dairy products." Mead interviewed Frank A. Oski, M.D., chief of pediatrics at Johns Hopkins School of Medicine, who stated:

At least 50 percent of all children in the United States are allergic
to cow's milk, many undiagnosed. Dairy products are the
leading cause of food allergy, often revealed by diarrhea,
constipation, and fatigue. Many cases of asthma and sinus
infections are reported to be relieved and even eliminated by
cutting out dairy. The exclusion of dairy, however, must be
complete to see any benefit. (5)

Three out of four humans suffer the most well-known allergic reaction to milk because they are unable to digest a milk sugar called lactose. These people's systems reject lactose. These individuals are termed "lactose intolerant." Symptoms of such intolerance include diarrhea, stomach bloating gas, cramps, flatulence, halitosis, and migraine headaches. Call the Lactose Intolerance Hotline at 800-HELP-KIT (1-800-435-7548) for a free health kit containing a test which will determine whether you are lactose intolerant.

What is an Allergy?

Like a tree falling in the forest with no one to hear, is there sound? If you have an allergic reaction to something but do not notice that reaction, do you still have an allergy? I would say that you do but many doctors, taught to treat symptoms, would diagnose no such allergy, despite the evidence of physiological reactions. An allergy is the reaction that your body makes to an unusual substance that "does not belong." That substance can be pollen from grass or trees which affect millions of people every spring. Different pollens like those from goldenrod affect different people in the autumn. People can have negative reactions to proteins in fruits or vegetables, smoke from cigarettes, perfumes, and iodine in seafood. Some people are allergic to fungi and molds, microscopic particles which enter the bloodstream and irritate the body's defenses which respond by creating antibodies to the irritants. Milk is a hormonal delivery system. After drinking milk, the liquid enters the stomach and should be digested. If FDA is correct, being allergic to milk is an impossibility because proteins are broken down in the stomach. Milk is loaded with protein hormones. Humans create antibodies to those proteins. All humans have allergic reactions by varying degrees to those "invaders." Some people have severe reactions, some barely none. However, antibodies are created by all humans who drink milk.

When an allergen enters the bloodstream it reacts with circulating white blood cells or mast cells which line the gastrointestinal tract. In either case, the mast cells or white blood cells secrete defensive drugs called histamines, which battle the invaders. When histamines are released there are many effects. In the lungs they release copious amounts of mucous which often results in coughing and congestion. They also can cause diarrhea and cramp the stomach. Most humans react to milk by creating various levels of mucous. Some humans react quite horribly, some not so bad. Many scientists and doctors have hypothesized that Sudden Infant Death Syndrome (SIDS) is actually an allergic reaction to milk hormones. Babies who drink formula are actually drinking milk which contains milk proteins. Some "formula!"

Is Sudden Infant Death Syndrome an allergic reaction? The medical literature contains many references suggesting that an allergy to milk is the primary cause of SIDS. In 1960, *The Lancet* implicated a milk allergy, hypersensitivity to milk, as the cause of sudden death in infancy. (6) The November 5, 1994, issue of *The Lancet* compared infants who breastfeed to infants who consume cow's milk or formula based on cow's milk. Those who consumed cows milk were fourteen times more likely to die from diarrhea-related complications and four times more likely to die of pneumonia than were breast-fed babies. This study implicated intolerance and allergy to cow's milk products as a factor in sudden infant death syndrome. (7)

The most shocking study, also reported in *The Lancet*, appeared on June 4, 1994. Histological analyses of 48 infants who had died from SIDS were compared with tissue samples of 30 infants who died from other nonpulmonary causes. The findings were that those infants who died of SIDS expressed inappropriate or inflammatory responses suggesting violent allergic reactions to "something foreign." Lung tissue and cells showed responses similar to bronchial wall inflammation in asthma. (8) These tiny infants were reacting to "something." It was not the role of the scientists to guess what that something was. Their job was to supply a clue. Do you suppose each of those babies enjoyed a cigar before retiring for the evening? How about a glass of cognac? These infants did not have pneumonia before going to bed, otherwise their death certificates would not have read SIDS.

Each and every child who died of SIDS probably had one thing in common. Each victim most likely ate his or her last meal in the hours preceding death. Each victim introduced a powerful allergen which initiated an allergic reaction. What do you suppose that meal was? In 1993, 4070 American infants died of SIDS. (9) In 1994, that number increased by more than 5 percent to 4290 infants. In 1994, milk consumption increased by over 4 percent. However, there is no coincidence when considering the relation between milk consumption, allergic reactions to cow's milk and Sudden Infant Death Syndrome.

The three most common milk proteins are casein, beta-lactoglobulin, and alpha-lactalbumin. These three "ingredients" have been identified as the major allergens in cow's milk. Authors of a study performed at the University of Brescia, Italy, developed a correlation between these three cow proteins and childhood allergies. At the conclusion of their article, the authors suggest a therapeutic strategy of soy protein as a substitute for cow's milk. (10) Warning: Monsanto is now marketing genetically engineered soy beans. Shall there be a sequel to this book entitled, "Don't Drink the Soy Milk?" This issue is front page news in Europe where citizens of many nations have been protesting and rejecting products containing these gene-altered soybeans.

Constipate Your Baby? (Hint) Got Milk?

Scientists at the University of Palermo discovered that constipation symptoms returned to a controlled group of infants 48 to 72 hours after they were placed on a regimen of cow's milk proteins. Their determination was that constipation in infants may have an allergic pathogenesis. (11) Researchers at the Department of Clinical Medicine, University of Tampere, Finland, indicated that diet has a significant effect on the developing immune system. They discovered that formula fed babies, at the age of 3 months, were secreting low levels of serum antibodies to bovine proteins contained in their formula. (12)

FDA believes this is not possible because, in theory, these proteins are destroyed by digestive processes. Message to FDA: Milk proteins survive digestion. Doctors at the Department of Pediatrics, Odense University Hospital in Denmark noted that most formula fed infants developed symptoms of allergic rejection to cow milk proteins before one month of age. The majority of infants tested had two or more symptoms. About 50-70 percent experienced rashes or other skin symptoms, 50-60 percent gastrointestinal symptoms, and 20-30 percent respiratory symptoms. The recommended therapy was to avoid cow's milk. (13)

Diabetes

Diabetes is classically characterized as a pancreatic disease; the inability of the pancreas to adequately produce insulin. This disease is characterized by excessive urinary secretions containing excessive amounts of sugar. America currently enjoys a popular diabetic "fad." "Hypochondriacs Anonymous" (join the club) seem to be relieved when they are diagnosed with diabetes. Finally, a disease which justifies their sugar cravings. Accommodating physicians recognize the potential cash flow represented by these patients who make monthly pilgrimages to their doctor's offices seeking routine blood tests which usually result in the diagnosis of diabetes.

True diabetes can be quite serious. More than 13 million Americans have diabetes. About 700,000 people have insulin-dependent diabetes. Six million Americans have non-insulin-dependent diabetes and do not know it. (14) It has been estimated that one out of 20 Americans are true diabetics. Of these, only about one or two must regularly inject insulin into their bodies. The others are diagnosed as "potential diabetics" and are advised to carefully watch their diets. Doctors suggest that their patients seek alternate sweeteners as substitutes for their cravings of sweets.

Milk and Aspartame

Aspartame is a neurotoxin, according to many doctors including Russell Blaylock, M.D., and Hymen Roberts, M.D., and is another example of most physician's inability to keep you informed of the poisons in your food. FDA receives more complaints from aspartame users than any other food product. Aspartame is made up of three ingredients: 10 percent methyl alcohol-a toxic, colorless, flammable liquid, 40 percent aspartic acid-a non-essential amino acid, and 50 percent phenylalanine-an essential amino acid. Never before have people ingested pure amino acids bonded by wood alcohol. Aspartame breaks down into formaldehyde. Aspartame is manufactured by the NutraSweet Company, a subsidiary of Monsanto. Users of aspartame have reported the following symptoms: headache, dizziness, change in mood quality, vomiting and nausea, abdominal pain, change in vision, diarrhea, seizures and convulsions, memory loss, fatigue, weakness, rash, sleep problems, hives, change in heart rate, change in menstrual pattern, change in activity level. Aspartame use often mimics symptoms of multiple sclerosis and Alzheimer's disease. FDA continuously asserts that there were no biological studies that aspartame caused problems in laboratory animals. If there had been, it would not have been approved. In approving aspartame, FDA reviewed 112 scientific studies from the manufacturer. Fifteen of those studies were deemed important by FDA and given the label, "pivotal."

The Rhesus Monkey Study

A study was performed at the University of Wisconsin on the affects of aspartame on rhesus monkeys. Monkeys, being close in their physiologies to humans, are excellent subjects for study. These monkeys, treated with aspartame, all experienced grand mal epileptic seizures after day 200 of a 52-week study. Blood samples from these primates revealed extremely high levels of phenylalanine in their blood serum. The researchers, noting that 50 percent of aspartame consisted of phenylalanine, attributed those seizures to aspartame ingestion. (15) After the study ended and the aspartame was removed from the animal's diets, no further seizure activity was observed.

Another Missing Link

In addition to laboratory tools and scientific literature, scientists must use one other tool to apply when making conclusions, so rarely lacking in their analyses of data. Common sense! FDA scientists did not comment on the epileptic seizures, nor did they comment on why humans did not experience similar effects. Human subjects took aspartame in either pill form or in orange juice. Monkeys took aspartame in milk-based formula. By now, you are aware that milk buffers the acidity in the stomach and allows simple proteins to survive digestion. So it is with aspartame, which like bovine proteins, is not destroyed by the stomach acids which have been weakened and made more basic by milk.

True diabetes can be a serious disease, leading to death. Diabetes results from either a failure of the pancreas to produce enough insulin or of the individual's inability to utilize insulin. It is usually characterized by an overabundance of glucose in the blood. An article titled, "More Evidence that Milk Causes Diabetes and Anemia" in *Prevention and Nutrition* revealed the following:

It has long been suspected that cow's milk proteins are a

principal cause of diabetes in children, and a new report in
the *New England Journal of Medicine* adds more support
for this explanation. In comparisons of different countries,
the prevalence of insulin dependent diabetes parallels the
consumption of cow's milk. (16)

The actual report being cited was published in Volume 327 of the *New England Journal of Medicine* in July of 1992. That journal article presented evidence implicating cow's milk as the cause of diabetes in every one of 142 diabetic children in the study. Each child produced antibodies to a bovine protein called bovine serum albumin. The antibodies which were naturally produced to fight this invader then turned on the children's own insulin-producing beta cells located in the pancreas. (17) This form of diabetes often leads to blindness, kidney disease and heart disease. The *Journal of the American Dietetic Association* supports the conclusion of the previous study and suggests that the avoidance of cow's milk products during the first few months of life may help reduce the incidence of insulin-dependent diabetes mellitus. (18) As a result of these reports, the American Academy of Pediatrics condemned the use of milk for children under one year of age. They did not include children over one year of age and all adults. Scientists have produced experimental evidence linking the development of diabetes directly to the consumption of dairy products. Researchers at the Institute for Pediatric Endocrinology in Sydney, Australia noted that the introduction of milk-based formula before the age of three months was associated with an increased risk of infant associated diabetes. (19)

Here's What Can Occur When a Baby Drinks Cow's Milk

S. M. Virtanen, M.D., at the University of Helsinki, Finland, discovered that early introduction of cow's milk in babies 3 months of age and younger, often resulted in complete insulin deficiency. This pathology occurred because naturally occurring beta cells were destroyed by the infant's allergic reaction created in response to the presence of milk proteins. (20) Scientists in Italy noted similar effects when they analyzed data from diabetic children. Their conclusion indicated an absolute cause and effect relationship between milk consumption and diabetes. (21)
Researchers at the University of Colorado published a paper in the July-August, 1994 issue of the *Journal of Endocrinology Investigations* which identified a bovine albumin peptide as a possible trigger of insulin-dependent diabetes mellitus. (22) Early exposure to cow's milk was linked to the development of diabetes in a carefully controlled rat experiment by scientists in Canada. They linked early exposure to bovine proteins in both rodents and humans as the cause of diabetes mellitus. Their work was published in the February 1994 issue of the

Journal of Immunology. (23) Other human and rat studies performed by the Department of Pediatrics at the University of Toronto suggest that the denial of dietary cow milk proteins early in life protects animals from later contracting insulin-dependent diabetes. (24)

These are the scientific studies that the milk industry and Dairy Coalition prefer you not read. The more knowledge you gain, the less ignorant you become. Ignorance is not bliss. Ignorance can be damned unhealthy. Armed with these facts, would you expose your infant to cow's milk? Now that you recognize that bovine hormones cause the body to react by producing antibodies which sometimes destroy insulin-producing cells, do you think that it is smart to drink the hormones from another animal species? Those hormones work. If you choose to believe the FDA, who assures us that these hormones do not work, you play with a dangerous loaded gun. If you choose to review the scientific evidence, then you arm yourself with ammunition which will protect you.

A Bone to Pick with Dairy

Common knowledge of osteoporosis is based upon false assumptions. American women have been drinking an average of two pounds of milk or eating the equivalent milk in dairy products per day for their entire lives. Doctors recommend calcium intake for increasing and maintaining bone strength and bone density which they call bone mass. According to this regimen recommended by doctors and milk industry executives, women's bone mass would approach that of pre-historic dinosaurs. This line of reasoning should be equally extinct. Twenty-five million American women have osteoporosis. Drinking milk does not prevent osteoporosis. Milk contains calcium. Bones contain calcium too. When we are advised to add calcium to our diets we tend to drink milk or eat dairy foods.

Calcium in Milk is Not Efficiently Utilized by the Body

In order to absorb calcium, the body needs comparable amounts of another mineral element, magnesium. Milk and dairy products contain only small amounts of magnesium. Without the presence of magnesium, the body only absorbs 25 percent of the available dairy calcium content. The remainder of the calcium spells trouble. Without magnesium, excess calcium is utilized by the body in injurious ways. The body uses calcium to build the mortar on arterial walls which becomes atherosclerotic plaques. Excess calcium is converted by the kidneys into painful stones which grow in size like pearls in oysters, blocking our urinary tracts. Excess calcium contributes to arthritis; painful calcium buildup often is manifested as gout. The USDA has formulated a chart of recommended daily intakes of vitamins and minerals. The term that FDA uses is Recommended Daily Allowance (RDA). The RDA for calcium is 1500 mg. The RDA for magnesium is 750 mg.

Society stresses the importance of calcium and, less frequently, magnesium. Yet, magnesium is vital to enzymatic activity. In addition to insuring proper absorption of calcium, magnesium is critical to proper neural and muscular function and maintains proper pH balance in the body. Magnesium, along with vitamin B6 (pyridoxine), helps to dissolve calcium phosphate stones which often accumulate from excesses of dairy intake. Good sources of magnesium include beans, green leafy vegetables like kale and collards, whole grains and orange juice. Non-dairy sources of calcium include green leafy vegetables, seafood, almonds, asparagus, broccoli, cabbage, oats, beans, parsley, sesame seeds and tofu. Salmon and sardines, eaten with the bones, are especially high in calcium.

Osteoporosis is **not** a problem that should be associated with lack of calcium intake. Osteoporosis results from calcium loss. The massive amounts of protein in milk result in a 50 percent loss of calcium in the urine. In other words, by doubling your protein intake there will be a loss of 1-1.5 percent in skeletal mass per year in postmenopausal women. The calcium contained in leafy green vegetables is more easily absorbed than the calcium in milk, and plant proteins do not result in calcium loss the same way as animal proteins do. A postmenopausal woman loses 1-1.5 percent bone mass per year. What will be the effect after 20 years? When osteoporosis occurs, levels of calcium in the blood are high. Milk only adds to these high levels of calcium which are excreted or used by the body to add to damaging atherscherosis, gout, kidney stones, etc.

Your bone mass does not increase after age 35. This is a biological fact that is not in dispute by scientists. However, this fact is ignored by marketing geniuses in the milk industry who make certain that women this age and older are targeted consumers for milk and dairy products. At least one in four women will suffer from osteoporosis with fractures of the ribs, hip or forearm. In 1994, University of Texas researchers published results of an experiment indicating that supplemental calcium is ineffective in preventing bone loss. Within 5 years of the initial onset of menopause, there is an accelerated rate of loss of bone, particularly from the spine. During this period of time, estrogen replacement is most effective in preventing rapid bone density loss. (25)

Bone Mass is Genetically Determined

In December 1994, another study, published in the *American Journal of Clinical Nutrition*, revealed that skeletal size and bone mass are genetically programmed. Optimal skeletal size is achieved through adequate calcium intake in an individual's youth. However, excess calcium has an effect upon bone mass. Once enough calcium is introduced, the excess is either excreted in the urine or absorbed by the kidneys, arteries and liver. This excess calcium can cause great damage. (26) The decrease in skeletal mass associated with osteoporosis in women is primarily caused by the age-dependent decrease in hormonal steroid secretion by the ovaries. While optimal calcium intake in childhood and adolescence is important for achieving proper bone density, calcium intake in adulthood has little significance.

An overview based upon recent findings regarding the pathogenesis of osteoporosis was published in Germany in 1994 and translated into English where the abstract appeared on Medline, a computer service containing scientific abstracts of research. The premise of this study is that osteoporosis is an unavoidable consequence of aging for which no prevention was previously possible. However, recent hormonal therapies have slowed down the process of rapid bone loss. The lack of estrogen plays an important role in the development of osteoporosis. (27)

Exercise, Vitamin D And Estrogen Prevent Osteoporosis

A *Journal of the American Medical Association* article reported a Tufts University study in which forty postmenopausal women, 50 to 70 years of age, were tested and measured by their participation in different levels of exercise. The conclusion of this study was that high intensity strength training exercises are an important effective and feasible means to preserve bone density. In other words, exercise prevented the onset of osteoporosis. (28) It is now recognized that insufficient levels of vitamin D are common in elderly people, especially those who are infirm and are not exposed to much sunlight. All animals including humans, receive most of their daily vitamin D, the sunshine vitamin, from outside exposure to the sun's rays. We drink milk which has lost its natural vitamin D through pasteurization and then been supplemented with artificial levels of vitamin D. Exercise and fresh air are better osteoporosis preventatives than milk containing calcium and added vitamin D.

Many factors are related to a decrease of bone mass. Scientists in Granada, Spain implicated the harmful effects of smoking cigarettes as being a causative factor in osteoporosis. Bone density was measured in two groups of premenopausal women (47 smokers, 54 nonsmokers). The results indicated that smoking was associated with decreased levels of bone mass density. (29) Effects of alcohol on osteoporosis were measured by researchers in Argentina who concluded that alcohol in an additional contributing factor to bone disease. (30) Milk is an excellent source of calcium. There is no food that is consumed in our society that contains more calcium. However, proteins in milk and lack of magnesium make milk an inefficient source for proper calcium absorption. Bone mass must be built before adulthood. Sufficient quantities of calcium are present in a normally balanced diet to satisfy the human need for calcium. Drinking milk can actually contribute to osteoporosis. Reliance upon milk as a preventive measure has allowed us to ignore the evidence and miss the true nature of osteoporosis.

Protein Inhibits Calcium Absorption

Protein inhibits calcium absorption. The FDA recommended dietary allowance for protein is less than two ounces per day. Many dietitians believe that half that amount is sufficient. The more protein you consume, the more calcium you lose. Vegetarians have significantly lower levels of osteoporosis than the general population. Nations in which protein consumption from meat is high, like the United States, have greater levels of osteoporosis than countries where meat consumption is low. Milk does not protect adults from getting osteoporosis. The dairy industry would like you to believe that milk is nature's perfect food, the perfect medicine. Milk is really the poison responsible for human disease.

In their best selling book, *Stop Osteoarthritis Now!*, the authors, one a medical doctor and the other a health writer, include no indexed reference to the word "milk." However, they do include one sentence, page 176, referenced in the index under dairy products. The authors note that when people with arthritis on low-fat vegetarian diets add dairy to their daily fare, their conditions worsen. Just one sentence for this earth-shattering news? I would have devoted an entire book to the subject. Actually, that's what I'm doing. For the most part, the medical establishment has ignored the obvious! (31)

Heart Disease: What a Doctor Won't Tell You

What Every Woman Must Know About Heart Disease provides everything you ever needed to know about America's number one killer. Dr. Siegfried J. Kra's no-nonsense approach to preventing this condition does not list one indexed reference to either milk or dairy products, yet he devotes entire chapters to cholesterol. (32) Perhaps Dr. Kra and others will wake up and smell the coffee (lightened by nondairy creamer) when he divides three into 159 and recognizes that the average American eats the equivalent cholesterol contained in fifty-three slices of bacon every day from milk and dairy products, understanding that there are three milligrams of cholesterol in each slice of bacon. The equivalent cholesterol of 19,000 slices of bacon are eaten every year by the woman for whom Kra wrote his book. By the time she's gone through her menopause, she's consumed the equivalent of more than a million slices of bacon. Kra should consider the cholesterol in dairy as a primary cause of heart disease.

So, Where Do Cows Get Their Calcium?

Where do cows get their calcium? Certainly not by drinking milk! In the summer, cows eat lots of "green stuff." Grass, weeds, vines, clover and rye. In the winter, they eat hay and different commercially prepared feeds. "Green stuff" contains chlorophyll. Red stuff (our blood) is very similar to chlorophyll. The basic difference between chlorophyll and hemoglobin, the major blood protein, is at the center of the molecule. Hemoglobin, the protein that makes our blood red, has iron as its center atom. Chlorophyll, the protein which makes plants green has as its center atom magnesium.

Hemoglobin and Chlorophyll are Nearly Identical

The magnificence of nature can be observed in the common bond between plants and humans. The active protein in our blood and the protein in the blood of plants are nearly identical. We live harmoniously, synergistically. Humans breathe in air containing oxygen and exhale carbon dioxide. Plants "breathe in" air containing carbon dioxide and exhale oxygen. The 1930 Nobel Prize for Chemistry was awarded to Dr. Hans Fischer who noted that chlorophyll and blood hemoglobin are nearly alike. Chlorophyll contains at its center a magnesium atom. Blood contains at its center an iron atom. Magnesium aids calcium absorption. Iron inhibits calcium absorption.

Mammals eating lots of green "stuff" containing calcium will efficiently use that calcium to build strong bones. Mammals eating calcium without the important magnesium atoms contained in chlorophyll will not efficiently use that calcium. Milk is loaded with calcium, but has almost no magnesium. Unless a diet also includes magnesium, that source of calcium is not efficiently used.

Thank you, R.P. Heaney, Ph.D. Thank you, M.S. Dowell, Ph.D. These two scientists found themselves with cases and cases of Italian bottled water (Sangemini) in 1994. What to do? They analyzed its essence. These two men of science measured the availability of the calcium contained in this popular Italian drink. They then recruited 18 healthy women and compared the levels of calcium in their blood from drinking milk with the levels from drinking the bottled water. Using sophisticated tracer techniques, Drs. Heaney and Dowell discovered that the calcium in bottled water was highly available, at least as available as the calcium in milk. (33)

IGF does not cause cancer. It releases the tight bonds which the immune system places on cancers which exist in the body and are quite common. IGF is like adding gasoline to a fire. Hundreds of lines of converging evidence meet to implicate IGF as the key factor in the growth and proliferation of cancer. The processes are well illustrated and are understood by the scientific community.

Why have they kept this information such a big secret? I would never have learned any of the things which I have related to you if milk had not been genetically engineered. Monsanto, seeking to profit from America's largest food industry, may very well have destroyed it. It is no wonder that the small American farmer did not welcome BST or the associated controversies which had the potential to educate American consumers.

Remember that countries with the highest rate of hip fractures also have the highest rate of breast cancer? Holland, Norway, Denmark and Sweden. These four countries also have the highest per capita consumption of milk. That Dutch milk maid carrying twin-yoked buckets of milk must be a warning signal to all. Many cultures, like the Japanese, consume less than one quarter of the recommended daily intake of calcium per day and yet these people have very low rates of osteoporosis. An American typically satisfies his calcium needs by eating the recommended portions of fruits, vegetables and protein contained on the Department of Agriculture's food pyramid. Eliminate milk and you still will satisfy all of your calcium requirements.

A single cup of milk contains 291 mg of calcium, while one cup of cooked collard greens contains nearly the same amount, 290 mg. If one considers that only one quarter of the milk calcium is utilized by the body because of a lack of magnesium and an overabundance of protein, then the calcium availability in one cup of cooked collards is equal to five cups of milk! There's plenty of calcium in milk, but it is not so easily absorbed.

Asthma

A recent column in *U.S. News and World Reports* titled "News You Can Use" reported that asthma deaths are on the rise. (34) Perhaps you can use this news. According to Alexandra Gorman, spokeswoman for the American Lung Association, 5487 people cannot because in 1994 they succumbed to fatal asthma attacks, more than twice the number of people who died (2598) in 1979. (35) Asthma is an inflammatory disease. The bronchial tubes become clogged with mucus. Asthma attacks are violent reactions to these clogged airways which become filled with a body's "glue." Why would the number of asthma cases double? As usual, doctors have no clue. If asthma is diet related, and if bovine proteins play a role in asthma then it would be easy to compare milk consumption rates between 1979 and 1995 and see what correlations, if any, exist.

Americans Changed Their Diet

Thanks to the Dairy Coalition, we changed our diets. We were told to drink no fat, low fat milk and skim milk. So, we followed the advice of the fluid milk processors and consumed less fat in fluid milk and, in doing so, drank a beverage with proportionately more protein.

Milk Proteins Cause Allergies

Milk proteins do not belong in human bodies. They are not injected directly into the bloodstream but they are eaten and they bypass digestive processes to enter blood serum by a circuitous route.

United States Department of Agriculture data reveal the incredible change in our diet over a fourteen-year period. In 1979, the average American consumed 149.3 pounds of high fat (low protein) liquid whole milk and 78.6 pounds of low fat (high protein) milk. By 1994, the average American drank 75.8 pounds of liquid whole milk and 124.4 pounds of low fat milk.

By converting pounds to ounces and dividing by 365 days per year, we can compare the daily intake in ounces of high fat/low protein milk consumption to low fat/high protein consumption. In 1979, two-thirds of the milk we drank was low protein/high fat. By 1994, over 62 percent of the milk we drank was high protein/low fat. Let's simplify the numbers. In 1994, the average American drank 6 1/2 ounces of the low protein "stuff" every day and 3 1/2 ounces of the high protein "stuff." By 1994, we had taken a 180 degree turn. We were now drinking only 3 1/3 ounces of the high protein stuff and 5 1/2 ounces per day of the high protein stuff. See a trend? The doctors and scientists do not!

	1979	1994
Asthma Deaths	2,598	5,487
Average Daily "LOW Protein" Milk Consumption in Ounces	6.54	3.32
Average Daily "HIGH Protein" Milk Consumption in Ounces	3.32	5.44

U.S. News and World Report reveals that the death rate has risen fastest for African-Americans. Aren't African Americans also more lactose intolerant than white Americans? Are African Americans more "allergic" to the vast array of bovine proteins?

Asthma can be prevented, although current medical philosophy is to focus upon treatment and not prevention. Asthma. What a dreadful human condition! Milk. What a shocking surprise!

What Have We Done to Milk?

We took wholesome milk with living vitamins and enzymes and boiled them away through pasteurization. We then homogenized the substance and decreased the size of the fat molecule so that it could safely carry hormones throughout the body. The FDA denies the possibility that this process of micronization of fat molecules could possibly work to protect and "deliver" IGF, yet, a food advisory committee within FDA will approve a new drug therapy this year, developed by NeXstar Pharmaceuticals. Capsules of a new drug intended to battle Kaposi's Sarcoma, the cancer associated with AIDS, will be encapsulated in microscopic fat bubbles, the same type of fat bubbles created by homogenization. These tiny fat globules will protect this potent drug from normal digestive processes much the same way that IGF-I is protected.

One group of scientists at FDA believe that milk hormones encased in miniature fat globules cannot survive digestion. This group should get together with the group of scientists at FDA who have approved a new drug delivery system based upon small fat globules protecting drugs from this natural breakdown process. Testimony that a process replicating homogenization (micronization of fat) works to protect hormones! Homogenization might be the key factor in the survival and absorption of milk hormones.

The most serious insult to "nature's perfect food" was genetically engineered milk. We created a new hormone. By attempting to decipher the genetic code Monsanto made a serious gene transcription error, detected nine years after all safety tests were completed on a different drug then the one that is now being used.

People have attempted to tame and control their universe and the result is that they created a hormone which has changed milk. I must have hope that things will change for the better. Here is my fantasy wish list.

When they see how dangerous genetically engineered bovine somatotropin is Monsanto will realize the errors of its ways and atone. When FDA recognizes that an entirely different hormone was tested then the one presently on the market, they'll require new studies, and apologize to the American people. One day Congress may realize that PAC donations are actually bribes and congressmen sacrifice their integrity by accepting such bribes. Perhaps they'll change their way of doing business, and ask for forgiveness for destroying a nation that was built on strong principles. Maybe one day the scientists will realize that human safety is more important then a few pieces of silver. Perhaps they'll be honest and do future research in an unbiased manner. When the Department of Agriculture and the Surgeon General recognize that more antibiotics are now in milk, they'll go back to the old safety standards, the ones in place before cows got increased levels of mastitis from BST making it necessary for FDA to raise the acceptable levels of antibiotics in all of our foods.

When the American medical establishment realizes that milk is poison, they'll care more about their patients and practice healthy preventive medicine instead of the kind of medicine where they get rich from overprescribing medications. Mothers all over America will spend 5 minutes more of quality time per day with their children, preparing a healthy breakfast, instead of routinely pouring a dose of hormonally laced milk into a bowl of cereal. The dairy coalition and the dairy farmers will find new careers, put out of business by educated consumers who realize that milk is poison. The mammography centers will close their doors and the cancer and leukemia clinics will go out of business, for want of patients.

Jewish delis will have to spread tofu on their bagels with lox, and Italian ices parlors will replace ice cream stores. Pizzerias will find new toppings for their pies and...we'll all adjust. We'll all survive. We'll cook with olive oil instead of butter and live healthier longer lives. Maybe all of these things will happen as a result of this book.

The Ills of Society and the Fountain of Youth

Where in the world would our society be if all milk and dairy products suddenly disappeared? Perhaps America would be a nation without cholesterol problems which contribute to our #1 killer, heart disease. We'd be a society with less cancer. Most certainly we'd experience a decrease in the incidence of the diagnosis of leukemia, encephalitis, meningitis, diabetes, osteoporosis and arthritis, and allergies. Our entire digestive processes would improve.

America would experience enormous unemployment. Everybody now employed in dairy, farmers, milkmen, the Dairy Coalition would be out of work. They'd all have to find employment elsewhere. We'd certainly destroy a few other industries including pharmacies which rely upon antacid and decongestants sales to booster cash flow by counteracting the harmful digestive consequences of milk consumption. Doctors would be standing on unemployment lines and hospitals might have to close. We'd be a lot healthier. Come to think of it, if we discontinued dairy, undertakers and morticians might face a grave situation...not enough caskets to lower into graves!

We would most certainly bankrupt our Social Security system which was not designed to support people living into their 100s. Pension funds would be challenged and cities and governments supporting those pensions would be paying unimagined increases. The current work force would be burdened, supporting four or five generations of retirees. The Federal Reserve would have to print more money and the resulting inflation would create havoc with our economic system. All because the fountain of youth currently exists. The answer lies in not what you do drink from that fountain, but what you do not drink. By eliminating milk we can eliminate the single most disease causing factor for all of humanity.

"He is sick, my Lord, of a strange fever."

William Shakespeare,
Measure for Measure, Act V, Scene 1

Chapter 13

Mad Cow Disease and Prions: A Frightening Biological Forecast

High school science classes teach lessons in organic biology. Students learn that cells are dynamic in their composition and function. Inside of cells are genetic blueprints for reproduction. Each cell in the human body contains a set of plans, located inside of its chromosomes. Each chromosome contains a genetically structured set of chemicals which determine how the cell is to replicate itself. The chemical substance which is the key to this entire process and which contains a double helical structure of coded chemicals is deoxyribonucleic acid, better know as DNA. Textbooks written before 1966 teach students that biological and cellular reproduction without DNA is not possible. These educators relying upon these books and previous knowledge teach incorrect science. They are ignorant of a newly revealed secret of nature. There is a group of chemicals, recently discovered, called prions which can reproduce themselves without DNA. Prions have been passed on from cows to humans. Mad Cow disease is a Prion disease. Americans laugh at the thought of mad cows. The British on the other hand, who have seen millions of cows destroyed, have a disparate sense of humor to ours. They recognize that there are diseases which turn bovine and human brains into sponge-like material. The scientific name for "Mad Cow" is "bovine spongiform encephalitis." After the first exposure to a prion, the onset of disease might take up to 20 years to develop. Prions are tiny crystals which replicate themselves and slowly destroy the human brain until Alzheimer-like symptoms develop.

Your 10-year-old child picks up the glass of milk and raises it to her lips. The "magic" crystals in that liquid are so small that they've been unobserved by pre-1994 scientists. You now know enough about milk to advise the child to stop, before she swallows, yet you do not. The tiny crystals are as immune to digestive acids as diamonds would be unaffected by liquid dish soap. They continue through the stomach into the upper gastrointestinal tract where they are passed through the intestinal mucosa and are absorbed into the bloodstream. They are "attacked" by antigens, by blood cells, the body sends line after line of "soldiers" against these invading crystals with no success. Could 98.6°F and cellular mechanisms succeed where two-thousand degree heat generated in laboratories could not?

The child laughs, wiping away her milk mustache, unaware that she has eaten the seed to a crippling disease that will end her life in thirty years. First it will turn her from a happy girl, perhaps a mother, in the prime of her life into a senile woman, at such a very young age, while it converts her brain into sponge-like material. The name spongiform will be used to identify the state and condition of her brain. When she can no longer dress herself, something that might very well occur 1 week after her first symptom, they will name this disease after the first doctors who treated such symptoms, Dr. Cruetzfeld and Dr. Jacob. Cruetzfeld-Jacob Disease.

In 1996, the European continent panicked, and one nation, Great Britain, killed 3 million cows and after the slaughter burned the carcasses, burying the remains deep underground. America laughed at a new generation of "mad-cow" disease jokes. That's because in America we are immune from such disaster, aren't we?

The crystal tumbles through the circulatory system of the little girl, too small to do any damage to the cell walls of the veins and arteries. Like a balloon bouncing slowly off a smooth plaster wall and then living room furniture, the crystal travels through the veins and into the lungs where blood is enriched by oxygen, then through the arteries and then around and around it goes. On one circuit it may travel to the tips of the fingers, on another to the nose. Hundreds of trips, thousands of voyages, an unlimited pass with free admission throughout the human amusement park which acts as host, until one day the crystal finds in a final resting place, the brain. There are perhaps 100 billion cells in the brain and 80 billion of these are protective bodies named glial cells. Like big fluffy pillows, these glials form a barrier, difficult but not impossible for most substances to pass through. Glial cells nourish and support the real workers of the brain, the neurons. Together, the glial cells form a wall called the "blood-brain barrier." The crystals, so small, a random voyage with no nucleus or intellect so instructing them, are fated to one day end up deep within the brain. How many trips will it take? That's of no importance to a crystal with "no brain," simply possessing magic. Can one crystal do damage, we wonder? Can something with no DNA, no genetic code, no set of instructions, can this something invade an organ like the brain and replicate itself? Biologists, chemists and physiologists unite! Certainly not. Impossible. Mother Nature smiles. The Gods on Olympus laugh at our lack of understanding, and our surety that we know everything there is to know. The crystal moves gently, with the neural tides, awash within a charged aqueous solution of protein, an electrical and chemical environment allowing that crystal to create its magic.

Mad Cow Disease

In 1990, a "new" disease was diagnosed among Great Britain's dairy cows. (1) This neurological disorder, Bovine Spongiform Encephalopathy (BSE), was appropriately named "Mad Cow Disease" by the British press. It is believed that cows contract BSE by eating protein including brains, blood meal, and bone meal from dead animals which are part of their feed. The disease affects the animal's central nervous system and is degenerative. The brain literally dissolves, a piece at a time, taking on a sponge-like consistency. Cattle with BSE appear to be crazy, or "mad." Actually, these animals are more sad. They often exhibit odd behavior such as twitching, convulsions, loss of muscular coordination and locomotive function. However, British people suspected for many years that the meat from their cattle was tainted. Government officials denied for many years that humans contracted diseases from cows. By May 1990, 25 percent of the English refused to eat beef. (2) Like dominos, the nations of the world soon began to ban British beef and milk products. The condition became so serious, epidemic, that in order to save what was left of the British meat and dairy industry, English regulators agreed to slaughter 3 million animals and incinerate the carcasses. (3) In 1996, Tim Lang, Professor of Food Policy at Thames University, commented:

> We are in a mass experiment which is killing us. Never
> before have diseased ruminants (sheep) been fed to other
> ruminants (cows) and then fed to humans. We have interfered
> with the whole process of nature and what is now happening
> is one of our worst nightmares...This is a tragedy on a
> massive scale. The government has been so totally stupid. (4)

United States Medical Officer Paul Brown was quoted in the same article:

> It now appears I was wrong. A great deal of work remains to
> be done...None of it will be of any help to those who may have
> been exposed to the infectious agent...Nor will it remedy the
> possible failure of the scientific pundits (including me) to
> foresee a potential medical catastrophe.

The Warning from Virgil Hulse, M.D.

As early as 1976, Virgil Hulse, M.D., began investigating neurological diseases from cows and their possible effects on humans. Dr. Hulse, author of *Mad Cows and Milk Gate*, recently wrote:

The case of the mad cow has not been exaggerated in the press, in fact, in many cases, the situation is much worse than has been told. Cows are being fed diseased sheep, chickens and other cows. These cows are then slaughtered, wrapped in plastic, priced and put out in your local grocery store as harmless for human consumption. Of these cows, 80 percent have the bovine leukemia virus and 50 percent have the bovine immunodeficiency virus -- the animal equivalent of AIDS. We are drinking milk and eating cheese with lymphocyte that are loaded with the proviral DNA of these viruses. It is only common sense that when consuming a fluid that has been emitted from an animal, or the actual flesh itself, we the consumers, are at risk for whatever ailed the animal. (5)

Hulse began working in the dairy industry as a milk inspector in 1952. He has experience in many areas of the dairy industry, having been a pasteurizer, milk and cream tester, butter and ice cream maker, milk plant supervisor and milk inspector for the state of California. In addition to his M.D. degree, Hulse received a master's degree in Public Health and Milk Technology and a master's degree in Food Technology. For 20 years Hulse has been dedicating his life to working within the dairy industry to insure the safety of America's milk supply. By writing his book he is now appealing directly to the American public. Hulse writes:

Despite increasing anecdotal (circumstantial) evidence linking bovine leukemia virus and bovine immunodeficiency virus to potential human health risks, the USDA has steadfastly refused to check slaughtered meat, milk and dairy products to see if they contain antibodies to these retroviruses. It seems that they just do not want to scare the milk consumer. Every day, Americans consume beef and dairy products from cows, some of which are infected with bovine leukemia virus and cow AIDS virus, without any assurance that the products are safe.

Mad Cow Disease: Is It in America?

Chicago area journalist, Barbara Mullarkey, recently reviewed the Mad Cow controversy. Writing in *Chicago Life*, Mullarkey quoted Oprah Winfrey:

It (Mad Cow) is the biggest health scare to hit Europe since the Chernobyl nuclear disaster. The fear it has generated may destroy an industry and dramatically alter the way we eat. (6)

Mullarkey attempted to determine whether Mad Cow Disease has been discovered in America's dairy and meat industry. She asked the question, "Has Mad Cow Disease been found in the U.S.?" Her answer includes an opinion by Richard Marsh, Ph.D., who was, before his recent death, a veterinary scientist at the University of Wisconsin, who felt that a version of Mad Cow may be linked to "Downer" Cow Syndrome. Such American cows do not go "mad" like their British counterparts; they simply lose all coordination, fall down and die. Howard Lyman, ex-cattleman and rancher who appeared on the Oprah show had this to say:

> Every year 100,000 U.S. cows appear healthy at night and are
> found dead in the morning.

Did the same "thing" that killed the cows find its way into the meat which we now eat or the milk and dairy products which we consume? That "thing" has been identified as a prion.

Is Alzheimer's a "Cow" Disease?

Mullarkey cited an article in the *Journal of Neurology* which reported that the autopsies of nearly six percent of Alzheimer deaths revealed Cruetzfeld-Jacob Disease (CJD) as the cause. (7) CJD is the human disease that has been directly linked to the bovine spongiform or Mad Cow Disease by scientists including Virgil Hulse and British Health Secretary Stephen Dorrell. On March 20, 1996, Dorrell went before the British House of Commons and reversed 10 years of government assurances by identifying ten cases of CJD in people under the age of 42 as having come directly as a result of ingesting milk or meat from infected cows. (8) An article appearing in the British journal *Nature* revealed that prion diseases are "...a group of neurodegenerative diseases that...can be transmitted between mammals...by dietary exposure." (9)

"Prion Diseases" by Stanley Prusiner

Stanley B. Prusiner, Ph.D., is a professor of biochemistry and neurology at the University of California School of Medicine in San Francisco, California. Prusiner, a man of great insight and courage, has taken a lot of criticism from his colleagues for his theories. Once considered a maverick, contentious of scientific dogma, Prusiner is now being given credit for one the most important biological discoveries of the twentieth century. At one time, scientists believed that in order for reproduction or replication to occur, a cell or virus or organism or group of amino acids needed DNA, a set of instructions. Prusiner coined the term, *prion* (pronounced: pree-on), as an acronym taken from the words, "protein-aceous infectious particles."

Prusiner published a review of prion diseases in the journal *Science* in which he described the molecular biology of neurologically caused prion diseases. According to Prusiner, these prions cause the brain to become riddled with holes. Prion diseases are always fatal. (10)   In January 1995, *Scientific American* published Prusiner's grand opus, "Prion Diseases." (11) This publication not only described how prion infections occurred in humans, but was timely enough to predict the outbreak of Mad Cow Disease in England.   Just a few months after *Scientific American* published Prusiner's paper, Mad Cow began to make world-wide front page news.

Prusiner reports that prions, crystalline in structure, are immune to normal digestive mechanisms which break protein substances down into their basic amino acids. He describes a process in which prions, finding their way into the human brain, begin a chemical process called "folding" in which these crystals replicate themselves. The *Scientific American* article revealed that, in 1984, Prusiner and his group of scientists identified the amino acid sequence of a prion protein. In the mid-1980s, Prusiner learned that ingestion of prions contained in one species of animal could infect another species. Today, the existence of Mad Cow Disease and universal agreement that humans have been directly affected by ingesting either milk or meat from cows is certification and tribute to Stanley Prusiner's prion theory, now a universally confirmed fact.

Recent Events

A front page headline in *The New York Times* screamed, "Britain Ties Deadly Brain Disease to Cow Ailment." (12) A recent study, cited by Hulse in *Mad Cows and Milk Gate*, reveals:

> Recent studies conducted with macaque monkeys provide the
> strongest evidence yet that the human form of mad cow disease may
> possibly come from cattle. Dr. Adrianno Aguzzi, chief of the
> National Survey Program for Cruetzfeldt-Jacob disease in Switzerland
> commented: 'In my view it ends the debate that it didn't come from
> cows. On one hand, now we can say this is something that can
> happen...the disease coming up in the monkeys is identical to the
> human disease found in Great Britain. (13)

Scientists noted that Mad Cow Disease showed a characteristic never seen before. It appeared to easily infect and affect animals of other species when transmitted orally. In August 1994, Howard Lyman, a cattleman who appeared on the Oprah Winfrey show, delivered a speech at the World Vegetarian Congress in The Hague, Netherlands. He remarked:

> If you think that Mad Cow Disease is an English problem, think
> again. About eight months ago there occurred the first case of
> Mad Cow Disease in Canada. Once more, we were told there was
> no problem. That cow - who had come from England, by the
> way - did not affect any other cow or the herd base. So confident
> were they this was true, that the government killed all 270 of the
> farmer's herd and burnt their bodies, promising they would find
> every cow with disease, kill her, and burn her. (14)

At that same conference, describing Downer Cow Syndrome, America's equivalent of Mad Cow Disease which kills at least 100,000 cows per year, Lyman said:

> When a farmer has a dead cow he has two choices. He can call
> the veterinarian who will come out and say, 'Hey Jack, you got a
> dead cow. You owe me $150.' Or the farmer can call the
> renderer who will come out and say, "Hey Jack, you got a dead cow.
> I can take it off your hands. Which is he going to choose? The
> renderer makes cows into feed, which is then fed back to cows or
> other animals. In this way one cow with Mad Cow Disease could
> infect thousands.

Indeed, that's just what happened to the cows in England. Many fear that Mad Cow Disease is affecting America's cows and, in turn, could be responsible for Cruetzfeld-Jacob Disease. These prions, tiny silent crystals, finding their way into our brains...laying dormant for decades. Then one day, many years later, they rapidly turn the human brain into a sponge.

On October 11, 1996, President Bill Clinton signed Public Law Number 104-294, the Economic Espionage Act of 1996. This act authorizes the United States Federal Bureau of Investigation (FBI) to investigate any incidences of illegal use of trade secrets. The Richard, Odaglia and Deslex study (in which laboratory animals got cancer from the new genetically engineered bovine protein) is such a trade secret. If unpublished data from that study were to be obtained and made public, the author/criminal would be in serious trouble. The act stipulates fines of $10 million dollars and 15 years imprisonment for each offense. America has a lot of secrets. Many state assemblies, successfully influenced by industry lobbyists, have also passed anti-food slander laws, called Agricultural Disparagement Acts, which make it a crime to criticize an agricultural product.

According to activist Ron Cummins of Pure Foods:

> Industry lobbyists admit that these laws are probably unconstitutional.
> The laws are intended to curtail the right to free speech, to make it illegal
> to hand out leaflets or to dump rbGH milk in the gutter. (15)

Alabama is one state that has passed a Food Slander Law. At the risk of placing myself in jeopardy, I am about to reveal a government secret and, furthermore, disparage an agricultural product. There is a farm in Vinemont, Alabama on which 17 beef cattle are currently quarantined by the United States Department of Agriculture. The farmer has asked me not to print his name and I will respect his request. He is seeking $25,000 per animal from the United States government, about $24,000 more per animal then they are worth as beef. Can you guess what "Old MacDonald's" real reason is? I imagine that our meat industry will "collapse" when America's carefully guarded secret reveals that we do indeed have Mad Cow Disease. The cow in Canada that was destroyed along with 270 other animals came from a herd of Charolais beef cattle in England. Seventeen of those animals from the same English herd were purchased by this farmer in Alabama and have been put under quarantine.

On August 23, 1997, a story appearing in the London Times revealed that a 24-year-old vegetarian had contracted Cruetzfeld-Jacob Disease. (16) The article discussed fears that milk and cheese might have been a source of infection. Richard Rhodes, writing in his brilliant chronicle, *Deadly Feasts*, reveals that bone meal from downer cows might also be a source for CJD. (17) He recounts his conversation with Carleton Gajdusek, the Nobel-laureate who knows more about transmissible spongiform disease than any man living. When asked whether one should use bone meal on roses, Gajdusek replied, "I wouldn't if I were you."

I recently received a letter from Gajdusek from his jail cell in Frederick, Maryland. I wonder how this very brilliant man was silenced at a time when the world so desperately needs his knowledge. What pressures were exerted on our society and FBI to illegally tap Gajdusek's telephones and to bribe one of his close associates so that Gajdusek be betrayed at a moment in history when the world is faced with a disease with such horrible implications? Gajdusek wrote to me:

> I thank you for reaching me at the bottom of my rabbit hole at the
> Mad Hatter's table...However, unlike Alice, I have little prospect
> of finding my way out of the hole into which I have fallen. I can do
> nothing in my current situation (about the things we have discussed)
> as I have no access to scientific papers or books. (18)

"Cow's milk is not suited for human consumption. Milk causes constipation, biliousness, coated tongue, headache, and these are the symptoms of intestinal auto-intoxication. Soybean milk, and nut milks are excellent substitutes, and have practically the same analyses, and the danger of disease is removed."

Jethro Kloss, "Back to Eden," 1939

Chapter 14

Alternatives to Milk

There is no better substance to nourish a human infant than the breast milk from its mother. Milk from cows should be consumed by calves, not humans. Milk from cats should be swallowed by kittens, not dogs. Each species of mammal has developed nature's perfect formula for its young. Most of the baby formulas sold in pharmacies and supermarkets are processed from cow's milk. Non-cow's milk alternatives exist. There are also soy-based formulas, developed for infants whose reactions to bovine proteins in traditional formulas are intolerable. There is no test or measure of tolerability. Infants who are fortunate enough to have discriminating parents able to note symptoms such as colic, congestion and discomfort discontinue the use of milk products at an early age. Many parents never make the connection between the many symptoms of milk intolerance.

Once children are weaned from the breast or the bottle of formula, parents seek healthy alternatives. Supermarkets have many types of juices available. There are 100 percent juice items like apple juice and mixed juices and products containing ten percent juice with sugar added. Water remains the cheapest drink of all. Most families have budgets and shop carefully for foods and beverages. One staple appearing on most shopping lists is milk. Breakfast in America is built around milk and dairy products. American meals are really quite boring when compared with other cuisines. The typical American breakfast preparation takes under 1 minute and involves a cereal box and a carton of milk. My children were surprised after a recent trip to New York City's Chinatown for breakfast. We enjoyed "congee," an exploded rice soup cooked with chicken and vegetables. There were also meat and fish-filled dumplings and fried bread. The taste, texture and variety of food was an Epicurean delight. The meal was enjoyed at the Silver Palace on the Bowery. The restaurant was filled with nearly 1000 diners, mostly Chinese, enjoying a total non-dairy breakfast.

"There's got to be something to put on my cereal," my kids used to yell. I no longer wanted milk in our household. When I first began to learn about dairy products my initial concern was about genetically engineered hormones. My solution was to find processors who would not accept milk from rBST-treated cows. My family enjoyed drinking milk from Ronneybrook Farms, a small dairy serving the New York metropolitan area. We visited the farm and saw the cows and bought the milk which was processed and put into attractive bottles, reminiscent of milk from "the good olde days." After coming to the realization that all milk contained hormones, we began to purchase dried milk. During the processing of powdered milk, I learned that the protein hormones were destroyed when milk was heated at the high temperatures necessary to turn liquid into powder quickly and efficiently.

I would mix a package of powdered milk with a quart of bottled water to yield a liquid appropriate for any cereal. Unfortunately, or fortunately, it just didn't taste the same. Soon, my family began eating different breakfasts. No longer did breakfast preparation take 15 seconds; bowl, spoon, open box of cereal, pour the milk, hurry up and eat, take the kids to school. We still have an open bowl of fruity shaped cereal left out on our kitchen table as an experiment. The bugs just won't eat that stuff. Neither will the bacteria, who are armed with an innate intelligence, which we seem to have lost.

I bake about 20 potatoes twice a week, add a little Parmesan cheese (I have not eliminated dairy entirely), add a touch of olive oil, then re-stuff the potato skins. I leave a large container of marinated beans in the refrigerator. Black, pinto, red, white, and kidney are marinated with spices in a dressing of oil and vinegar, liberally salted. These two items stay in the refrigerator until used. At any given time, there are homemade soups which all three of my children eat for after school snacks and supper. Two children also eat soup for breakfast. I have a large freezer filled with enormous quantities and varieties of soup, which I prepare 5 gallons at a time. We have fresh fruit every morning. How many mothers have time to cut the cantaloupes and peel the bananas? It only adds 5 minutes more to our sometimes hectic morning routine. When spontaneous, it can be a problem. When properly planned, it becomes a welcome ritual.

I usually rise a few hours before everybody else in my home and it's no trouble at all to put the ingredients for fresh bread or rolls into my bread maker. We occasionally put mozzarella on our chicken covered with marinara sauce. We buy a container of sour cream for vegetable or onion dip when we entertain. Occasionally, we buy a pint of ice cream for the girls to share. We cook with olive oil or chicken fat when necessary. We spread cream cheese on our bagels.

Dairy products are a part of our life, although they've been minimized and are now "condiments," not main dishes. Where we once fit into the profile of the average American consuming 2 1/2 pounds a day of milk and dairy, each member of our family now averages less than one ounce per day. Sometimes I am asked one or two questions by panicky mothers or friends. The most frequently occurring query is, "What do you use instead of milk?" I answer, "What do you mean, 'instead of milk'?" I drink water, or juice.

Sometimes the question is clarified. "What do you do for calcium?" I then try to explain that the research shows that dietary calcium does not play as large a role in determining bone density as the dairy industry would have one believe. I go on to tell the questioner that dairy products most certainly are responsible for osteoporosis and cite the nations with the highest osteoporosis rates, the Scandinavian dairy consumers. Some people just do not want to listen, and find change of routine too traumatic. These people would deny all of the overwhelming scientific evidence and for them, dairy products will forever fill their cupboards and bodies.

These people should realize that America has actually discovered the fountain of youth. By avoiding milk and dairy products, people can live longer and healthier. Isn't that what Ponce DeLeon was trying to discover in looking for his "fountain of youth?" We most certainly have the potential to live many more years than we do. What a remarkable effect dairy has had on keeping us from reaching that potential. Heart disease, cancer, allergies, fat and cholesterol leading to overweight and out of shape bodies, growing old before their time. Without milk would we live an extra decade or two? I believe so, but such controlled studies are impossible to perform. There have been no formal studies but I'd like to propose one for the next millennium. A review of the scientific evidence is certainly convincing. Milk and dairy products cause many health problems. We'd be better off without them!

Here's What We Drink: "Substitutes" for Milk

What does my family drink? Primarily water. There have been books written about water and I don't intend to get involved with a discussion of the many water issues and controversies. Just drink water. Our bodies need water. It cleanses and refurbishes cells. We could get water from juice or fruit or soda or beer. Why not just plain water? It's the best drink I know of. The water supplied by our water company comes from the nearby reservoir where we go fishing for catfish, carp and bass. There is an abundance of wildlife that shares the water with the residents of my county. The water, which used to be purified with chlorine, is now treated and made purer with ozone, a very reactive form of oxygen. The water does not smell of chemicals and tastes sweet, right from the tap. Occasionally I buy bottled water which I use on rare occasions when mixing up a quart of powdered milk, but I would have trouble noticing a difference in taste between the two, especially when it is ice-cold.

I also make smoothies. I'll freeze trays of ice cubes from various juices. Sometimes I'll freeze a half gallon of orange juice into small cubes, then take seven cubes, fill a glass with another juice, pour both into a blender, and have an incredible drink that doubles as a rich dessert by adding more juice cubes. In the summer I peel and seed a cantaloupe or honeydew and put the entire fruit into the blender, the liquid goes into an ice cube tray and the result is a low calorie nutritious snack. The ice cubes are closer in consistency to hard ice cream than ice cubes made from just water. We have a juicer and occasionally make our own cider. However, it's easier to buy fresh apple cider without preservatives from the local supermarket.

The Health Food Store

A visit to the health food store reveals many milk alternatives. The question is, which one to buy? Why not buy one of each and submit them to a test audience? That's just what I did. Thank you to Mrs. Simmons and her sixth grade class at New Jersey's Oradell Public School. In a not-so-scientific test, no double blind study, no placebos, four different milk alternatives were tested. The children (9 boys and 10 girls) were asked to put their names on a piece of paper and answer a few basic questions after sampling each product.

The four products were:

1)   Almond Milk, manufactured by Pacific Foods of Oregon, Inc. Each 8 ounce serving contains 90 calories, no cholesterol and 2.5 gr of fat.
2)   Rice Dream, manufactured by Imagine Foods, Palo Alto, California. Each 8 ounce serving contains 130 calories, no cholesterol and 2 gr of fat.
3)   EdenSoy, manufactured by Eden Foods, Clinton, Michigan. Each 8 ounce serving contains 150 calories, no cholesterol and 3 gr of fat.
4)   Oat Drink, manufactured by Mill Milk, Sweden. Each 8 ounce serving contains 110 calories, no cholesterol and 2.5 gr of fat.

The children were also asked to rate natural cow's milk, of which each 8 ounce portion contains 150 calories, 8.4 gr of fat and 25 mg of cholesterol. (1) In the interest of keeping this test simple, each question asked the sixth grade reviewer to rate each product on a scale of from 1 to 3.

1 = I like it a lot
2 = It's okay
3 = It doesn't thrill me

The first question was, "Do you enjoy drinking regular milk?" The four products were then tasted and the students asked the same question for each product, as well as for cow's milk. Here are the results. With 1 being the highest and best score and 3 being the lowest and worst score, the students overall grade for milk was 1.68. The girls rated milk at 1.80, the boys, 1.60. The milk substitute showing the strongest preference was rice milk at 2.37. The children were nearly unanimous in their dislike for oat milk, giving it a 2.84 rating. The results, according to this group of sixth grade children, demonstrate that alternative milk products do not compare in taste to good old fashioned "wholesome" milk.

I then thought to myself, why not take this nonscientific study to another level. Sure, it's a little work, but why not? I opened up my copy of our PTA book of names and addresses and found the numbers for each of the households of the children from the tested class. I spoke to one parent in each household and asked them to rank, in order of preference, their child's partiality to each of four products: juice, milk, soda and water.

Results: The Beverage Sixth Grade Children Prefer to Drink

In tabulating the results, I assigned 5 points to every first place vote, three points to every second, one point to every third, and no points for a fourth place finish. Nineteen children would total 171 points. According to their parents, children prefer to drink soda, which just edged out water by a few drops, over the other choices. Soda took first place with 57 points and water recorded 56 points. Juice finished third with 51 points and milk, America's favorite drink, finished a dismal fourth with only 7 points.

One luxury afforded senior authors of scientific studies is the opportunity to wander from pure scientific data and conclude the paper with a few guesses and, of course, the safety line, "More study is needed..." As the author of this study and this book, I am the one who gets to make the final observation and conclusion. And the conclusion, as well as the data, is clear. To this group of sixth graders, there are a lot of alternatives which measure up to their least favorite drink, milk. In other words, given the choice, milk is the last beverage that would be consumed. However, grain and nut milks seem to be poor alternatives to cow's milk.

Years of hearing from their parents the phrase, "Drink your milk, it's good for you," will probably result in these children saying the same thing to their children. Wordsworth wrote, "The child is the father of the man." We will repeat the same phrases, mistakes, positive imprinting on our children that we received from our parents and that they received from our grandparents. Parents tell their kids to drink milk because their parents told them to drink milk. All because one day somebody got the carefully marketed message that milk was good for you. These kids, when given the choice, drink anything but milk at home. Yet, the average American consumes more milk and dairy products than any other food. As the great philosopher and comic, W.C. Fields stated:

> My illness is due to my doctor's insistence that I drink milk, a
> whitish fluid they force down helpless babies.

Isn't that what we do to ourselves and our children. We do it because our parents did it to us. We do it because we believe that milk is healthy for us. We do it because we are continuously sold a bill of goods by the milk manufacturers of America. Do they need to spend hundreds of millions of dollars marketing this message to us every year? There really hasn't been a competitor marketing the message that milk was not healthy. By the time you've reached this page, you should have an altogether different perspective about milk and dairy products than you had before your inauguration into the beauty of milk mustaches in Chapter One.

We had taken milk for granted. We drank milk and ate cheese and never imagined that there were so many problems associated with dairy products. If not for the genetic engineering controversy, we might never have explored milk's true composition. We most certainly would never had suspected that milk contained powerful growth hormones. We most certainly would never have made the connection between milk consumption and cancer and heart disease and dozens of other human miseries.

Got milk? Not after reading this book!

Get milk? No way!

Milk? What a surprise!

References and Notes

Chapter 1 - Wholesome Milk: The Dairy Industry Message

1) Judith Jones Putnam and Jane E Allshouse. *Food Consumption, Prices, and Expenditures.* Annual Data published by the United States Department of Agriculture, 1997.
2) National Fluid Milk Processor Promotion Board. *Milk: What a Surprise!*, 1995.
3) National Fluid Milk Processor Promotion Board, *Real Men Drink Milk,* 1996.
4) EMAIL letter from Dr. Susan Barr to Robert Cohen, December 19, 1996.
5) Estelle Mongeau. NIN (National Institute of Nutrition) Review, #24. Summer, 1995.
6) EMAIL letter from Dr. Suzanne Oparil to Robert Cohen, December 12, 1996.
7) National Fluid Milk Processor Promotion Board. *Milk: What a Surprise!*, 1995.
8) Judith Jones Putnam and Jane E. Allshouse. *Food Consumption, Prices, and Expenditures.* Annual Data published by the United States Department of Agriculture, 1997.

Chapter 2 - A Brief History of Milk in America

1) Vernon Heaton. *The Mayflower.* New York: Mayflower Books, 1980, p. 72.
2) *Pictorial History of American History*, vol. 1. Chicago: Davco Publishing, 1962, p.45.
3) *Bradford's History of Plymouth Plantation.* New York: Charles Scribner's Sons, Inc., 1908, p. 166.
4) Will Durant and Ariel Durant. *The Story of Civilization,* Part IV: *The Age of Faith.* New York: Simon and Schuster, 1950, p. 645.
5) *The 1997 World Almanac and Book of Facts.* K-III Reference Corporation, p. 610.
6) *The World Book Encyclopedia.* 1995 edition, "Milk."
7) Samuel Eliot Morison. *Old Colony of New Plymouth.* Alfred A. Knopf, 1956, p. 47.
8) William Bradford. *Of Plymouth Plantation.* NewYork: Random House, 1952, p. 49.
9) *Ibid.,* pP. 50-51.
10) Jane Heimlich Column. *Health and Healing Newsletter.* Published by Julian Whitaker, July, 1994, p. 3.
11) Jane, Heimlich. *What Your Doctor Won't Tell You.* New York: Harper Collins, 1990.

Chapter 3 - Milk Has Changed: Genetic Engineering

1) Letter from Robert Cohen to Dr. Robert Collier, August 25, 1994.

2)   Judith C. Juskevich and C. Greg Guyer. "Bovine Growth Hormone: Human Food Safety Evaluation." *Science*, vol. 249. August 24, 1990, pp. 875-884.

3)   Background information on the American Association for the Advancement of Science, FAXED to Robert Cohen on June 12, 1995.

4)   Ann Gibbons letter. *Science*, vol. 249. August 24, 1990, p. 852.

5)   Monsanto's INAD application to FDA. Figure 1, p. 114.

6)   Bernard Violand. "Isolation of Escherichia Coli synthesized recombinant eukaryotic proteins that contain epsilon-N-acetyllysine." *Journal of Protein Science*, July, 1994, pp. 1089-1097.

7)   Letter from Richard Teske to Robert Cohen, August 10, 1995.

8)   Kurt A. Oster, M.D. and Donald J. Ross, Ph. D. *The X-O Factor*. New York: Park City Press, 1983.

9)   P.V. Malvern. "Prolactin and other protein hormones in milk." *J. Dairy Science* 45. 1977, pp. 609-616.

10)   P.V. Malvern, H.H. Head, R.J. Collier, F.C. Buonomo. "Periparturient Changes in secretion and mammary uptake of insulin and in concentrations of insulin and insulin-like growth factors in milk of dairy cows." *J. Dairy Science* 70. 1987, pp. 2254-2265.

11)   B.G. Hammond, R.J. Collier, et al. "Food safety and pharmakinetic studies which support a zero (0) meat and milk withdrawal time for use of sometribove in dairy cows." Originally presented at a conference of Pharmakinetics of Veterinary Drugs, October 11-12, 1989, Fougeres, France.

12)   D. Richard, G. Odaglia, P. Deslex, unpublished report. Department of Product Safety Assessment, Searle Research and Development, prepared for Monsanto Co., St. Louis, MO., 1989.

13)   Jerome A. Moore, et al. "Equivalent Potency and Pharmacokinetics of Recombinant Human Growth Hormones with or without an N-Terminal Methionine." *Endocrinology* 122. 1988, pp. 2920.

14)   Telephone call from Robert Cohen to Judy Jeskevich, September 15, 1994.

15)   Genetics class taught by Professor William Burke. Southampton College, Long Island University, 1970.

16)   D.E. Bauman, B.W. McBride, J.L.Burton, K. Sejrsen. *Somatotropin (BST): International Dairy Federation Technical Report*. Bulletin of the IDF. 293:2, February, 1994.

17)   "Effect of heat treatment, enzymatic, and microbial processing and quantification of peptide hormones in milk and dairy products." *Proceedings of the NIH Technology Assessment Conference: Bovine Somatotropin. December 5-7, 1990.* National Institutes of Health, Bethesda, Maryland.

18)   Telephone conversations between Robert Cohen and Paul Groenewegen, April 28, 1995.

19)   Paul P. Groenewegen, Brian W. McBride, John H. Burton, Theodore H. Elsasser. "Bioactivity of Milk from bST-Treated Cows." *J. Nutrition* 120, 1990, pp. 514-519.

20)   Anthony F. Philipps, et al."Fate of Insulin-Like Growth Factors I and II Administered Orogastrically to suckling rats." *Pediatric Research*, vol. 37,

no. 5, 1995, pp. 586-592.

21) Frystyk K, et al. "Free Insulin-like growth factors (IGF-I and IGF-II) in human serum." *FEBS-lett.*, July 11, 1994, 348 (2), pp. 185-191.

22) Portions of the insert warning label on Monsanto's rbST product sold under the trade name of Posilac.

Starred References Contained in Juskevich & Guyer *Science* Paper

1*) D.E. Bauman *et al.*, in *Proceedings of the 7th International Conference on Production Disease in Farm Animals*, F.A. Kallfelz, Ed. (Cornell Univ., Ithaca, NY, 1989), pp. 306-323.

2*) FDA's Center for Veterinary Medicine has approved the use for human consumption of milk from investigational herds treated with rbGH, based on its conclusion about the safety of the drug. The Center has not yet taken final action on the pending new animal drug applications for use of rbGH in dairy cows.

3*) Code of Federal Regulations, Title 21, Part 514, revised as of 1 April 1989.

4*) Food and Drug Administration, *Fed. Regist.*, 52FR49583 (1986).

5*) Code of Federal Regulations, Title 21, Part 58, revised as of 1 April 1989.

6*) D.M. Matthews, *Physiol. Rev.* 55, 537 (1975).

7*) A.S. McNeish, *Ann. Allergy* 53, 643 (1984); E. Lebenthal, P.C. Lee, L.A. Heitlinger, *J. Pediatr.* 102, 1 (1983); E. Lebenthal and Y.K. Leung, *Pediatr. Ann.* 16, 211 (1987).

8*) I.G. Morris, in *Handbook of Physiology*, sect. 6, *Alimentary Canal*; vol. 5, *Bile; Digestion; Ruminal Physiology*; C.F. Code, Ed. (American Physiology Society, Washington, DC, 1968), pp. 1491-1512.

9*) A.L. Warshaw, W.A. Walker, R. Cornell, K.J. Isselbacher, *Lab. Invest.* 25, 675 (1971); W.A. Walker, R. Cornell, L.M. Davenport, K.J. Isselbacher, *J. Cell Biol.* 54, 195 (1972).

10*) A.L. Warshaw, W.A. Walker, K.J. Isselbacher, *Gastroenterology* 66, 987 (1974).

11*) R.J. Levinsky, *Proc. Nutr. Soc.* 44, 81 (1985).

12*) J.C. Leissring, J.W. Anderson, D.W. Smith, *Am. J. Dis. Child.* 103, 160 (1962).

13*) E.J. Eastham, T. Lichauco, M.I. Grady, W. A. Walker, *J. Pediatr.* 93, 561 (1978).

14*) D.M. Roberton, R. Paganelli, R. Dinwiddie, R.J. Levinsky, *Arch. Dis. Child.* 57, 369 (1982).

15*) M.C. Reinhardt, *Ann. Allergy* 53, 597 (1984).

16*) J.G. Lece, *Environ. Health Perspect.* 33, 57 (1979).

17*) I. Jakobsson, T. Lindberg, L. Lothe, I. Axelsson, B. Benediktsson, *Gut* 27, 1029 (1986).

18*) T. Vukavic, *J. Pediatr. Gastroenterol Nutr.* 2, 248 (1983).

19*) _____, *ibid.* 3, 700 (1984).

20*) A. de la Cruz et al., *Fertil. Steril.* 26, 894 (1975); I. Yamazaki et al., *J. Takeda Res. Lab.* 38, 64 (1977); J.A. Thomas and M.G. Mawhunney, in *Synopsis of Endocrine Pharmacology* (University Park Press, Baltimore, 1973), pp. 9-11; M. Amoss, J. Rivier, R. Guillermin, *Clin. Endocrinol. Metab.* 35, 175 (1972); N. Nishi, A. Arimura, D.H. Cov, J.A. Vilchez-Martinez, A.V. Schally, *Proc. Soc. Exp. Biol. Med.* 148, 1009 (1975).

21*) W.H. Daughaday, in *Endocrine Control of Growth*, W.H. Daughaday, Ed. (Elsevier, Amsterdam, 1981), pp. 1-24.

22*) S.L. Davis, *J. Anim. Sci.* 66 (suppl. 3) 84 (1988).

23*) O.G.P. Isaksson, A. Lindahl, A. Nilsson, J. Isgaard, *Aeta Paediatr. Scand. Suppl.* 343, 12 (1988).

24*) S.A. Kaplan, *Am. J. Dis. Child.* 110, 232 (1965).

25*) J.L. Kostyo, *Metabolism* 23, 885 (1974).

26*) F. Matsuzaki and M.S. Raben, *Annu. Rev. Pharmacol.* 5,137 (1965); G.P. Talwar et al., in *Recent Progress in Hormone Research*, G. Pincus, Ed. (Academic Press, New Yrk, 1975), vol. 31, pp. 141-174; O.G. P. Isakson , S. Eden, J.O. Jansson, *Annu. Rev. Physiol.* 47, 483   (1985); R.D. Boyd and D.E. Bauman in *Annual Growth Regulation*,   D.R. Campion, G. J. Hausman, R.J. Martin, Eds. (Plenum, New York, 1989), pp. 257- 293.

27*) H. Green, M. Morikawa, T. Nixon, *Differentiation* 29, 195 (1985).

28*) E. Knobil and R.O. Greep, in *Recent Progress in Hormone Research*, G. Pancus, Ed. (Academic Press, New York, 1959), vol. XV, pp. 1-69.

29*) M.S. Raben, *ibid.*, pp. 71-114.

30*) N. Yamasaki, M. Kikutani, M. Sonenberg, *Biochemistry* 9, 1107   (1970).

31*) D.M. Bergenstal and M.B. Lipsett, *J. Clin. Endocrinal Metab.* 20,   1427 (1960).

32*) J.B. Mills, S.C. Howard, S, Scapa, A.E. Wilhelmi, *J. Biol. Chem.* 245, 3407 (1970).

33*) C.A. Baile and D.H. Krestel-Rickert, *Feed Manage*, 36, 26 (1985).

34*) W.V. Moore, S. Draper, C.H. Hung, *Horm. Res.* 21, 33 (1985).

35*) M. Sonenberg et al., in *Growth and Growth Hormone*, A. Pecile and E.F. Muller, Eds. (Excerpta Medica, Amsterdam, 1972), pp. 75-90.

36*) L. Graf and C.H. Li, *Biochemistry* 13, 5408 (1974).

37*) K. Hara, C.J.H. Chen, M. Sonenberg, *ibid.* 17, 550 (1978).

38*) M. Sonenberg, M. Kikutani, C.A. Free, A.C. Nadler, J.M. Dellacha, *Ann. N.Y. Acad. Sci.* 148, 532 (1968).

39*) A.C. Nadler, M. Sonenberg, M.I. New, C.A. Free, *Metabolism* 16, 830 1967); M. Sonenberg et al., *ibid.* 14, 1189 (1965).

40*) J.L. Nappier and G.A. Hoffman, unpublished report (Agricultural   Research and Development Laboratories, Union Co., Kalamazoo, MI, 1986); W.J. Seaman and P.J. Skinner, unpublished report (Pharmaceutical Research and Development, Upjohn Co., Kalamazoo, MI, 1986).

41*) D.G. Serota, N.G. Phipps, R.D. Alsaker, J.F. Carter, B. Colpean, unpublished report (Hazelton Laboratories America, Inc., prepared for   Monsanto Co., St. Louis, MO, 1984).

42*) D. Richard, G. Odaglia, P. Deslex, unpublished report (Department of Product Safety Assessment, Searle Research and Development, prepared for Monsanto Co., St. Louis, MO 1989).

43*) J.E. Fischer, R.L. Depew, C.A. Lowe, J. Panfili, unpublished report (Agricultural Research Division, American Cynanamid Co., Wayne, NJ, 1984).

44*) L.F. Fisher, unpublished report (Toxicology Division, Lilly Research Laboratories, Eli Lilly & Co., Indianapolis, IN, 1985).

45*) Note: Organs weighed included, at a minimum, the following: adrenals, brain, heart, kidneys, liver, ovary, spleen, and testes. Histopathological examination included, at a minimum, the following organs: adrenals, bone, bone marrow, brain, colon, duodenum, esophagus, heart, ileum, jejunum, kidneys, liver, lung, lymph nodes, mammary gland, ovary, pancreas, parathyroid, prostate, salivary gland, skeletal muscle, skin, spinal cord, spleen, stomach, testes, thymus, thyroid, trachea, urinary bladder, uterus, and all gross lesions.

46*) B.K. Birmingham et al., *J. Dairy Sci.* 71, 227 (1988).

47*) J.A. Moore et al., *Endocrinology* 122, 2920 (1988).

48*) K.L. Simkins, in *Proceedings of the California Animal Nutrition Conference on Nutrient Partitioning*, E. Robb, Ed. (Fresno, California, 1987), pp. 36-45.

49*) P.P. Groenewegen, B.W. McBride, J.H. Burton, T.H. Elasser, *J. Nutr.* 120, 514 (1990).

50*) G. Van den Berg, in *Use of Somatotropin in Livestock Production*, K. Sejrsen, M. Vestergaard, A. Neimann-Sorensen, Eds. (Elsevier, Science, New York, 1989), pp. 178-191; R.J. Baer et al., *J. Dairy Sci.* 72, 1424 (1989).

51*) A.J. D'Ercole, L.E. Underwood, J.J. Van Wyk, *J. Pediatr.* 90, 375 (1977); R.W. Furlanetto, L.E. Underwood, J.J. Van Wyk, A.J. D'Ercole, *J. Clin. Invest.* 60, 648 (1977).

52*) J.F. Perdue, *Can. J. Biochem. Cell Biol.* 62, 1237 (1984).

53*) D. Matier, L.E. Underwood, M. Maes, M.L. Davenport, J.M. Ketelslegers, *Endocrinology* 123, 1053 (1988); K.C. Copeland, L.E. Underwood, J.J. Van Wyk, *J. Clin. Endocrinol. Metab.* 50, 690 (1980); M.B. Grant et al., *ibid.* 63, 981 (1986).

54*) J.J. Van Wyk, M.E. Svoboda, L.E. Underwood, *J. Clin. Endocrinol. Metab.* 50, 206 (1980).

55*) J. Zapf and E.R. Froesch, *Horm. Res.* 24, 121 (1986).

56*) K. Hall and V.R. Sara, in *Vitamins and Hormones* (Academic Press, New York, 1983), vol. 40, pp. 175-233; L.E. Underwood, A.J. D'Ercole, D.R. Clemmons, J.J. Van Wyk, *Clin. Endocrinol. Metab.* 15, 59 (1986); R.C. Baxter, *Adv. Clin. Chem.* 25, 49 (1986).

57*) A.J. D'Ercole, A.D. Stiles, L.E. Underwood, *Proc. Natl. Acad. Sci. U.S.A.* 81, 935 (1984).

58*) C.C. Orlowski and S.D. Chernausek, *Endocrinology* 123, 44 (1988); J. Isgaard et al., *ibid.* 122, 1515 (1988); J. Isgaard, A. Nilsson, K. Vikman, O.G.P. Isaksson, *J. Endocrinol.* 120, 107 (1988); N.L. Schlechter, S.M. Russell, E.M. Spencer, C.S. Nicoll, *Proc. Natl. Acad. Sci. U.S.A.* 83, 7932 (1986).

59*) J. Zapf, C. Hauri, M. Waldvogel, E.R. Froesch, *J. Clin. Invest.* 77, 1768 (1986).

60*) A. Skottner, R.G. Clark, I.C.A.F. Robinson, L. Fryklund, *J. Endocrinol.* 112, 123 (1987).

61*) E. Schoenle, J. Zapf, C. Hauri, T. Steiner, E.R. Froesch, *Acta Endocrinol.* 112, 123 (1987).

62*) K. Hall and V.R. Sara, *Clin. Endocrinol. Metab.* 13, 91 (1984).

63*) R.C. Baxter, Z. Zaltsman, J.R. Turtle, *J. Clin. Endocrinol. Metab.* 58, 955 (1984).

64*) A.N. Corps, K.D. Brown, L.H. Rees, J. Carr, C.G. Prosser, *ibid.* 67, 25 (1988).

65*)   A. Honegger and R.E. Humbel, *J. Biol. Chem.* 261, 569 (1986).

66*)   L.F. Fisher and E.L. Russell, unpublished report (Toxicology Division, Lilly Research Laboratories, Eli Lilly & Co., Indianapolis, IN, 1989).

67*)   J.B. Terrill, unpublished report (Hazelton Laboratories of America, Inc., prepared for Monsanto Agricultural Co., St. Louis, MO 1989).

68*)   T.C. White et al., unpublished report MSL 8671 (Monsanto Agricultural Co., St. Louis, MO, 1989).

69*)   R.J. Collier et al., unpublished report MSL 8531 (Monsanto Agricultural Co., St. Louis, MO, 1988).

70*)   D. Schams and H. Karg, unpublished Elanco report, Eli Lilly & Co., dated 23 September 1988 (Institute of Physiology, Technische Universitat Munchen, D-8050 Freising-Weihenstephan, FRG, 1988); unpublished Elanco report, Eli Lilly & Co. (Insitute of Physiology, Technische Universitat Munchen, D-8050 Freising-Weihenstephan, FRG, 1988).

71*)   S.R. Davis, P.D. Gluckman, A.M. Bryant, unpublished Elanco report, Eli Lilly & Co. (Ruakura Agricultural Centre, Hamilton, New Zealand, 1989).

72*)   T.C. White et al., unpublished report MSL 8633 (Monsanto Agricultural Co., St. Louis, MO, 1989).

73*)   M.A. Miller et al., unpublished report MSL 8673 (Monsanto Agricultural Co., St. Louis, MO, 1989).

74*)   M.A. Miller, T.C. White, R.J. Collier, unpublished report (Monsanto Agricultural Co., St. Louis, MO, 1989).

75*)   We thank S. Sechen for her contributions to the manuscript.

Chapter 4 - Scientific Proof: Milk Hormones Are Hazardous to Your Health

1)   D. Richard, G. Odaglia, P. Deslex. Unpublished report, Department of Product Safety Assessment, Searle Research and Development, prepared for Monsanto Monsanto Co., St. Louis, MO., 1989.

2)   Letter from Dr. Richard Teske to Robert Cohen, August 10, 1995.

3)   Reference #45 of the Juskevich and Guyer paper. (See **45*** in the list of references contained in chapter 3).

4)   Telephone call from Robert Cohen to Robert Collier, Ph.D., September 15, 1994.

5)   Freedom of Information Act Request, reference # 94-39274.

Chapter 5 - The Domino Effect: How FDA Misled America

1)   *Science News*, vol. 138, August 25, 1990, p. 116.

2)   Barbano, Lynch, Bauman, Hartnell. "Influence of sometribove (recombinant methionyl bovine somatotropin) on general milk composition." *J. Dairy Science*, 71 Suppl 1:101, 1988.

3)   Daughaday & Barbano. "Bovine Somatotropin supplementation of dairy cows, Is the Milk Safe?" *JAMA*, 264(8), August 22, 1990, pp. 1003-1005.

4)   Monsanto Press Release, June, 1992.

5)   Shari Roan. "Despite Bad Report, Milk Still Does a Body Good." *Los Angeles Times*, November 18, 1992, pp. E-1.
6)   Ronald E. Kleinman, et al. "The Use of Whole Cow's Milk in Infancy." *Pediatrics*, vol. 89, no. 6, June, 1992, pp. 1105-1109.
7)   Dr. Neal Barnard. "Doctors File Complaint With FTC Over 'Milk Mustache' Ads." *Physicians Committee for Responsible Medicine News Release*, April, 1995.
8)   Harvey and Marilyn Diamond. *Fit For Life*. Warner Communications, 1994.
9)   Devra Lee Davis. "Decreasing cardiovascular disease and increasing cancer among whites in the United Staes from 1973 through 1987." *JAMA*, vol. 271, no. 6, September 9, 1994, pp. 431-437.
10)   Reference #42 of the Juskevich and Guyer paper. (See **42*** in the list of references contained in chapter 3).
11)   *Executive Branch Report on BST issues*. Issued February 9, 1994.

Chapter 6 - The Plot Thickens: Collusion Between Monsanto, FDA and Congress

1)   Neal Barnard. "Good Medicine," *Physician's Committee for Responsible Medicine*, vol. 2, no. 4, Autumn, 1993.
2)   Letter from Ann Beagley of Freedom of Information Clearinghouse to Robert Cohen, July 11, 1995.
3)   James Bovard. "First Step to an FDA Cure: Dump Kessler." *Wall Street Journal*, vol. CCXXIV, no. 112, December 8, 1994, p. A18.
4)   "Mother Nature is Lucky Her Products Don't Need Labels" (advertisement). *National Geographic*, vol. 158, no. 3, September, 1980, p. 433.
5)   http://www.monsanto.com/MonPub/Environment/MonsantoPledge.
6)   McDermott. *Journal of The American Veterinary Association*, May 15, 1994.
7)   *The Fifth Estate*, September 9, 1994. Broadcast on Canadian Television.
8)   The Congressional Record, vol. 131, no. 58, May 7, 1985.
9)   Michael R. Taylor. "The De Minimus Interpretation of the Delaney Clause: Legal and Policy Rationale." *Journal of the American College of Toxicology*, vol. 7, no. 7, Nov. 4, 1988.
10)   James Ridgeway. "Robocow: How Tomorrow's Farming is Poisoning Today's Milk." *The Village Voice*, March 14, 1995.
11)   Margaret Miller's Application for Federal Employment, Form SF 171.
12)   Robert Collier, Margaret Miller, et al. "Nutrient balance and stage of lactation effect response of Insulin, Insulin-like growth factor I and II and the insulin-like binding proteins 2 to somatotropin administration in dairy cows." *American Institute of Nutrition*, December, 1990.
13)   Dale Bauman, Margaret Miller, et al. "Response of Somatomedins (IGF-I and IGF-II) in Lactating Cows to Variations in Dietary Energy and Protein and Treatment with Recombinant n-Methionyl Bovine Somatotropin." *Journal of Animal Science*.

14) Linda Grasse, ed. *FDA Veterinarian,* May/June, 1994.
15) Statement by Stephen Sundloff to Congress, September 28, 1994.
16) Statement by Mr. Michael Taylor to Congress, September 28, 1994.

Starred References Contained in Cohen's Presentation to FDA on 4/21/95

(1*) B.N. Violand, et al. "Isolation of Escherichia coli synthesized recombinant eukaryotic proteins that contain epsilon-N-acetyllysine." (Animal Sciences Division, Monsanto Corporation, St. Louis, Missouri.) *Protein Sci.,* 1994 July 3, 1994,pp.1089-1097.

(2*) J.C. Juskevich; C.G. Guyer. "Bovine growth hormone: Human Food Safety Evaluation." *Science,* volume 249, August 24, 1990, pp. 875-884.

(3*) C.E. Rogler, et al. "Altered body composition and increased frequency of diverse malignancies in insulin-like growth factor-II transgenic mice." Marion Bessin Liver Research Center, Albert Einstein College of Medicine, Bronx, New York. *J Biol Chem,* May 13, 1994, p. 269.

(4*) B.G. Hammond, et al. "Food safety and pharmacokinetic studies which support a zero (0) meat and milk withdrawal time for use of sometribove in dairy cows." Monsanto Agricultural Company, Animal Sciences Division, St. Louis, Missouri. *Pharmacokinetics of Veterinary Drugs,* October 11-12, 1989.

(5*) D. Kleinman, et al. "Regulation of endometrial cancer cell growth by insulin-like growth factors and the luteinizing hormone-releasing hormone antagonist SB-75." Clinical Biochemistry Department, Faculty of Health Sciences, Ben-Gurion University of the Negev, Sokora Medical Center of Kupat Holim, Beer-Sheva, Israel. *Regul-Pept.,* October 20, 1993, 48(1-2), pp. 91-98.

(6*) A. D'Errico, et al. "Expression of insulin-like growth factor II (IGF-II) in human hepatocellular arcinomas: An immunohistochemical study." Institute of Pathological Anatomy, University of Bologna, Italy. *Pathol-Int.,* February, 1994, 44(2), pp. 131-137.

(7*) C.F. Kwok, et al. "Insulin-like growth factor-I receptor increases in aortic endothelial cells from diabetic rats." Department of Medicine, Veterans General Hospital-Taipei, Republic of China. *Metabolism,* November, 1993, 42(11), pp. 1381-1385.

(8*) J. Wimalasena, et al. "Growth factors interact with estradiol and gonadotropins in the regulation of ovarian cancer cell growth and growth factor receptors." Department of Obstetrics/Gynecology, Graduate School of Medicine, University of Tennessee Medical Center, Knoxville, Tennessee. *Oncol-Res.,* 1993, 5(8), pp. 325-337.

(9*) D.D. DeLeon, et al. "Effects of insulin-like growth factors (IGFs) and IGF receptor antibodies on the proliferation of human breast cancer cells." Department of Pediatric Endocrinology, Stanford University Medical School, California. *Growth Factors,* 1992, 6(4), pp. 327-336.

(10*) D.M. Martin, et al. "IGF receptor function and regulation in autocrine human neuroblastoma cell growth." Department of Neurology, University of Michigan, Ann Arbor. *Regul. Pept.,* October 20, 1993, 48(1-2), pp. 225-232.

(11*) D. Ambrose, et al. "Growth regulation of human glioblastoma T98G cells by insulin-like growth factor-I and its receptor." Department of Pathology, Jefferson Medical College, Philadelphia, Pennsylvania. *J-Cell-Physiol.*, April, 1994 159(1), pp. 92-100.

(12*) F.C. Nielsen, et al. "Insulin-like growth factor IImRNA, peptides, and receptors in a thoracopulmonary malignant small round cell tumor. Department of Clinical Biochemistry, Rigshospitalet, Copenhagen, Denmark. *Cancer*, February 15, 1994, 73(4), pp.1312-1319.

(13*) D. Prager, et al. "Dominant negative inhibition of tumorigenesis in vivo by human insulin-like growth factor I receptor mutant." Department of Medicine, Cedars-Sinai Medical Center, University of California, Los Angeles School of Medicine, Los Angeles, California. *Proc-Natl-Acad-Sci-USA*, March 15, 1994, 91(6), pp. 2181-2185.

(14*) K. Raile, et al. "Human osteosarcoma (U-2 OS) cells express both insulin-like growth factor-I (IGF-I) receptors and insulin-like growth factor-II/mannose-6-phosphate (IGF-II/M6P) receptors synthesize IGF-II: autocrine growth stimulation by IGF-II via the IGF-I receptor." Department of Pediatric Endocrinology, Children's Hospital, University of Munich, Germany. *J-Cell Physiol.*, June, 1994, 159(3), pp. 531-541.

(15*) K.S. Langford, et al. "The insulin-like growth factor-I/binding protein axis: physiology, pathophysiology and therapeutic manipulation." Academic Department of Medicine, King's College School of Medicine and Dentistry, London, UK. *Eur-J- Clin-invest.*, September, 1993, 23(9), pp. 503-516.

(16*) H. Olanrewaju, et al. "Trophic action of local intraileal infusion of insulin-like growth factor-I: polyamine dependence." *Am-J-Physiol.*, 263:E282-286, 1992.

(17*) Baumrucker, C.R., et al. "Effects of dietary recombinant human insulin-like growth factor-I on concentrations of hormones and growth factors in the blood of newborn calves." Department of Dairy and Animal Science, Pennsylvania State University, University Park, Pennsylvania. *J-Endrocrinol.*, January, 1994, 140(1), pp. 15-21.

(18*) R.G. Taylor, et al. "Hormonal regulation of intestinal adaptation." Department of Surgery, Royal Children's Hospital, Parkville, Victoria, Australia. *Baillieres-Clin-Endocrinol-Metab.*, January, 1994, 8(1), pp.165-183.

(19*) R.J. Playford, et al. "Effect of Luminal growth factor preservation on intestinal growth." *The Lancet*, 1993, 2, pp. 843-848.

(20*) R.K. Rae, et al. "Presence of multiple forms of peptidase inhibitors in rat milk.". Department of Pharmacology, Steele Memorial Children's Research Center, University of Arizona, Tucson. *J-Pediatr-Gastroenterol-Nutr.*, November 17, 1993, (4), pp.414-420.

(21*) K.A. Oster, et al. "Liposomes as a proposed vehicle for the persorption of bovine xanthine oxidase." *Proc. Soc. Exper. Bio. & Med.*, January, 1980, 163(1).

(22*) J. Frystyk, et al. "Free insulin-like growth factors (IGF-I and IGF-II) in human serum." Institute of Experimental Clinical Research, Asrhus University Hospital, Denmark. *FEBS-Lett.*, July 11, 1994, 348(2), pp. 185-191.

(23*) Z. Kachra, et al. "The augmentation of insulin-like growth factor-I messenger ribonucleic acid in cultured rat hepatocytes: activation of protein kinease-A and -C is necessary, but not sufficient." Polypeptide Hormone Laboratory, Royal Victoria Hospital, Montreal, Quebec, Canada. *Endocrinology*, February, 1994, 134(2), pp. 702-708.

(24*) M. Frodin, et al. "Insulin-like growth factors act synergistically with basic fibroblast growth factor and nerve growth factor to promote chromaffin cell proliferation." Department of Clinical Chemistry, Bispebjerg Hospital, Copenhagen, Denmark. *Proc-Natl-Acad-Sci-USA*, March 1, 1994, 91(5), pp. 1771-1775.

(25*) D. Romagnono, et al. "Lactogenic hormones and extracellular matrix regulate expression of IGF-I linked to MMTV-LTR in mammary epithelial cells." Department of Dairy Science, Virginia Polytechnic Institute and State University, Blacksburg, Virginia. *Mol-Cell-Endocrinol.*, October, 1993, 96(1-2), pp. 147-157.

(26*) J. Gillespie, et al. "Inhibition of pancreatic cancer cell growth in vitro by the tyrphostin group of tyrosine kinase inhibitors." Academic Surgical Unit, St. Mary's Hospital Medical School, Imperial College of Science, Technology and Medicine, London, UK. *Br.-J-Cancer*, December, 1993, 68(6), pp. 1122-1126.

(27*) R.P. Glick, et al. "Identification of insulin-like growth factor (IGF) and glucose transporter-I and -3 mRNA in CNS tumors." Department of Neurology, University of Illinois at Chicago, Cook County Hospital. *Regul-Pept.*, October, 20,1993, 48(1-2), pp. 251-256.

(28*) F. Atiq, et al. "Alterations in serum levels of insulin-like growth factors and insulin-like growth-factor-binding proteins in patients with colorectal cancer." Labor d'Immunologie, Faculte de Medecin, Marseille, France. *Int-J-Cancer*, May 15, 1994, 57(4), pp. 491-497.

(29*) T. Yashiro, et al. "Increased activity of insulin-like growth factor-binding protein in human thyroid papillary cancer tissue." Department of Sirgery, Tsukuba University, Ibaraki, Japan. *Jpn-J-Cancer-Res.*, January, 1994, 85(1), pp. 46-52.

(30*) K. Robbins, et al. "Immunological effects of insulin-like growth factor---enhancement of immunoglobulin synthesid." Department of Immunology, Genetech, Inc., South San Francisco, California. *Clin-Exp-Immunol.*, February, 1994, 95(2), pp. 337-342.

(31*) K. Yun, et al. "Insulin-like growth factor II messenger ribonucleic acid expression in Wilms tumor, nephrogenic rest, and kidney." Department of Pathology, University of Otago Medical School, Dunedin, New Zealand. *Lab-Invest.*, November, 1993, 69(5), pp. 603-615.

(32*) C.P. Minniti, et al. "Specific expression of insulin-like growth factor-II in rhabdomyosarcoma tumor cells." Institutes of Health, Bethesda, Maryland. *Am-J-Clin-Pathol.*, February, 1994, 101(2), pp. 198-203.

(33*) C.C. Kappel, et al. "Human osteosarcoma cell lines are dependent on insulin-like growth factor I for in vitro growth." Molecular Oncology Section, National Cancer Institute, Bethesda, Maryland. *Cancer-Res.*, May 15, 1994, 54(10), pp. 2803-2807.

(34*) M. Lippman. "Growth factors, receptors and breast cancers." (IGF-I and related growth factors are critically involved in aberrant growth of human breast cancer cells.) *J. Natl. Inst. Health Res.*, 1991, 3, pp. 59-62.

(35*) A.V. Lee, et al. "Processing of insulin-like growth factor-II (IGF-II) by human breast cancer cells." Imperial Cancer Research Fund, Breast Biology Group, School of Biological Sciences, University of Surrey, Guildford, UK. *Mol-Cell-Endocrinol.*, March, 99(2), pp. 211-220.

(36*) J.C. Chen, et al. "Insulin-like growth factor-binding protein enhancement of insulin-like growth factor-I (IGF-I)-mediated DNA synthesis and IGF-I binding in human breast carcinoma cell line." Department of Medicine, University of Maryland School of Medicine, Baltimore, Maryland. *J-Cell-Physiol.*, January, 1994, 158(1), pp. 69-78.

(37*) J.A. Figueroa, et al. "Recombinant insulin-like growth factor binding protein-1 inhibits IGF-I serum, and estrogen-dependent growth of MCF-7 human breast cancer cells." Department of Medicine, University of Texas Health Science Center, San Antonio, Texas. *J-Cell-Physiol.*, November, 1993, 157(2), pp. 229-236.

(38*) X.S. Li, et al. "Retinoic acid inhibition of insulin-like growth factor I stimulation of c-fos mRNA levels in breast carcinoma cell lines." Department of Medicine, University of Maryland School of Medicine, Baltimore, Maryland. *Exp-Cell-Res.*, March, 1994, 211(1), pp. 68-73.

(39*) A. Krasnick, et al. "Insulin-like growth factor-I (IGF) and IGF-binding protein-2 are increased in cyst fluids of epithelial ovarian cancer." Institute of Endocrinolgy, Chaim Sheba Medical Center, Tel-Hashomer, Israel. *J-Clin-Endocrinol-Metab.*, February, 1994, 78(2).

(40*) E.A. Musgrove, et al. "Acute effects of growth factors on T-47D breast cancer cell cycle progression." Cancer Biology Division, Garvan Institute for Medical Research, St. Vincent's Hospital, Darlinghurst, NSW, Australia. *Eur-J-Cancer*, 29A (16), 1993, pp. 2273-2279.

(41*) Gina Kolata. "New Ability to Find Earliest Cancers: A Mixed Blessing?" *The New York Times*, Science Section, November 8, 1994, p. C1.

Chapter 7 - The Fourth Estate: What America Was Told About the "New" Milk

1) Judith Blake. "Some Milk Labeling Called Improper." *The Seattle Times*, September, 1, 1994.

2) Bob Walter. "Biotech Milk Hormone Weathers a Challenge." *The Sacramento Bee*, August 30, 1994.

3) *Redbook*, vol. 178, January, 1992, p. 116.

4) A bibliography of BST-related issues, HHS Document # 90-13.

5) Marian Burros. "The Debate Over Milk and an Artificial Hormone." *The New York Times*, Section C4, May 18, 1994.

6) Ellen Ferguson. *The Burlington Free Press*, February 24, 1994, p. 7B.

7) *Ibid.*

8)   Senate Bill #234, 89th General Assembly, State of Illinois (LRB8900063FNsb).
9)   *Vegetarian Times*, February, 1994.
10)   Joel McNair. "FDA: 9,500 Cows Had Problems with BGH." *Agri-View*, March 23, 1995, Section 2, p. 1.
11)   Bob Arnot. "The Great American Milk War." *Good Housekeeping*, June, 1994, p. 50.
12)   Keith Schneider. *The New York Times*, Business Section, March 9, 1994.
13)   "Cash Cow." *Newsweek*, December 6, 1993.
14)   Philip Elmer-Dewitt. "Udder Insanity." *Time*, May 17, 1993, p. 52.
15)   Philip Elmer-Dewitt. "Brave New World of Milk." *Time*, February 14, 1994, p 31.
16)   Staff Editorial. "The Milk Lobby." *The Wall Street Journal*, March 14, 1994.
17)   Peter Hubber. "In Praise of the Bionic Cow." *Forbes*, August 6, 1990, vol. 146, p.108.
18)   *Science* Editorial. December 14, 1990, p. 1506.
19)   Sam Epstein. BST Article. *The Los Angeles Times*, March 20, 1994.
20)   Dennis Bier's 3 page letter to David Kessler, February 25, 1994.
21)   Bill Haworth. Dairy Coalition's (undated) response to Sam Epstein.
22)   Sam Epstein. "Insulin-like Growth Factor 1 in Biosynthetic Milk is a Potential Risk Factor for Breast Cancer and Gastrointestinal Cancers."A copy of which I reviewed for Dr. Epstein.
23)   Michael Hansen's testimony before the joint meeting of the Food Advisory Committee and the Veterinary Medicine Advisory Committee, Consumers Union, May 6, 1993.
24)   Philip Hager. "Courts Get Health Alert Authority." *The Los Angeles Times*, March 20, 1993, p. A3.
25)   Michael Hansen's testimony before the Veterinary Advisory Committee on rbGH use, March 31, 1993.
26)   "Milk Prices Raised." *The Los Angeles Times*, November 17, 1993.
27)   Eric Millstone. "Plagiarism or Protecting Public Health." *Nature*, vol. 371, October 20, 1994, p. 647.

Chapter 8 - (Not So) Wholesome Milk

1)   Alika Brandenberg. *Green Grass and White Milk*. New York: Crowell, 1974.
2)   Rod Serling's introduction to each episode of *The Twilight Zone*, recorded and transcribed from a 1960 episode.
3)   Michael McMenamin and Walter McNamara. *Milking the Public*. Chicago: Nelson-Hall, 1980.
4)   D. Bauman. *International Dairy Federation Bulletin*, December, 1993.
5)   *Ibid.*
6)   "Which Milk to Choose?" *Consumers Union*, September, 1991, vol. 56, p. 627.
7)   James Payne. "The Culture of Spending: Why Congress Lives Beyond Our Means." *National Review*, April 27, 1992.

Chapter 9 - Milk Consumption: A Second Opinion from the Medical Establishment

1) "The use of whole cow's milk in infancy." *Pediatrics*, American Academy of Pediatrics, Committee on Nutrition, 1992, 89, pp. 1105-1109.

2) J.A.T Pennington and H.N Church. "Food values of portions commonly used." New York: Harper and Row, 1989.

3) E.E. Ziegler, S.J. Fomon, S.E. Nelson, et al. "Cow milk feeding in infancy: further observations on blood loss from the gastrointestinal tract." *J Pediat.*, 1990, 116, pp. 11-18.

4) F.W. Scott. "Cow milk and insulin-dependent diabetes mellitus: is there a relationship?" *Am J Clin Nutr*, 1990, 51, pp. 489-491.

5) J. Karjalainen, J.M. Martin, M. Knip, et al. "A bovine albumin peptide as a possible trigger of insulin-dependent diabetes mellitus." *N Engl J Med.* 1992, 327, pp. 302-307.

6) D.M. Robertson, R. Paganelli, R. Dinwiddie, R.J. Levinsky. "Milk antigen absorption in the preterm and term neonate." *Arch Dis Child*, 1982, 57, pp. 369-372.

7) G.J. Bruining, J. Molenaar, C.W. Tuk, J. Lindeman, H.A. Bruining, B. Marner. "Clinical time-course and characteristics of islet cell cytoplasmatic antibodies in childhood diabetes." *Diabetologia*, 1984, 26, pp. 24-29.

8) D.W. Cramer, et al. "Galactose consumption and metabolism in relation to the risk of ovarian cancer." *The Lancet*, 1989, 2, pp. 66-71.

9) F.J. Simoons. "A geographic approach to senile cataracts: possible links with milk consumption, lactase activity, and galatose metabolism." *Digestive Diseases and Sciences*, 1982, 27, pp. 257-264.

10) C. Couet, P. Jan, G. Debry. "Lactose and cataract in humans: a review." *J Am Coll Nutr*, 1991, 10, pp. 79-86.

11) M.F. Holick, Q. Shao, W.W. Liu, T.C. Chen. "The vitamin D content of fortified milk and infant formula." *New Engl J Med.*, 1992, 326, pp. 1178-1181.

12) C.H. Jacobus, M.F. Holick, Q. Shao, et al. "Hypervitaminosis D associated with drinking milk." *New Engl J Med.*, 1992, 326, pp.1173-1177.

13) B.L. Riggs, H.W. Wahner, J. Melton, L.S. Richelson, H.L. Judd, M. O'Fallon. "Dietary calcium intake and rates on bone loss in women.' *J Clin Invest.*, 1987, 80, pp. 979-982.

14) B. Dawson-Hughes "Calcium supplementation and bone loss: a review of controlled clinical trials." *Am J Clin Nutr.*, 1991, 54, pp. 274S-280S.

15) B. Dawson-Hughes, P. Jacques, C. Shipp. "Dietary calcium intake and bone loss from the spine in healthy postmenopausal women." *Am J Clin Nutr.*, 1987, 46, pp. 685-687.

16) R.B. Mazess, H.S. Barden. "Bone density in premenopausal women: effects of age, dietary intake, physical activity, smoking, and birth-control pills." *Am J Clin Nutr.*, 1991, 53, pp. 132-142.

17) G. Kolata. "How important is dietary calcium in preventing osteoporosis?" *Science*, 1986, 233, pp. 519-520.

18)   R.P. Heaney, C.M. Weaver. "Calcium absorption from kale." *Am J Clin Nutr.*, 1990, 51, pp. 656-657.
19)   M.J. Nicar, C.Y.C. Pak. "Calcium bioavailability from calcium carbonate and calcium citrate." *J Clin Endocrinol Metab.*, 1985, 61, pp. 391-393.
20)   M.E. Nelson, E.C. Fisher, F.A. Dilmanian, G.E. Dallal, W.J. Evans. "A 1-y walking program and increased dietary calcium in postmenopausal women: effect on bone." *Am J Clin Nutr.*, 1991, 53, pp. 1304-1311.
21)   F.H. Nielsen, C.D. Hunt, et al. "Effect of dietary boron on mineral, estrogen, and testosterone metabolism in postmenopausal women." *FASEB*, 1987, 1, pp. 394-97.
22)   M.B. Zemel. "Role of the sulfur-containing amino acids in protein-induced hypercalciuria in men." *J Nut.*, 1981,111, p. 545.
23)   M. Hegsted, et al. "Urinary calcium and calcium balance in young men as affected by level of protein and phosphorus intake." *J Nutr.*, 1981, 111, p. 553.
24)   A.G. Marsh, T.V. Sanchez, O. Mickelsen, J. Keiser, G. Mayor. "Cortical bone density of adult lacto-ovo-vegetarian and omnivorous women." *J Am Dietetic Asso.*, 1980, 76, pp. 148-151.

Chapter 10 - An Analysis: What is in Milk

1)   *Handbook of the Nutritional Contents of Foods.* USDA, New York: Dover Publications, 1995, p. 38.
2)   Barbara Kraus. *The Dictionary of Sodium, Fats and Cholesterol.* New York: Grosset & Dunlap, 1974, p. 212.
3)   Freedom of Information Adverse Reaction Report of humans, accidentally (and intentionally) injected with rbGH (Posilac), January 14, 1995.
4)   Scott Veggeberg. "Beyond Steroids." *New Scientist*, vol. 14, no. 2012, January 13, 1996.
5)   *Ibid.*
6)   Barbara Kraus. *The Dictionary of Sodium, Fats and Cholesterol.* New York: Grosset & Dunlap, 1974, p. 212.
7)   H.D. Belitz, W. Grosch. *Food Chemistry.* Translated from 2nd. German Edition by D. Hadziyev, Pub. Springer-Verlag, Berlin, 1987, p. 379.
8)   Clark E. Grosvenor, et. al. "Hormones and Growth Factors in Milk." *Endocrine Reviews*, vol. 14, no. 6, 1992.
9)   Ratsimamanga, et al. *C.R. Soc. Biol* (France) 150, pp. 2179-2182.
10)   Klagsburn, M. "Human milk stimulates DNA synthesis and cellular proliferation in cultured fibriblasts." *Proceeds of Natl. Acad. Sci.* 1978, 75, pp. 5057-61.
11)   Kurt A. Oster, M.D., and Donald J. Ross, Ph. D. *The X-O Factor.* New York: Park City Press, 1983

Chapter 11 - Cancer: The Link Between Growth Hormones in Milk and Dairy Consumption

1) Cancer Facts & Figures - 1994. American Cancer Society, Atlanta, Georgia, (Inside cover-Incidence).

2) Cancer Treatment Centers Brochure, 1-800-FOR-HELP (367-4357).

3) Carlos Arteaga. "Interference of the IGF system as a strategy to inhibit breast cancer growth." Breast Cancer Research and Treatment, 1992, 22, pp. 101-106.

4) Andreas Friedl, et al. "Suppression of serum insulin-like growth factor-1 levels in breast cancer patients during adjuvant tamoxifen therapy." *European Journal of Cancer*, 1993, 29A (10), pp. 1368-1372.

5) J. Gillespie, et al. "Inhibition of pancreatic cancer cell growth in vitro by the tyrphostin group of tyrosine kinase inhibitors." *Br.-J-Cancer*, December, 1993, 68(6), pp. 1122-1126.

6) R.P. Glick, et al. "Identification of insulin-like growth factor (IGF) and glucose transporter-I and -3 mRNA in CNS tumors." *Regul-Pept.*, October 20, 1993, 48(1-2), pp. 251-256.

7) F. Atiq, et al. "Alterations in serum levels of insulin-like growth factors and insulin-like growth-factor-binding proteins in patients with colorectal cancer." *Int-J-Cancer*, May 15, 1994, 57(4), pp. 491-497.

8) T. Yashiro, et al. "Increased activity of insulin-like growth factor-binding protein in human thyroid papillary cancer tissue." *Jpn-J-Cancer-Res.*, January, 1994, 85(1), pp. 46-52.

9) K. Robbins, et al. "Immunological effects of insulin-like growth factor--- enhancement of immunoglobulin synthesid." *Clin-Exp-Immunol.*, February, 1994, 95(2), pp. 337-342.

10) Yun, K, et al. "Insulin-like growth factor II messenger ribonucleic acid expression in Wilms tumor, nephrogenic rest, and kidney." *Lab-Invest.*, November, 1993, 69(5) pp. 603-615.

11) C.C. Kappel, et al. "Human osteosarcoma cell lines are dependent on insulin-like growth factor I forin vitro growth." *Cancer-Res.*, May 15, 1994, 54(10), pp. 2803-2807.

12) M. Lippman. "Growth factors, receptors and breast cancers." *J. Natl. Inst. Health*, Res. 3, 1991, pp. 59-62.

13) A.V. Lee, et al. "Processing of insulin-like growth factor-II (IGF-II) by human breast cancer cells." *Mol-Cell-Endocrinol.*, March, 99(2), pp. 211-220.

14) J.C. Chen, et al. "Insulin-like growth factor-binding protein enhancement of insulin-like growth factor-I (IGF-I)-mediated DNA synthesis and IGF-I binding in human breast carcinoma cell line." *J-Cell-Physiol.*, January, 1994, 158(1), pp. 69-78.

15) J.A. Figueroa, et al. "Recombinant insulin-like growth factor binding protein-1 inhibits IGF-I serum, and estrogen-dependent growth of MCF-7 human breast cancer cells." *J-Cell-Physiol.*, November, 1993, 157(2), pp. 229-236.

16) X.S. Li, et al. "Retinoic acid inhibition of insulin-like growth factor I stimulation of c-fos mRNA levels in breast carcinoma cell lines." *Exp-Cell-Res.*, March, 1994, 211(1), pp. 68-73.

17) A. Krasnick, et al. "Insulin-like growth factor-I (IGF) and IGF-binding protein-2 are increased in cyst fluids of epithelial ovarian cancer." *J-Clin-Endocrinol-Metab.*, February, 1994, 78(2).

18) E.A. Musgrove, et al. "Acute effects of growth factors on T-47D breast cancer cell cycle progression." *Eur-J-Cancer*, 1993, 29A (16), pp. 2273-2279.

19) Gina Kolata. "New Ability To Find Earliest Cancers: A Mixed Blessing?" *The New York Times*, Science Section, November 8, 1994, p. C1.

20) *Cure 2000*, Leukemia Society Update, March, 1994.

21) Letter from Shaw Watanabe (Epidemiology Division of the Japan Leukemia Study Group) to *The Lancet*, February, 1988.

22) *Growth Hormone Treatment and Leukemia.* Press Release of the Lawson Wilkins Pediatric Endocrine Society, May 6, 1968.

23) R. Weiss. *Science News*, May 18, 1988, vol. 133, p. 308.

24) J.A. Moore, et al. *Endocrinology*, 1988, 122, p. 2920.

25) Reprinted with permission of the *Dick Davis Digest*, 1080 S. 3rd Ave., Ft. Lauderdale, FL. 33316, (954)-467-8500, vol.16, no. 369, October 13, 1997, p. 8.

Chapter 12 - The Truth About Calcium, Osteoporosis and Milk Allergies

1) John E. Priestly, M.D., with Janet Barton. *The Allergy Discovery Diet.* New York: Doubleday, 1990, p. 29.

2) Harvey and Marilyn Diamond. *Fit For Life.* New York: Warner Books, 1985, pp. 80-87.

3) Myron Lipowitz, M.D., Tova Navarra, RN. *Allergies: A-Z.* New York: Facts on File, 1994, p. 174.

4) Julie Klotter. *Townsend Medical Newsletter*, May, 1995.

5) Nathaniel Mead. "Don't Drink Your Milk." *Natural Health*, July/August, 1994, p. 70.

6) W.E. Parish et al. "Hypersensitivity to Milk and Sudden Death in Infancy." *The Lancet*, vol. 2, 7160, November 19, 1960, pp. 1106-1110.

7) "Cow Milk Allergies and Sudden Infant Death." *The Lancet*, vol. 344, November 5, 1994,

8) W.J. Howatt, et al. "Pulmonary Immunopathology of Sudden Infant Death Syndrome." *The Lancet*, vol. 343, June 4, 1994, pp. 1390-1392.

9) Facts About SIDS, Sudden Infant Death Syndrome 1-800-221-7437, SIDS ALLIANCE, Baltimore, Maryland.

10) Cavagni, et al. "Allergy to cow's milk proteins in childhood: The author's personal experience and new diagnostic and therapeutic proposals." *Pediatr-Med-Chir.*, September/October, 1994, 16(5), pp. 413-419.

11) Iacono, et al. "Chronic Constipation as a Symptom of Cow Milk Allergy." *J. Pediatr.*, January, 1995, 126(1), pp. 34-39.

12)   Kaila, et al. "A Prospective Study of Humoral Immune Response to Cow Milk Antigens in the First Year of Life." *Pediatr-Allergy-Immunol.*, August, 1994, 5(3) pp. 164-169.

13)   Host. "Cow's Milk Protein Allergy and Intolerance in Infancy. Some Clinical, Epidemiological and immunological aspects." *Pediatr.-Allergy-Immunol.*, 1994, 5(5 Suppl), pp. 1-36.

14)   "What You Need To Know About Diabetes." The American Diabetes Association, 1994.

15)   Rao, et al. "SC-18862 (ASPARTAME) 52 Week Oral Toxicity Study in the Infant Monkey," pp. 3179-3218 of an application made by Searle Pharmaceutical to FDA for Aspartame approval.

16)   "More Evidence that Milk Causes Diabetes and Anemia," *Prevention and Nutrition*, Autumn, 1992, p. 13.

17)   Karjalainen. "A bovine albumin peptide as a possible trigger of insulin-dependent diabetes mellitus." *N Engl J Med.*, 1992, 327, pp. 302-307.

18)   "Cow's Milk: Environmental Factor in IDDM (Insulin Dependent Diabetes Mellitus)." *Journal of the American Diabetic Association.* vol. 16, December, 1993.

19)   Verge, et al. "Environmental Factors in Childhood IDDM, A Population-Based Case-Control Study." *Diabetes Care.* December, 1994, 17(12), pp. 1381-1389.

20)   Virtanen and Aro. "Dietary factors in the aetiology of diabetes." *Ann-Med. Dec.*, 1994, 26(6), pp. 469-478.

21)   Fava, et al. "Relationship between dairy product consumption and the incidence of IDDM in childhood in Italy." *Diabetes Care*, December, 1994, 17(12), pp. 1488-1490.

22)   Norris and Pietropaolo. "A bovin albumin peptide as a possible trigger of insulin-dependent diabetes mellitus." *J. Endocrinological Invest.*, July/August, 17(7), pp. 565-72.

23)   Miyazaki, et al. "T Cell Activation and Anergy to Islet Cell Antigen in Type-I Diabetes." *J. Immunol.*, February, 1995, 154(3), pp. 1461-1469.

24)   Cheung, et. al. "T Cells From Children With IDDM are Sensitized to Bovine Serum Albumin." *J. Immunol.*, December, 1994, 40(6), pp. 623-628.

25)   Breslau. "Calcium, Estrogen and Progestin in the Treatment of Osteoporosis," *Rheum-Dis-Clin-North-Am.*, August, 1994, 20(3), pp. 691-716.

26)   Holick. "Environmental Factors that Influence the Cutaneous Production of Vitamin D." *Am-J-Clin-Nutr.*, March, 1995, 61(3 Suppl). pp. 638S-645S.

27)   Schacht. "Differential Therapy of Osteoporosis--An Overview Based on Recent Findings Regarding the Pathogenesis." *Z-Rheumatol.*, September/October, 1994, 3(5), pp. 274-298.

28)   Nelson, et al. "Effects of High-Intensity Strength Training on Multiple Risk Factors for Osteoporotic Fractures. A Randomized Controlled Trial." *JAMA*, December 28, 1994, 272(24), pp. 1909-1914.

29)   Ortego, et al. "Bone Mineral Density, Sex Steroids, and Mineral Metabolism in Premenopausal Smokers." *Calcif-Tissue-Int.*, December, 1994, 55(6), pp. 403-407.

30)   Sarli, et al. "Alcoholic Osteopathy." *Medicina-B-Aires,* 1994; 54(4), pp.363-370.
31)   Harris H. McIlwain, M.D., and Debra Fulghum Bruce. *Stop Osteoarthritis Now!* New York: Simon & Schuster, 1996, p. 176.
32)   Siegfried Kra, M.D. *What Every Woman Must Know About Heart Disease.* New York: Warner Books, 1996.
33)   Heaney and McDowell. "Calcium in Milk vs. Calcium in Bottled Water." University of Omaha Study, November, 1994.
34)   *U.S. News and World Report.* January 12, 1997, p. 22.
35)   Phone conversation with Alexandra Gorman, January 15, 1997.

Chapter 13 - Mad Cow Disease and Prions: A Frightening Biological Forecast

1)   *Food Microbiology,*1990, 7, pp. 253-279.
2)   *British Food Journal,* 1992, 94 (9), pp. 23-26.
3)   Steve Sternberg. *Science News,* vol. 150, October 12, 1996.
4)   John Stauber and Sheldon Rampton. "Toxic Sludge is Good For You." Email: 74250.735@ compuserve.com.
5)   Virgil Hulse. *Mad Cows and Milk Gate.* Phoenix, Oregon: Marble Mountain Publishing, 1996.
6)   *Chicago Life,* July/August, 1996.
7)   *Journal of Neurology,* January, 1989.
8)   *Mad Cows and Milk Gate, ibid.,* p. 67.
9)   John Collinge, et al. "Molecular analyses of prion Stran variation and the aetiology of 'new variant' CJD." *Nature,* vol. 24, October, 1996, p. 685
10)   S. B. Prusiner. "Molecular biology of Prion diseases." *Science,* vol. 252, June 14, 1991, pp. 1515-1522,
11)   Stanley Prusiner. "Prion Diseases." *Scientific American,* January, 1995, pp. 48-57.
12)   John Darnton. "Britain Ties Deadly Brain Disease to Cow Ailment." *The New York Times,* vol. CXLV, no. 50,373, March 21, 1996, p. 1 & A7.
13)   Virgil Hulse. *Mad Cows and Milk Gate.* Phoenix, Oregon: Marble Mountain Publishing, 1996.
14)   Howard Lyman, transcript of speech given at the World Vegetarian Congress in the Hague, Netherlands, August, 1994.
15)   Evan Halper. "Food Fight." *In These Times,* Chicago, Il., 8/11/97, pp. 24-25.
16)   Michael Hornsby. "New CJD Strain Threatens Thousands." *London Times,* August 23, 1997.
17)   Richard Rhodes. *Deadly Feasts.* New York: Simon & Schuster, 1997.
18)   Letter from Dr. Carleton Gajdusek to Robert Cohen, May 4, 1997.

Chapter 14 - Alternatives to Milk

1)   *Handbook of the Nutritional Content of Foods*, Prepared for the USDA, New York: Dover Publications Inc., 1975.

Index